Before We Are Born

Basic Embryology and Birth Defects

KEITH L. MOORE, M.Sc., Ph.D., F.I.A.C.

Professor of Anatomy and Associate Dean, Basic Sciences
University of Toronto, Faculty of Medicine,
Toronto, Ontario, Canada

Formerly Head of Anatomy at the University of Manitoba and
Chairman of the Department at the University of Toronto

Third Edition

1989
W. B. SAUNDERS COMPANY
Harcourt Brace Jovanovich, Inc.
Philadelphia   London   Toronto   Montreal   Sydney   Tokyo

W. B. SAUNDERS COMPANY
Harcourt Brace Jovanovich, Inc.

The Curtis Center
Independence Square West
Philadelphia, PA 19106

Library of Congress Cataloging-in-Publication Data

Moore, Keith L.
Before we are born: basic embryology and birth defects /
Keith L. Moore.—3rd ed.

p. cm.
Includes index.

ISBN 0–7216–2207–0

1. Embryology, Human.   2. Fetus—Abnormalities.   I. Title.

[DNLM: 1. Abnormalities.   2. Embryology.   QS 604 M822b]

QM601.M757   1989

612'.64—dc19

DNLM/DLC   88–37926

Listed here are the latest translated editions of this book, together with the language of each translation and the publisher.

Japanese—Ishiyaku Publishers Inc., Tokyo, Japan

Greek—C. Litsas Medical Books & Publications, Athens, Greece

Portuguese—Editora Guanabara S.A., Rio de Janeiro, Brazil

Spanish—Nueva Editorial Interamericana SA de CV, Mexico 06450 D.F., Mexico

Cover: A human embryo, about 28 days. (Courtesy of Professor Hideo Nishimura,
          Kyoto University, Kyoto, Japan.)

Editor: Martin Wonsiewicz

Designer: Terri Siegel

Production Manager: Bob Butler

Manuscript Editor: Ann Houska

Illustration Coordinator: Lisa Lambert

Indexer: Victoria Boyle

Before We Are Born: Basic Embryology and Birth Defects   ISBN   0–7216–2207–0

Last digit is the print number: 9   8   7   6   5   4   3   2   1

To my wife Marion
who has been my closest friend and
colleague for many years. Her suggestions and constructive criticism during the
preparation of this book have been of
enormous help.

Preface

The international acceptance of the previous two editions of *Before We Are Born*, reflected by its many adoptions and several translations, indicates that the book fills a need for beginning students in medicine, dentistry, and the other health professions. This textbook presents the prerequisites for understanding normal human development and for explaining the congenital abnormalities that are commonly encountered. When more information is desired, it may be obtained from my larger text, *The Developing Human: Clinically Oriented Embryology*, 4th edition, W. B. Saunders Company, 1988.

Before We Are Born resulted from an expressed need for a less detailed textbook of embryology. The material has been carefully selected in order to present the basic concepts of human embryology and the causes for abnormal development, in the belief that this material constitutes a realistic expectation of what a beginning student is capable of assimilating in a relatively short period of time. Because it emphasizes basics, it provides an overview of the subject, which many students find helpful to read before they attempt to study more detailed textbooks. Some students use it for review because it presents the basic information needed to pass the National Board and other examinations.

The illustrations and the summaries, at the ends of the chapters, provide a rapid way of reviewing embryology. A third edition of the *Study Guide and Review Manual of Human Embryology* is available for those wishing an opportunity to test their knowledge in preparation for multiple-choice type examinations. As a further help for students, I have included a new feature, *Commonly Asked Questions* along with their answers, at the end of each chapter.

Several new color illustrations have been prepared for this edition and others have been modified, because in many cases drawings present concepts more clearly than words. The illustrations in the first two editions were prepared mainly by Glen Reid in the University of Manitoba. Angela Cluer and Jean Calder in the Division of Instructional Media Services, University of Toronto, and Megan Thompson have prepared all the new illustrations. I am indebted to these and other artists for their skill in presenting difficult concepts in a clearly understandable way.

I should like to thank Professors Anne Agur and Michael Wiley in the Department of Anatomy, University of Toronto, for their suggestions for improving this edition. The comments of other teachers and students who use this book would be greatly appreciated. To Karen Bell and Sylvia Genders, I owe many thanks for typing the changes and additions to the manuscript for the third edition. My wife, Marion, has spent many hours reading the proofs and listening to me as my ideas for improving this edition developed. As in previous editions, I owe much to Marty Wonsiewicz, medical editor, and to the production staff of the W. B. Saunders Company for producing such a high-quality textbook.

KEITH L. MOORE

Contents

Introduction

Human development begins when an ovum from a female is fertilized by a sperm from a male. Development is a long process of change that transforms a single cell, the fertilized ovum or *zygote*, into a multicellular human being.

Most developmental changes occur before birth, that is, during the embryonic and the fetal periods, but important changes also occur during the later periods of development: infancy, childhood, adolescence, and adulthood.

Human embryology is the science that is concerned with the *origin and development of the human being* from fertilization of the ovum to the birth of an infant.

STAGES OF DEVELOPMENT

Development can be divided into *prenatal* and *postnatal* periods, but it is important to understand that *human development is a continuous process that begins at fertilization*. Birth is a dramatic event during development, and important developmental changes occur after birth (e.g., in the teeth and female breasts). Most developmental changes are completed by the age of 25.

The developmental stages occurring before we are born are illustrated in the *Timetables of Human Prenatal Development* (Figs. 1–1 and 1–2). The following list explains the terms used in these timetables and other commonly used names.

Zygote. This cell, formed by the union of an ovum and a sperm, represents the *beginning of a human being*. The expression "fertilized ovum" refers to the zygote.

Cleavage. Division or cleavage of the zygote by mitosis[1] forms daughter cells called *blastomeres*. The blastomeres become smaller at each succeeding cell division.

Morula. When 12 to 16 blastomeres have formed, the ball of cells resulting from division of the zygote is called a morula. It resembles the berry-like fruit known as a mulberry (L. *morus,* mulberry). The morula stage is reached about three days after fertilization, just as the developing human is about to enter the uterus.

Blastocyst. After the morula passes from the uterine tube into the uterus, a cavity forms in it known as the *blastocyst cavity.* This converts the morula into a blastocyst.

Embryo. The cells of the blastocyst that give rise to the embryo appear as an *inner cell mass,* often referred to as the embryoblast (Gr. *blastos,* germ). The term embryo is not usually used until the *bilaminar embryonic disc* forms during the second week. The *embryonic period* extends until the end of the eighth week, by which time the beginnings of all major structures are present. By the eighth week, characteristics are present that mark the embryo as distinctly human.

Conceptus. This term is used when referring to the embryo and its membranes, i.e., the *products of conception.* The term refers to all the structures that

Text continued on page 6

---

[1]A method of division of a cell by means of which two daughter cells receive identical complements of chromosomes. For details of this process, see a histology or biology textbook.

TIMETABLE OF HUMAN PRENATAL DEVELOPMENT
1 to 6 weeks

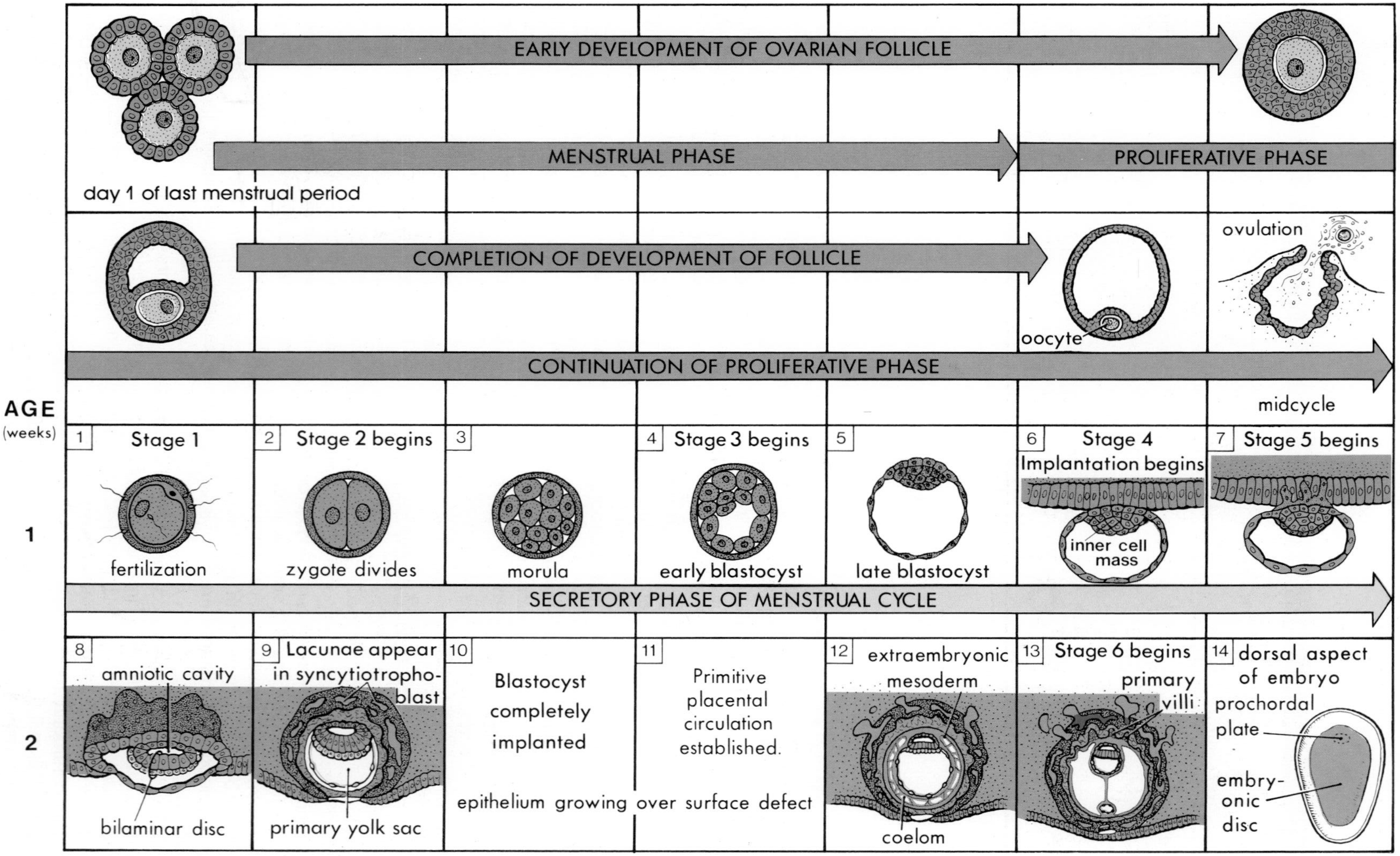

EARLY DEVELOPMENT OF OVARIAN FOLLICLE

PROLIFERATIVE PHASE

MENSTRUAL PHASE

COMPLETION OF DEVELOPMENT OF FOLLICLE

CONTINUATION OF PROLIFERATIVE PHASE

SECRETORY PHASE OF MENSTRUAL CYCLE

day 1 of last menstrual period

ovulation

oocyte

midcycle

AGE (weeks)

1

1	Stage 1	2	Stage 2 begins	3		4	Stage 3 begins	5		6	Stage 4 Implantation begins	7	Stage 5 begins
	fertilization		zygote divides		morula		early blastocyst		late blastocyst		inner cell mass		

2

8	amniotic cavity	9	Lacunae appear in syncytiotrophoblast	10	Blastocyst completely implanted	11	Primitive placental circulation established.	12	extraembryonic mesoderm	13	Stage 6 begins primary villi	14	dorsal aspect of embryo
	bilaminar disc		primary yolk sac		epithelium growing over surface defect				coelom				prochordal plate / embryonic disc

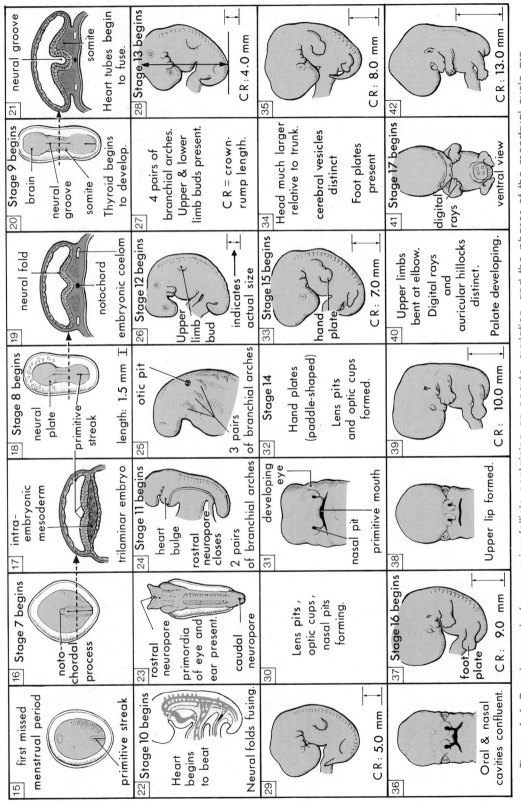

Figure 1–1. Development of an ovarian follicle containing an oocyte, ovulation, and the phases of the menstrual cycle are illustrated first. *Human development begins at fertilization*, about 14 days after the onset of the last menstruation. Cleavage of the zygote in the uterine tube, implantation of the blastocyst, and early development of the embryo are also shown. The main features of developmental stages in human embryos are illustrated. For a full discussion of embryonic development, see Chapter 6. Students should make no attempt to memorize these tables or the periods of the stages (e.g., that stage 3 begins on day 4 and stage 4 on day 6).

15 first missed menstrual period — primitive streak

16 Stage 7 begins — notochordal process

17 intraembryonic mesoderm — trilaminar embryo

18 Stage 8 begins — neural plate — primitive streak — length: 1.5 mm

19 neural fold — notochord — embryonic coelom

20 Stage 9 begins — brain — neural groove — somite — Thyroid begins to develop.

21 neural groove — somite — Heart tubes begin to fuse.

22 Stage 10 begins — Heart begins to beat. Neural folds fusing.

23 rostral neuropore — primordia of eye and ear present. — caudal neuropore

24 Stage 11 begins — heart bulge — rostral neuropore closes — 2 pairs of branchial arches

25 otic pit — 3 pairs of branchial arches

26 Stage 12 begins — Upper limb bud — indicates actual size

27 4 pairs of branchial arches. Upper & lower limb buds present. — CR = crown-rump length.

28 Stage 13 begins — CR: 4.0 mm

29 CR: 5.0 mm

30 Lens pits, optic cups, nasal pits forming.

31 developing eye — nasal pit — primitive mouth

32 Stage 14 — Hand plates (paddle-shaped) — Lens pits and optic cups formed.

33 Stage 15 begins — hand plate — CR: 7.0 mm

34 Head much larger relative to trunk. — cerebral vesicles distinct — Foot plates present

35 CR: 8.0 mm

36 Oral & nasal cavities confluent.

37 Stage 16 begins — foot plate — CR: 9.0 mm

38 Upper lip formed.

39 CR: 10.0 mm

40 Upper limbs bent at elbow. Digital rays and auricular hillocks distinct. Palate developing.

41 Stage 17 begins — digital rays

42 CR: 13.0 mm — ventral view

3

4

5

6

TIMETABLE OF HUMAN PRENATAL DEVELOPMENT
7 to 38 weeks

AGE (weeks)

7
- 43 — CR: 16.0 mm
- 44 — Stage 18 begins
- 45 — Tip of nose distinct. Digital rays appear in foot plates.
- 46 — Loss of villi. Smooth chorion forms.
- 47 — genital tubercle, urogenital membrane, anal membrane — ♀ or ♂
- 48 — Stage 19 begins. Trunk elongating and straightening.
- 49 — CR: 18 mm

8
- 50 — Upper limbs longer & bent at elbows. Fingers distinct.
- 51 — Anal membrane perforated. Urogenital membrane degenerating. Testes and ovaries distinguishable.
- 52 — Stage 21 begins. CR: 17.0 mm
- 53 — Stage 21. External genitalia still in sexless state but have begun to differentiate.
- 54 — Stage 22 begins. genital tubercle, urethral groove, anus — ♀ or ♂
- 55 — Beginnings of all essential external and internal structures are present.
- 56 — Stage 23. CR: 30 mm

9
- 57 — Beginning of fetal period.
- 58 —
- 59 — Genitalia show some ♀ characteristics but still easily confused with ♂.
- 60 — phallus, urogenital fold, labioscrotal fold, perineum — ♀
- 61 — Genitalia show fusion of urethral folds. Urethral groove extends into phallus.
- 62 — phallus, urogenital fold, labioscrotal fold, perineum — ♂
- 63 — CR: 50 mm

10
- 64 — Face has human profile. Note growth of chin compared to day 44.
- 65 —
- 66 — Face has human appearance.
- 67 — clitoris, labium minus, urogenital groove, labium majus — ♀
- 68 — Genitalia have ♀ or ♂ characteristics but still not fully formed.
- 69 — glans penis, urethral groove, scrotum — ♂
- 70 — CR: 61 mm

The Fetal Period

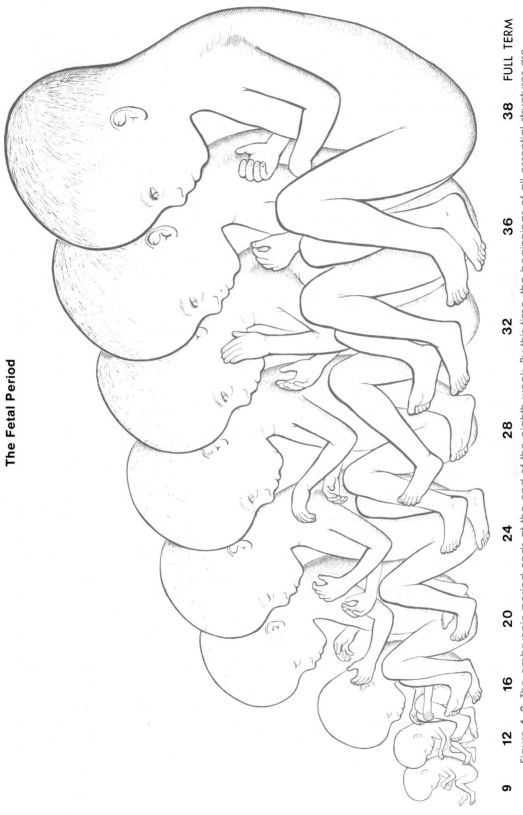

9   12   16   20   24   28   32   36   38   FULL TERM

Figure 1–2. The embryonic period ends at the end of the eighth week. By this time, the beginnings of all essential structures are present. The fetal period, extending from the ninth week until birth, is characterized by growth and elaboration of structures. Sex is clearly distinguishable by 12 weeks. The above 9- to 38-week fetuses are about half actual size. For more information about fetal development, see Chapter 7.

develop from the zygote, both embryonic and extraembryonic.

Fetus. After the embryonic period, the developing human is called a fetus. During the *fetal period* (ninth week to birth), many systems develop further. Although developmental changes are not as dramatic as those occurring during the embryonic period, they are very important. The rate of body growth is remarkable, especially during the third and fourth months, and weight gain is phenomenal during the terminal months.

Abortion (L. *abortio, miscarriage).* This term refers to the birth of an embryo or a fetus before it is viable (mature enough to survive outside the uterus). All terminations of pregnancy that occur before 20 weeks are called *abortions.*

About 15 per cent of all recognized pregnancies end in *spontaneous abortions* (ones that occur naturally), usually during the first 12 weeks. Legally *induced abortions* are brought on purposefully (often for social reasons), usually by *suction curettage* (evacuation of the embryo and its membranes from the uterus).

Therapeutic abortions are induced owing to the mother's poor health, or to prevent the birth of a severely malformed child (e.g., one without a brain).

Abortus. This term describes any product or all products of an abortion. *An embryo or a nonviable fetus and its membranes* weighing less than 500 gm is called an *abortus.* More commonly, one refers to an aborted embryo or fetus.

Primordium (L. *primus,* first + *ordior,* to begin). This term refers to the first trace or indication of an organ or structure, i.e., its earliest stage of development. The term *anlage* has a similar meaning. For example, the *primordium* or anlage of the upper limb appears on about day 26 (see Fig. 1–1).

Miscarriage. This word is used colloquially to refer to any interruption of pregnancy that occurs in the late fetal period, that is, before a fetus is viable (i.e., a spontaneous abortion of a mature fetus). In description, it is most accurate to use the term *spontaneous abortion* for the birth of an embryo or a fetus prior to about 20 weeks; thereafter the event should be referred to as a *premature birth.*

Trimesters. Obstetricians commonly divide the nine calendar months, or period of gestation (stages of intrauterine development) into three 3-month periods called *trimesters.* The **critical period of development** occurs during the first trimester. Birth occurs at the end of the third trimester.

THE IMPORTANCE OF EMBRYOLOGY

The study of prenatal stages of development, especially those occurring during the embryonic period, helps us to understand the normal relationships of adult body structures and the causes of congenital malformations. In other words, *embryology illuminates anatomy* and explains how abnormalities develop.

The embryo is extremely vulnerable during the third to eighth weeks to large amounts of radiation, viruses, and certain drugs (see Chapter 9). The physician's knowledge of normal development and the causes of congenital malformations aid in giving the embryo the best possible chance of developing normally. Much of the modern practice of obstetrics involves what might be called "applied developmental biology."

The significance of embryology is readily apparent to pediatricians because some of their patients have disorders resulting from maldevelopment, e.g., spina bifida and congenital heart disease. Progress in surgery, especially in the pediatric age group, has made knowledge of human development more clinically significant. The understanding of most congenital malformations (e.g., cleft palate and cardiac defects) depends upon an understanding of normal development and the deviations that may occur.

HISTORICAL HIGHLIGHTS

If I have seen further, it is by standing on the shoulders of giants.

SIR ISAAC NEWTON
English mathematician, 1643–1727

This statement emphasizes that each new study of a problem rests on a base of knowledge established by earlier investigators. Every age gives explanations according to the knowledge and experience of its people, and so we should be grateful for their ideas and neither sneer at them nor consider ours as final.

A brief *Sanskrit treatise* on ancient Indian embryology is thought to have been written in 1416 B.C. This scripture of the Hindus, called *Garbha Upanishad,* described ancient ideas concerning the embryo. It states:

From the conjugation of blood and semen the embryo comes into existence. During the period favorable for conception, after sexual intercourse, (it) becomes a kalada (one-day-old embryo). After remaining for seven nights, it becomes a vesicle. After a fortnight it becomes a spherical mass. After a month it becomes a firm mass. After two months the head is formed. After three months the limb regions appear.

Although the dates of appearance of the structures are inaccurate, the sequence is correct.

The Greeks made important contributions to the science of embryology. The first recorded embryo-

logical studies are in a book by **Hippocrates,** the famous Greek physician of the fifth century B.C. In the fourth century B.C., **Aristotle** wrote the first known account of embryology, in which he described development of the chick and other embryos. **Galen** (second century A.D.) wrote a book entitled *On the Formation of the Foetus* in which he described the development and nutrition of fetuses.

Growth of science was slow during the Middle Ages, and no embryological investigations are known to us, but it is cited in the *Koran,* or *Qur'an,* The Holy Book of the Muslims, that human beings are produced from a *mixture of secretions* from the male and female. Several references are made to the creation of a human being from a *droplet,* and it is also suggested that the resulting organism settles in the woman like a seed, six days after its beginning. (The human blastocyst begins to implant in the lining or endometrium of the uterus about six days after fertilization.) Reference is also made to the leechlike appearance of the early embryo. (The embryo of 22 to 24 days resembles a leech, or bloodsucker.) The embryo is also said to resemble "a chewed substance" like gum or wood. (The somites of the embryos shown in Chapter 6 somewhat resemble teethmarks in a chewed substance.)

In the 15th century, **Leonardo da Vinci** made accurate drawings of dissections of the pregnant uterus and associated fetal membranes (Fig. 1–3).

In 1651 **Harvey** studied chick embryos with simple lenses and made observations on the circulation of blood. Early microscopes were simple (Fig. 1–4), but they opened a new field of observation. In 1672 **de**

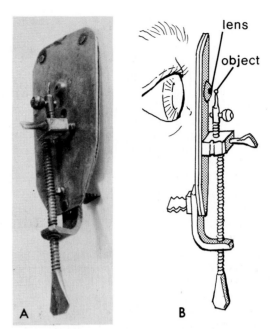

Figure 1–4. *A,* Photograph of a 1673 Leeuwenhoek microscope. *B,* Drawing of a lateral view illustrating its use. The object was held in front of the lens on the point of the short rod, and the screw arrangement was used to adjust the object under the lens. After the development of this crude instrument, embryologists were able to observe the early stages of development.

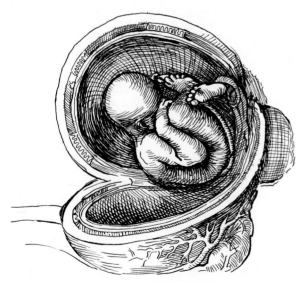

Figure 1–3. Reproduction of Leonardo da Vinci's drawing (15th century A.D.) showing a fetus in a uterus that has been incised and opened.

Graaf observed little chambers (undoubtedly what we now call blastocysts) in the rabbit's uterus and concluded that they came from organs he called ovaries.

Malpighi, in 1675, studying what he believed to be unfertilized hen's eggs, observed early embryos. As a result, he thought the egg contained a miniature chick. Despite this, his observations on the developing chick were very good.

In 1677 **Hamm and Leeuwenhoek,** using an improved microscope, first observed the human sperm, but they did not understand the sperm's role in fertilization. They thought it contained a miniature human being (Fig. 1–5).

In 1775, **Spallanzani** showed that both the ovum and the sperm were necessary for initiation of a new individual. From his experiments, he concluded that the sperm was the fertilizing agent.

Great advances were made in embryology when the *cell theory* was established in 1839 by **Schleiden and Schwann.** The concept that the body was composed of cells and cell products soon led to the realization that the embryo developed from a single cell, called the zygote. They discovered and demonstrated the cellular nature of tissues.

The *principles of heredity* were developed in 1865

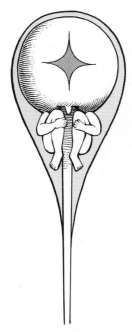

Figure 1–5. Copy of a drawing of a sperm by Hart-soeker. The miniature human being within it was thought to enlarge after it entered an ovum. Other embryologists in the 17th century thought the oocyte contained a miniature human being that enlarged when it was stimulated by a sperm.

by an Austrian monk named **Mendel,** but biologists did not understand the significance of these principles in the study of mammalian development for many years.

Flemming observed chromosomes in 1878 and suggested their probable role in fertilization. The first significant observations on human chromosomes were made by **von Winiwarter** in 1912. In 1923 **Painter** concluded that there were 48 chromosomes. This number was accepted until 1956, when **Tjio and Levan** reported finding only 46 chromosomes. This number is now universally accepted.

DESCRIPTIVE TERMS

In anatomy and embryology, several terms of position and direction are used, and various planes of the body are referred to in sections. All descriptions of the adult are based on the assumption that the body is erect, with the upper limbs by the sides and the palms directed anteriorly (Fig. 1–6A). This is called the **anatomical position.**

The terms *anterior* or *ventral* and *posterior* or *dorsal* are used to describe the front or back of the body or limbs, and the relations of structures within the body to one another. In embryos, dorsal and ventral are always used (Fig. 1–6B).

Superior or *cranial* (cephalic) and *inferior* or *caudal* are used to indicate the relative levels of different structures. In embryos, cranial and caudal are used to denote relationships to the head and tail ends, respectively. Distances from the source of attachment of a structure are designated as *proximal* or *distal;* e.g., in the lower limb the knee is proximal to the ankle and the ankle is distal to the knee.

The *median plane* is a vertical plane passing through the center of the body, dividing it into right and left halves (Fig. 1–6C). The terms *lateral* and *medial* refer to structures that are respectively farther from or nearer to the median plane of the body. A *sagittal plane* is any vertical plane passing through the body parallel to the median plane (Fig. 1–6C).

A *transverse* or *horizontal plane* refers to any plane that is at right angles to both the median and frontal planes (Fig. 1–6D). A *frontal* or *coronal plane* is any vertical plane that intersects the median plane at a right angle; it divides the body into front (anterior or ventral) and back (posterior or dorsal) parts (Fig. 1–6E).

Commonly Asked Questions

1. Should I learn to reproduce the timetables and stages of human development?
2. What is the difference between the terms *conceptus* and *embryo*?
3. Why are we asked to study human embryology?
4. I have heard that animal and human embryos look alike. Is this true?
5. Doctors date a pregnancy from the first day of the last menstrual period, but the embryo does not start to develop until about two weeks later. Why do they do this?
6. Is the zygote a human being?

Answers

1. No. You should not attempt to learn how to reproduce the timetables of development. They are presented as an overview of human development before birth. Neither should you try to memorize the stages (e.g., that stage 3 begins on day 4). These stages are used by embryologists when referring to embryos they are describing in detail. You should, however, be able to describe human development to a lay person and some of the sketches in the timetables would be helpful. You could even *use the timetables to describe human development.*

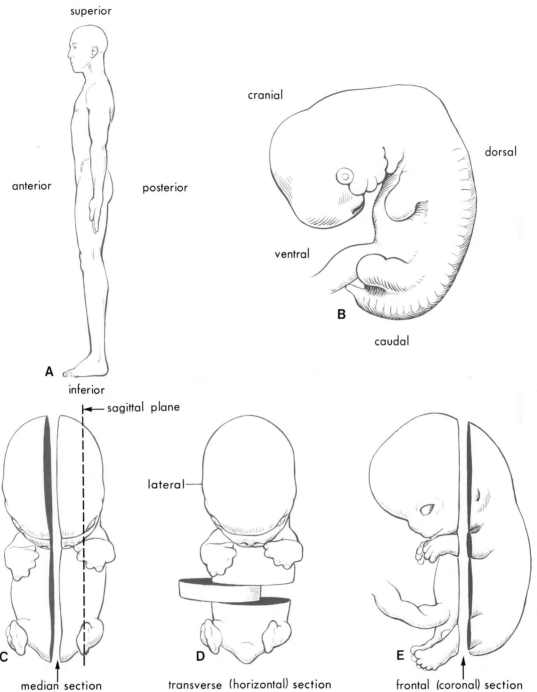

superior

anterior

posterior

A

inferior

cranial

dorsal

ventral

B

caudal

sagittal plane

lateral

C

median section

D

transverse (horizontal) section

E

frontal (coronal) section

Figure 1–6. Drawings illustrating descriptive terms of position, direction, and planes of the body. *A,* Lateral view of a human adult in the anatomical position. *B,* Lateral view of a five-week embryo. *C* and *D,* Ventral views of six-week embryos. *E,* Lateral view of a seven-week embryo.

2. The term *conceptus* is used to refer to the embryo and its membranes (e.g., amnion and chorion). Some people refer to the conceptus as the products of conception, that is, everything that develops from the fertilized ovum or zygote.

3. Everyone should know about conception, contraception, and how people develop (normally and abnormally). People in the health professions are expected to give answers to the questions people ask. For example, when does the baby's heart start to beat? When does it look like a human being?

4. Animal and human embryos look very much alike for the first few weeks (e.g., they both have branchial arches and tails). After the seventh week, human embryos do not resemble animal embryos, mainly because the head starts to look human and the tail begins to disappear (see Fig. 6–16).

5. *Doctors date pregnancies from the last menstrual period (LMP)* because it is a time that is easily remembered by the woman. It is not possible to detect the precise time of ovulation and fertilization, but there are tests that can be done to detect when ovulation is likely to occur and when pregnancy has occurred. These tests are not routinely performed owing to the costs involved. When dating pregnancies by using LMP, doctors are aware that the age of the developing human is about two weeks less than the "menstrual age" and base their decisions on this (e.g., concerning its vulnerability to drugs and so forth).

6. *The zygote has the potential to develop into a human being,* just as the acorn has the potential to develop into an oak tree. The zygote is a single cell, whereas a human being consists of millions of cells. No one knows when an embryo becomes a human being, but many people consider seven- to eight-week old embryos to be developing human beings.

Human Reproduction

Human beings have a limited life span. Consequently, for humankind to survive there must be a mechanism for the production of new individuals. Human reproduction, like that of most animals, involves the fusion of germ cells or gametes—an ovum from the female and a sperm from the male. Each cell brings to the union a half share of genetic information so that the united cell or **zygote** receives the full amount of genetic information that is required for directing the development of a new human being. The reproductive system in both sexes is designed to ensure the successful union of the sperm and the ovum, a process known as *fertilization.*

Puberty. Before puberty, male and female children are not strikingly different, except for their genitalia. The sexual maturation that normally occurs during puberty results in considerable differences in appearance, so that the sexually mature male is very masculine and the female is unmistakably feminine.

Puberty encompasses the period of years during which the child, who is incapable of reproduction, is transformed into a person who is capable of reproduction. These changes involve the gross appearance, as well as alterations in the reproductive organs and the psyche. The time period of puberty varies, as does the age of onset.

Puberty in females is usually between the ages of 12 and 15 years, but **menarche** (the first menstruation) sometimes occurs in 11-year-old girls.

Puberty in males usually begins later (13 to 16 years), but signs of sexual maturity may appear in 12-year-old boys.

Puberty begins when secondary sex characteristics first appear in either sex (e.g., the development of breasts in females and the increase in the size of the testes in males), and ends when the person is fully capable of reproduction.

THE REPRODUCTIVE ORGANS

Each sex has reproductive or *sex organs,* which produce and transmit the *germ cells* or gametes from the *sex glands* or gonads (Fig. 2–1). The sex organ in the male, called the *penis,* deposits the sperms (spermatozoa), produced by the *testes,* in the female genital tract (see Fig. 2–10). In the female the *vagina* is a receptacle for the sperms and the *uterus* nourishes the embryo and protects it until birth.

The Female Reproductive Organs

The *ova* (female germ cells) are produced by two oval-shaped *ovaries* located in the superior part of the pelvic cavity, one on each side of the uterus (Fig. 2–1A). When released from the ovary at *ovulation* (see Fig. 2–8), the secondary oocyte, often called an ovum, passes into one of two trumpet-shaped *uterine tubes* (Figs. 2–1A and 2–2A). These tubes open into the pear-shaped *uterus* (womb), which contains and nourishes the embryo and fetus until birth.

Structure of the Uterus (Fig. 2–2). The uterus is a thick-walled, pear-shaped organ. It varies considerably in size but is usually 7 to 8 cm in length, 5 to 7 cm in width at its superior part, and 2 to 3 cm in thickness.

The uterus consists of two main parts, the **body** and the **cervix.** The *fundus* is the rounded superior part of the uterine body.

The wall of the body of the uterus consists of three layers: (1) a very thin outer layer of peritoneum called the *perimetrium;* (2) a thick smooth-muscle layer or *myometrium;* and (3) a thin, inner lining layer, the mucosa or *endometrium.*

The Vagina (Figs. 2–1A and 2–2A). The vagina is a muscular tube that passes to the exterior from the inferior end of the uterus, called the *cervix.* The vagina is the female organ that receives the male organ or penis during *sexual intercourse* (see Fig. 2–10). It also

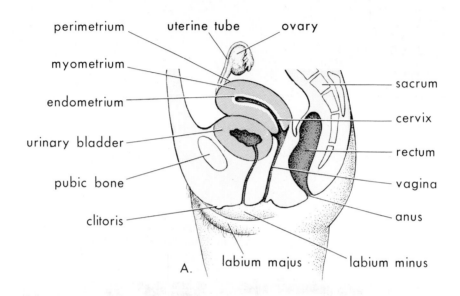

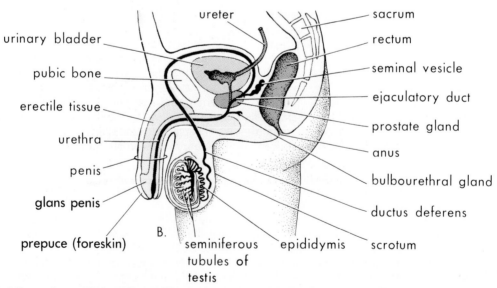

Figure 2–1. Schematic sagittal sections of the pelvic region showing the reproductive organs. *A,* Female. *B,* Male. The ovary is the sex gland of the female, and the testis (testicle) is the sex gland of the male. There are two ovaries in the normal female, both located in the pelvis. There are two testes in the normal male, both located in the scrotum. The vagina, the female copulatory organ, is an elastic tube (7 to 9 cm long) that leads from the uterus to the outside of the body. It stretches during sexual intercourse and during childbirth. The penis is the male copulatory organ and the organ for urination. Sperms leave the urethra during sexual intercourse and are deposited in the vagina (see Fig. 2–10).

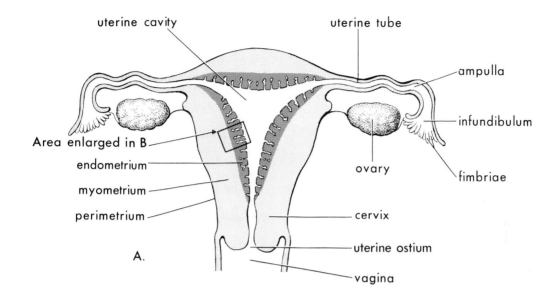

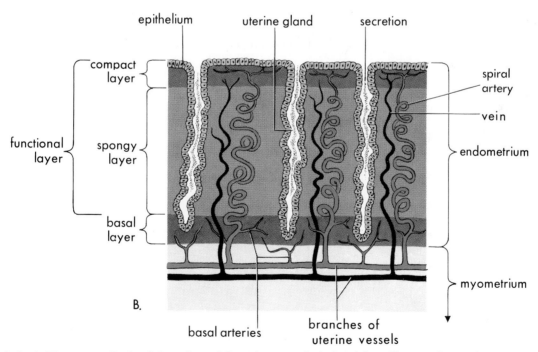

Figure 2–2. *A,* Diagrammatic frontal section of the uterus and uterine tubes. The ovaries and vagina are also indicated. *B,* Detail of the area outlined in *A.* The endometrium (lining of the uterus) is composed of three layers (compact, spongy, and basal) which are subject to cyclic changes in response to ovarian secretory activity (see Fig. 2–7). The functional layer of the endometrium is sloughed off during menstruation, the monthly endometrial shedding and discharge of bloody fluid from the uterus.

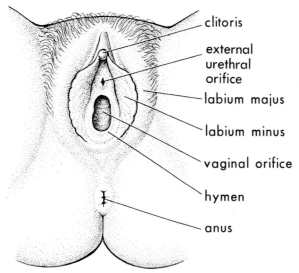

clitoris

external urethral orifice

labium majus

labium minus

vaginal orifice

hymen

anus

Figure 2–3. The female external genital organs, known collectively as the vulva. The opening at the inferior end of the alimentary canal, the anus, is also shown. In most women the labia majora are opposed and usually conceal the labia minora. The labia have been spread apart in this drawing to demonstrate the parts of the vulva. The hymen is a thin incomplete fold of mucous membrane that surrounds the vaginal orifice. The labia majora are fatty folds of skin, whereas the labia minora are thin folds of pink mucous membrane. The clitoris, 2 to 3 cm in length, is homologous with the penis in the male. Unlike the penis, the clitoris is not traversed by the urethra. The clitoris is composed of erectile tissue and, like the penis, is capable of enlargement upon tactile stimulation. It is highly sensitive and important in the sexual excitement of the female.

serves as a temporary receptacle for the sperms before they begin their passage through the uterus and uterine tubes.

The External Sex Organs (Figs. 2–2 and 2–3). The external genitalia or sex organs of the female are known collectively as the *vulva* or pudendum. Two external folds of skin, called the *labia majora* (large lips), conceal the opening of the vagina. Inside these folds are two smaller folds of mucous membrane called the *labia minora* (small lips).

The *clitoris* is at the junction of these folds; it is a small erectile organ. The vagina and urethra open into a cavity known as the *vestibule* (the cleft between the labia minora). The clitoris is the morphological equivalent of the penis. It is important in the sexual excitement of a female.

The Male Reproductive Organs

The parts of the male reproductive system (see Fig. 2–1B) include the testis, epididymis, ductus deferens,

prostate gland, seminal vesicles, bulbourethral glands, ejaculatory ducts, urethra, and scrotum.

The *sperms* (male germ cells) are produced in the *testes,* two oval-shaped glands which are suspended in the *scrotum,* a loose pouch of skin (Fig. 2–1B). Each testis consists of many highly coiled *seminiferous tubules* which produce the sperms. The sperms pass into a single, complexly coiled tube, the *epididymis,* where they are stored. The sperms are not mature (i.e., capable of fertilizing ova) when they leave the testes. It takes days for the sperms to mature in the epididymis, located alongside the testis in the scrotum (see Fig. 2–1B).

From the inferior end of the epididymis, a long straight tube, the *ductus deferens* (vas deferens) carries the sperms from the epididymis to the ejaculatory duct. The ductus deferens passes from the scrotum through the inguinal canal into the abdominal cavity. It then descends into the pelvis where it fuses with the duct of the *seminal vesicle* to form the *ejaculatory duct* which enters the urethra.

The *urethra* is a tube leading from the urinary bladder to the outside of the body; its spongy part runs through the *penis.* Within the penis the urethra is surrounded by three columns of spongy erectile tissue. During sexual excitement, this tissue becomes filled with blood under increased pressure. This causes the penis to become erect and thus able to enter the vagina. Ejaculation of *semen* (sperms mixed with seminal fluid produced by various glands, e.g., the seminal vesicles and prostate gland) occurs when the penis is further stimulated.

Consequently, the urethra transports both urine and semen, but not at the same time. Urine cannot be passed during sexual arousal.

GAMETOGENESIS

Gametogenesis (gamete formation) is the process of formation and development of specialized generative cells, called gametes or germ cells (see Fig. 2–5). This process, which involves the chromosomes and the cytoplasm of the gametes, prepares these sex cells for *fertilization* (union of male and female gametes or sex cells, i.e., the sperm and ovum).

During gametogenesis, the chromosome number is reduced by half, and the shape of the cells is altered.

THE GAMETES

The *sperm* (spermatozoon) and the *ovum,* the male and female germ cells or gametes, are highly *specialized sex cells* (Figs. 2–4 and 2–5). They contain half the usual number of chromosomes (i.e., 23 instead

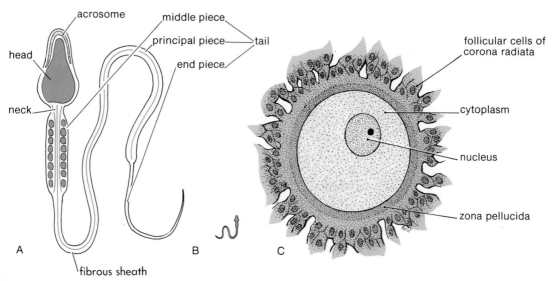

Figure 2–4. *A*, Drawing showing the main parts of a human sperm or spermatozoon (× 1250). The head, composed mostly of the nucleus, is covered by the acrosome, which contains enzymes that are released during fertilization. *B*, A sperm drawn to about the same scale as the ovum. *C*, Drawing of a human ovum (secondary oocyte) (× 200), surrounded by the zona pellucida, an elastic membrane, and the corona radiata, composed of follicular cells that accompany it during ovulation (see Fig. 2–8).

of 46 as in most cells). The number of chromosomes is reduced by the process of *meiosis* or reduction division, a special type of cell division which occurs during the formation of gametes (*gametogenesis*). The gamete-forming process is known as *spermatogenesis* in males and *oogenesis* (*ovogenesis*) in females (Fig. 2–5).

Meiosis consists of two cell divisions during which the chromosome number is reduced to half (23, the *haploid number*) that is present in other cells in the body (46, the *diploid number*). During the final stages of maturation, the two chromosomes in each of the 23 pairs separate from each other and are distributed to different cells. Therefore, each mature germ cell (sperm or ovum) contains one member of each pair of the chromosomes present in the immature germ cell (primary spermatocyte or primary oocyte). In summary, meiosis halves the number of chromosomes and re-sorts the genes received from the mother and the father.

The significance of meiosis is that it provides for constancy of the chromosome number from generation to generation by producing *haploid germ cells*. It also allows the independent assortment of maternal and paternal chromosomes and genes among the gametes. *Crossing over,* by relocating segments of the maternal and paternal chromosomes, "shuffles" the genes and thereby produces a recombination of genetic material.

Consequently, each gamete carries a mixture of maternal and paternal genes. Fertilization then results in a new cell, the zygote, which has a mixture of genes from the maternal and paternal parents and grandparents.

Spermatogenesis

The term *spermatogenesis* refers to the entire sequence of events by which primitive germ cells called *spermatogonia* are transformed into spermatozoa (called *sperms* for brevity). This maturation process begins at *puberty* (13 to 16) years and continues into old age (see Fig. 2–5).

The mature sperm (spermatozoon) is a free-swimming, actively motile cell consisting of a *head* and a *tail* (Fig. 2–4A). The head, forming most of the bulk of the sperm, contains the nucleus with its 23 chromosomes. The anterior two thirds of the nucleus is covered by the *acrosome,* a caplike organelle containing enzymes that facilitate sperm penetration during fertilization (see Chapter 3).

The tail of the sperm consists of three segments: the *middle piece,* the *principal piece,* and the *end piece.* The tail provides the motility of the sperm, assisting with its transport to the site of fertilization in the ampulla of the uterine tube (see Fig. 2–2A). The middle piece of the tail contains the energy-producing cytoplasmic and mitochondrial apparatus. The junction between the head and the tail is called the *neck* of the sperm (Fig. 2–4A).

The early germ cells, called *spermatogonia,* which

NORMAL GAMETOGENESIS

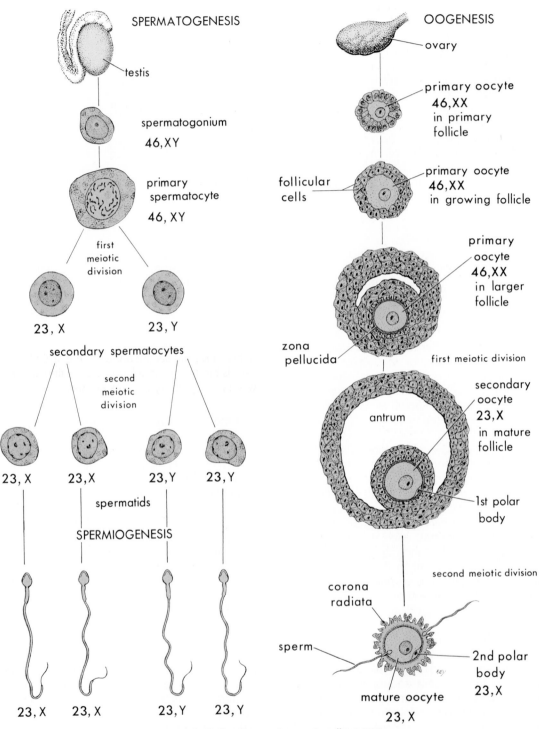

SPERMATOGENESIS

OOGENESIS

ovary

testis

spermatogonium
46,XY

primary oocyte
46,XX
in primary
follicle

follicular
cells

primary oocyte
46,XX
in growing follicle

primary
spermatocyte
46, XY

first
meiotic
division

primary
oocyte
46,XX
in larger
follicle

zona
pellucida

23, X

23, Y

first meiotic division

secondary spermatocytes

second
meiotic
division

antrum

secondary
oocyte
23,X
in mature
follicle

1st polar
body

23, X

23, X

23, Y

23, Y

spermatids

SPERMIOGENESIS

second meiotic division

corona
radiata

sperm

2nd polar
body
23,X

mature oocyte
23, X

23, X

23, X

23, Y

23, Y

Figure 2–5 *See legend on opposite page*

have been dormant in the seminiferous tubules of the testes since the fetal period, begin to increase in number at *puberty* (13 to 16 years). After several mitotic cell divisions, the spermatogonia grow and undergo gradual changes which transform them into *primary spermatocytes* (Fig. 2–5), the largest germ cells in the seminiferous tubules of the testes.

Each primary spermatocyte subsequently undergoes a reduction division,[1] called the *first meiotic division*, to form two haploid[2] *secondary spermatocytes* which are about half the size of primary spermatocytes. Subsquently, the secondary spermatocytes undergo a *second meiotic division* to form four haploid *spermatids*, which are about half the size of secondary spermatocytes. During this division, there is no further reduction in the number of chromosomes.

The spermatids are gradually transformed into *mature sperms* by a process known as *spermiogenesis*. During this metamorphosis (change in form), the nucleus condenses, the acrosome forms, and most of the cytoplasm is shed (Fig. 2–6). Spermatogenesis, including spermiogenesis, requires many days for completion and normally continues throughout the reproductive life of a male.

Oogenesis

The term *oogenesis* (ovogenesis) refers to the sequence of events by which oogonia are transformed into ova. This maturation process begins before birth, but is not completed until after *puberty* (12 to 15 years). Oogenesis is a recurring process that is *part of the ovarian cycle* (Fig. 2–7). Except during pregnancy, these cycles occur during the reproductive period of females.

---

[1]This process of chromosome reproduction by an atypical method of cell division is called *meiosis*; it consists of two specialized divisions called the first and second meiotic divisions (see Fig. 2–5).

[2]In humans, body cells and early sex cells have 46 chromosomes (the *diploid number*). Mature sex cells have 23 chromosomes (the *haploid number*).

During early fetal life, primitive ova called *oogonia* proliferate by mitotic division. These oogonia enlarge to form *primary oocytes* before birth (see Fig. 2–5). By the time of birth all the primary oocytes have completed the prophase of the first meiotic division. The primary oocytes remain in prophase until puberty.

Shortly before ovulation the primary oocyte completes the *first meiotic division*. Unlike the corresponding stage of spermatogenesis, however, the division of cytoplasm is unequal. The *secondary oocyte* receives almost all the cytoplasm and the *first polar body* receives hardly any (see Fig. 2–5); this small nonfunctional cell soon degenerates.

At ovulation the nucleus of the secondary oocyte begins the *second meiotic division,* but progresses only to metaphase, where division is arrested. If the secondary oocyte is penetrated by a sperm (see Figs. 2–5 and 3–1), the second meiotic division is completed. Again most cytoplasm is again retained by one cell, the *mature ovum* (see Fig. 2–5). The other cell, called the *second polar body,* is very small; it soon degenerates.

The ovum released at ovulation is surrounded by a covering of amorphous material known as the *zona pellucida* and a layer of follicular cells called the *corona radiata* (see Fig. 2–4C). Compared with ordinary cells, the secondary oocyte is truly large and is just visible to the unaided eye as a tiny speck. Up to two million primary oocytes are usually present in the ovaries of a newborn female infant. Most of these regress during childhood so that by puberty no more than 40,000 remain. Of these, only about 400 mature and are expelled at ovulation during the reproductive period (about 30 years).

It is important to realize that primary oocytes that develop toward the end of the reproductive period have been dormant in arrested first meiotic division for at least 30 years. As it is known that the incidence of children with malformations resulting from chromosomal abnormalities (e.g., the Down syndrome) increases with maternal age, it appears that the extended first meiotic division makes the primary oocyte susceptible to damage by environmental factors (e.g., radiation).

Figure 2–5. Drawings comparing spermatogenesis and oogenesis (formation of sperms and ova, respectively). Oogonia are not shown in this figure because all oogonia differentiate into primary oocytes before birth. The chromosome complement of the germ cells is shown at each stage. The number designates the total number of chromosomes, including the sex chromosome(s) shown after the comma. Note that (1) following the two meiotic divisions, the diploid number of chromosomes, 46, is reduced to the haploid number, 23; (2) *four sperms* form from one primary spermatocyte, whereas only *one* mature ovum results from maturation of a primary oocyte; and (3) the cytoplasm is conserved during oogenesis to form one large cell, the mature oocyte or ovum. The polar bodies, nonfunctional cells that soon degenerate, also contain the haploid number of chromosomes.

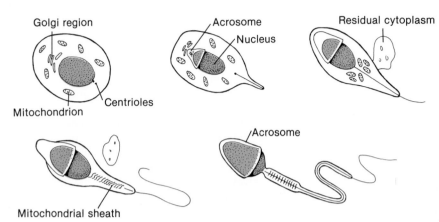

Golgi region · Acrosome · Nucleus · Residual cytoplasm · Centrioles · Mitochondrion · Acrosome · Mitochondrial sheath

Figure 2–6. Drawings illustrating the last phase of spermatogenesis, known as *spermiogenesis*. During this process the rounded spermatids are transformed into elongated sperms (spermatozoa). Note the loss of cytoplasm, the development of the tail, and the formation of the acrosome (acrosomal cap). The acrosome, derived from the Golgi region of the spermatid, contains enzymes that are released at the beginning of the fertilization process and assist the sperm in penetrating the corona radiata and zona pellucida surrounding the secondary oocyte. Note that the excess cytoplasm is shed during spermiogenesis.

Comparison of the Sperm and Oocyte

The sperm and secondary oocyte (ovum) are dissimilar in several ways because of their adaptation for specialized roles in reproduction. The ovum is massive compared to the sperm (see Fig. 2–4) and is immotile, whereas the microscopic sperm is highly motile. The ovum has an abundance of cytoplasm; the sperm has very little. The sperm bears little resemblance to an ovum or to any other cell because of its specialization for motility.

With respect to sex chromosome constitution, *there are two kinds of normal sperm* (see Fig. 2–5): 22 autosomes plus an X chromosome (i.e., 23,X); and 22 autosomes plus a Y chromosome (i.e., 23,Y). *There is only one kind of normal ovum:* 22 autosomes plus an X chromosome (i.e., 23,X). This difference in sex chromosome complement forms the basis of primary sex determination (see Chapter 3).

Abnormal Gametes

The ideal maternal age for reproduction is considered to be from 18 to 35 years. The likelihood of chromosomal abnormalities in the ova and the embryo increases significantly after the age of 35. It is also undesirable for the father to be old because the likelihood of gene mutation (alteration) increases with paternal age. The older the father at the time of conception, the more likely he is to have accumulated mutations that the embryo might inherit. This relationship does not hold for all dominant mutations and is not present, or at least has not been recognized, in older mothers.

Ionizing radiation is a strong *mutagen* (producer of mutations). Therefore it is wise to reduce as much as possible the exposure of the gonads (ovaries or testes) to radiation during the usual reproductive period (e.g., from diagnostic and therapeutic x-rays).

Chromosomal Abnormalities in Gametes. During meiosis, homologous chromosomes sometimes fail to separate and go to opposite poles of the cell. As a result of this error of cell division, known as *nondisjunction* (nonseparation), some germ cells have 24 chromosomes and others have only 22.

If a gamete with 24 chromosomes fuses with a normal one during fertilization, a zygote with 47 chromosomes forms. This condition is called *trisomy* because of the presence of three representatives of a particular chromosome, instead of the usual two. For example, people with *Down syndrome* have 47 chromosomes owing to the presence of three number 21 chromosomes.

If a gamete with only 22 chromosomes fuses with a normal one, a zygote with 45 chromosomes forms. This condition is known as *monosomy* because only one representative of the particular chromosome pair is present. For example, people with the Turner syndrome have 45 chromosomes owing to absence of one sex chromosome. For photographs of patients with these syndromes, see Chapter 9.

Morphological Abnormalities of Sperms. Up to 10 per cent of the sperms in a sample of semen may be grossly abnormal (e.g., two heads or two tails), but it is generally believed that they do not fertilize oocytes owing to their lack of normal motility.

Most, if not all, morphologically abnormal sperms are unable to pass through the mucus in the cervical canal. X-rays, severe allergic reactions, and certain antispermatogenic agents are believed to increase the percentage of abnormally shaped sperms. Such sperms are not believed to affect fertility unless their number exceeds 20 per cent.

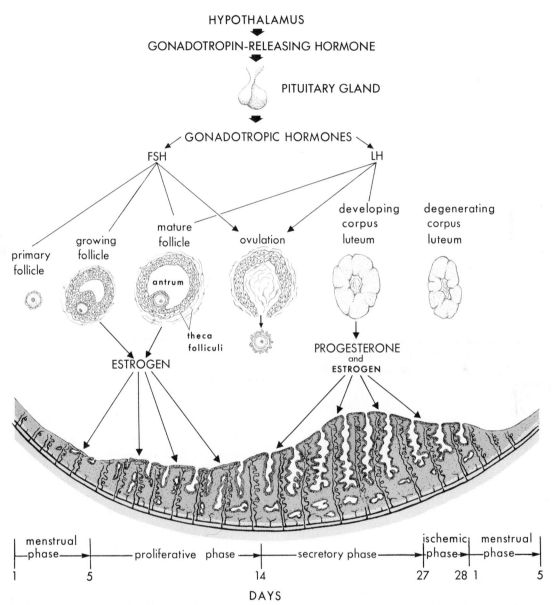

HYPOTHALAMUS

GONADOTROPIN-RELEASING HORMONE

PITUITARY GLAND

GONADOTROPIC HORMONES

FSH   LH

primary   growing   mature   developing   degenerating
follicle   follicle   follicle   ovulation   corpus   corpus
                                                                        luteum   luteum

antrum

theca
folliculi

ESTROGEN   PROGESTERONE
                                                      and
                                                   ESTROGEN

menstrual	proliferative phase	secretory phase	ischemic	menstrual
phase			phase	phase
1 5	14	27 28 1	5

DAYS

Figure 2–7. Schematic drawing illustrating the interrelations of the hypothalamus of the brain, hypophysis cerebri (pituitary gland), ovaries, and endometrium. One complete menstrual cycle and the beginning of another are shown. Changes in the ovaries, called the ovarian cycle, are promoted by the gonadotrophic hormones (FSH and LH). Hormones from the ovaries (estrogens and progesterone) then promote changes in the structure and function of the endometrium, called the endometrial or uterine cycle. Thus, the cyclical activity of the ovary is intimately linked with changes in the uterus. The ovarian cycles are under the rhythmic endocrine control of the adenohypophysis, the anterior part of the pituitary gland, and this, in turn, is dominated by the influence of neurosecretory cells in the hypothalamus of the brain.

FEMALE REPRODUCTIVE CYCLES

Commencing at puberty and normally continuing throughout the reproductive years, *human females undergo monthly reproductive or sexual cycles* involving the hypothalamus, pituitary gland (hypophysis cerebri), ovaries, and uterus (Fig. 2–7).

Cyclic changes in structure and function also occur in the uterine tubes, vagina, and mammary glands. The reproductive cycles prepare the female reproductive system for pregnancy.

Small blood vessels carry *gonadotropin-releasing hormones* (GnRH) from neurosecretory cells in the hypothalamus to the anterior pituitary gland which regulates this gland's production of gonadotropins (gonad-stimulating hormones): *follicle-stimulating hormone* (FSH) and *luteinizing hormone* (LH).

The Ovarian Cycle

The gonadotropins (FSH and LH) produce cyclic changes in the ovaries (development of follicles, ovulation, and corpus luteum formation). Collectively, these changes constitute the *ovarian cycle* (Figs. 2–7 and 2–8). In each cycle, FSH promotes growth of 5 to 12 primary follicles; however, usually only one of them develops into a mature follicle and ruptures through the surface of the ovary, expelling its oocyte (Fig. 2–8). Hence, most follicles begin to develop and then degenerate (i.e., they never mature).

Follicular Development (see Figs. 2–5 and 2–7). Development of an ovarian follicle is characterized by (1) growth and differentiation of the primary oocyte, (2) proliferation of follicular cells, and (3) development of a connective tissue capsule, the *theca folliculi.*

The ovarian follicle soon becomes oval in shape and the ovum eccentric in position because the follicular cells proliferate more rapidly on one side. Subsequently fluid-filled spaces appear around the follicular cells that soon coalesce to form a large fluid-filled cavity, the *follicular antrum*. When the antrum has formed, the ovarian follicle is called a *secondary or vesicular follicle*. The oocyte is located at one side of the follicle, where it is surrounded by a mound of follicular cells, the *cumulus oophorus*, that projects into the antrum (Fig. 2–7).

The development of ovarian follicles is initially induced by FSH, but final stages of maturation require LH as well. Growing follicles produce *estrogen,* a female sex hormone which regulates development and function of the reproductive organs.

Ovulation (Fig. 2–8). Ovulation (expulsion of an oocyte from the ovary) usually occurs about two weeks before the next expected menstrual period, i.e., about 14 days after the first day of the menstrual period in the typical 28-day cycle (Fig. 2–7).

Under FSH and LH influence, the follicle undergoes a sudden growth spurt, producing a swelling on the surface of the ovary. A small oval avascular spot, the *stigma,* soon appears on this swelling (Fig. 2–8A). Soon the ovarian surface ruptures at the stigma and the oocyte is expelled with the follicular fluid from the follicle and the ovary. The released secondary oocyte is surrounded by the *zona pellucida* and follicular cells of the *corona radiata* (Figs. 2–4C and 2–8C).

Ovulation is triggered by a surge of LH production, which is induced by the high level of estrogen in the blood. Some women do not ovulate owing to an inadequate release of gonadotropins (FSH and LH); as a result they are unable to become pregnant. In some of these patients *ovulation can be induced* by the administration of FSH and LH or drugs that stimulate their production. Multiple births frequently result from overstimulation of ovulation in these patients.

Oral administration of estrogen, with or without progesterone, in the form of *birth control pills* suppresses ovulation by inhibiting the release of FSH and LH. As a result, the midcycle surge of LH that triggers ovulation does not develop.

The Corpus Luteum (Figs. 2–7 and 2–8). At ovulation the walls of the ovarian follicle collapse and, under LH influence, develop into a glandular structure known as the corpus luteum. It secretes *progesterone* and estrogen. These hormones, particularly progesterone, cause the endometrial glands to secrete and prepare the endometrium for the implantation of a blastocyst (Chapter 3). If the ovum is fertilized, the corpus luteum enlarges to form a *corpus luteum of pregnancy* and increases its hormone production. If the ovum is not fertilized, the corpus luteum begins to degenerate 10 to 12 days after ovulation (Fig. 2–7).

The Menstrual Cycle

The hormones produced by the ovaries (estrogen and progesterone) produce changes in the endometrium of the uterus (Fig. 2–7). These cyclic changes constitute the endometrial or *uterine cycle*, commonly referred to as the menstrual cycle because menstruation is an obvious event.

The length of the cycle illustrated in Figure 2–7 is 28 days, but the length of cycles varies from individual to individual (23 to 35 days).

Ovarian hormones cause cyclic changes in the structure of the reproductive tract, notably the endometrium. Although divided into phases (see Fig. 2–7), it must be stressed that *the menstrual cycle is a*

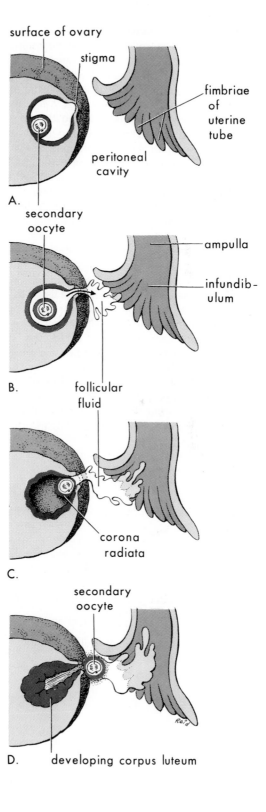

Figure 2–8. Diagrams illustrating ovulation. The stigma ruptures and the oocyte is expelled with the follicular fluid. Note that the mature follicle produces a bulge on the surface of the ovary. Increasing distention results in rupture of the follicle and the surface of the ovary at the stigma (an area of degeneration). As this rupture occurs the oocyte is expelled from the follicle and the ovary with the follicular fluid.

continuous process, during which each phase gradually passes into the next one.

The Menstrual Phase (see Fig. 2–7). The first day of menstruation is counted as the beginning of the menstrual cycle. The functional layer of the uterine wall (see Fig. 2–2B) is sloughed off and discarded during menstruation, which typically occurs at 28-day intervals and lasts three to five days.

The Proliferative Phase. During the proliferative (estrogenic or follicular) phase, estrogen causes regeneration of the epithelium, lengthening of the glands, and multiplication of connective tissue cells. There is a twofold to threefold increase in the thickness of the endometrium during this phase of repair and proliferation. During this phase, the glands increase in number and in length, and the spiral arteries elongate (see Fig. 2–7).

The Secretory Phase. During the secretory (progestational or luteal) phase, progesterone induces the glands to become tortuous (see Fig. 2–7) and to secrete profusely, and the connective tissue to become edematous (a condition in which there are large amounts of fluid in the intercellular spaces).

When fertilization does not occur, the secretory endometrium enters an *ischemic phase* during the last day or two of the menstrual cycle (see Fig. 2–7). The ischemia (localized deficiency of blood) gives the endometrium a pale appearance and results from the spiral arteries constricting intermittently. This constriction of the spiral arteries results from the decreasing secretion of hormones by the degenerating corpus luteum.

Toward the end of the ischemic part of the secretory phase, the spiral arteries become constricted for longer periods. Eventually, blood begins to seep through the ruptured walls of the spiral arteries into the surrounding stroma. Small pools of blood soon form and break through the endometrial surface, resulting in bleeding into the uterine lumen. This indicates the beginning of another menstrual phase. As small pieces of the endometrium detach and pass into the uterine cavity, the ends of the arteries tear and bleed into this cavity, resulting in an average loss of 35 ml of blood. Eventually, over three to five days, the entire compact layer and most of the spongy layer of the endometrium are discarded in the menstrual flow. The remnants of the spongy layer and the basal layer remain to undergo regeneration during the subsequent proliferative phase of the endometrium. Consequently, *the cyclic hormonal activity of the ovary is intimately linked with cyclic histological changes in the endometrium* (see Fig. 2–7).

If pregnancy does not occur, the menstrual cycles normally continue until the end of a woman's reproductive life, usually between the ages of 47 and 52. *Menstruation ceases at the menopause.*

If pregnancy occurs, the menstrual cycles stop and the endometrium passes into a pregnancy phase. With the termination of pregnancy, the ovarian and menstrual cycles resume after a variable period of time.

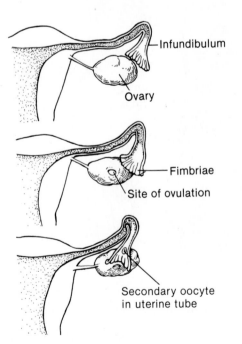

Infundibulum

Ovary

Fimbriae

Site of ovulation

Secondary oocyte in uterine tube

Figure 2–9. Schematic frontal sections of the uterus and uterine tubes, illustrating the movement of the uterine tubes that occurs during ovulation. Note that the funnel-shaped infundibulum of the tube becomes closely applied to the ovary and that its finger-like fimbriae move back and forth over the ovary. They "sweep" the secondary oocyte into the infundibulum as soon as it is expelled from the ovarian follicle in the ovary (see Fig. 2–8).

TRANSPORT OF GAMETES

Oocyte Transport. At ovulation the secondary oocyte leaves the ovarian follicle and the ovary with the escaping follicular fluid (Fig. 2–8). The fimbriated end of the uterine tube becomes closely applied to, and partially covers, the ovary at ovulation (Fig. 2–9). The finger-like *fimbriae* of the uterine tube (Fig. 2–8) move to and fro over the ovary and "sweep" the ovum into the tube. The ovum passes into the *ampulla* of the tube (Fig. 2–8*B*). Movement of the secondary oocyte to the ampulla of the tube results mainly from the gentle *waves of peristalsis* that pass down the tube toward the uterus.

Sperm Transport. From 200 to 600 million of the sperms stored in the epididymis are deposited in the vagina during the process of *ejaculation* (Fig. 2–10). The sperms pass by movements of their tails into the cervical canal, but passage of the sperms through the remainder of the uterus and the uterine tubes results mainly from contractions of the walls of these organs. It takes the sperms about five minutes to reach the fertilization site. Only a few hundred sperms reach the fertilization site in each uterine tube. Most sperms degenerate and are absorbed by the female genital tract. The main sites of reduction in the number of sperms are in the cervix and uterine tubes.

VIABILITY OF GAMETES

Oocytes. Studies on early stages of development indicate that ova are usually fertilized within 12 hours after expulsion of the secondary oocytes at ovulation. Unfertilized oocytes die within 12 to 24 hours.

Sperms. Most sperms probably do not survive for more than 24 hours in the female genital tract. However, some sperms retain their fertilizing power for two to three days.

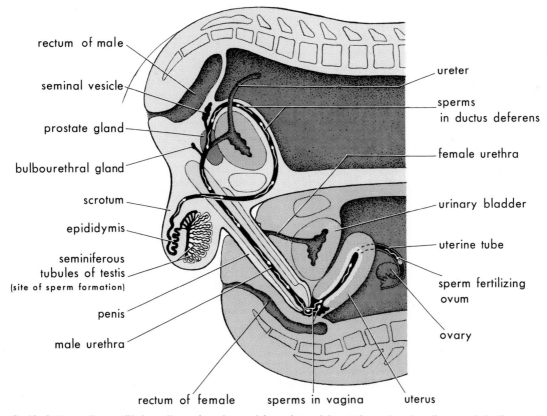

Figure 2–10. Schematic sagittal section of male and female pelvic regions showing the penis in the vagina. The sperms are produced in the seminiferous tubules of the testis and stored in the epididymis. During ejaculation the sperms pass along the ductus deferens and ejaculatory duct and enter the urethra, where they mix with secretions from the seminal vesicles, prostate, and bulbourethral glands. This mixture, called semen, is deposited in the superior portion of the vagina, close to the external opening of the uterus. The sperms pass through the cervix and the cavity of the uterus into the uterine tubes, where fertilization occurs (see Figs. 2–1 and 2–2).

SUMMARY

Fertilization (conception) involves the fusion of an ovum from a female and a sperm from a male. The reproductive system in both sexes is designed to ensure the union of these gametes.

The secondary oocyte, developed in the ovary, is expelled from it at ovulation. It is carried into the uterine tube by the sweeping motions of the fimbriae of the uterine tube.

The sperms are produced in the seminiferous tubules of the testis and stored in the epididymis. During the process of ejaculation, occurring during sexual intercourse, the semen is deposited in the vagina. Although there are several million sperms in the semen, only a few thousand pass through the cervical canal, the uterine cavity, and along the uterine tube. Only a few hundred sperms reach the ampulla where fertilization occurs if a secondary oocyte is present.

Commonly Asked Questions

1. Does a ruptured hymen indicate that a woman is not a virgin?
2. I have heard that woman can have an erection. Is this true?
3. I know of a woman who menstruated throughout her pregnancy. How could this happen?
4. If a woman forgets to take a birth control pill and then takes two, will she become pregnant?
5. What is coitus interruptus? I have heard that it is a safe method of birth control. Is this true?
6. I have been told that an IUD (intrauterine device) is a contraceptive. Is this correct?

Answers

1. The hymen usually ruptures during the perinatal period, forming the vaginal orifice. This opening usually enlarges during childhood as the result of physical activity. Contrary to popular myth, the rupture of this fold of mucous membrane surrounding the vaginal orifice (see Fig. 2–3), or the absence of bleeding owing to tearing of it during the initial intercourse, is not necessarily an indication of the loss of virginity. The vaginal orifice in virgins will usually admit the tip of a finger and in some cases has to be dilated to prevent painful tearing during subsequent intercourse.
2. The term *erection* is rarely used when referring to the sexual excitement of the female, but it is true that the clitoris (homologous to the penis) enlarges (''erects'') when it is stimulated and the female is sexually aroused. It is a highly sensitive and important organ related to the sexual excitement of a female.
3. Pregnant women do not menstruate in the usual sense, even though there may be some bleeding at the usual time of the menstrual period. This blood leaks from the intervillous space of the placenta (see Chapter 8), owing to partial separation of the placenta. As there is no shedding of the endometrium, this is not typical menstrual fluid.
4. It depends on when she forgets to take the pill. If it was around midcycle, ovulation might occur and pregnancy could result. The taking of two pills the next day would not likely prevent ovulation. Failure to take a pill later in the cycle is not as serious (i.e., if pregnancy is undesirable).
5. *Coitus interruptus* is the term applied to withdrawal of the penis from the vagina before ejaculation occurs. It depends on the self-discipline of the couple to part before orgasm. Not only is this difficult to do, it is neither reliable nor psychologically acceptable. Often a few sperms are expelled from the penis with the secretions of one of the auxiliary sex glands (e.g., the seminal vesicles) before ejaculation occurs. One of these sperms could fertilize an ovum.
6. The IUD may inhibit the capacitation of sperms and their transport through the uterus to the fertilization site in the uterine tube. In this case it would be a *contraceptive device*. More likely the IUD produces endometrial changes that present a hostile environment for the blastocyst. As a result it does not implant. In this case it would be a *contraimplantation device,* which results in the death and absorption of the embryo when it is a week or so old.

The First Week of Human Development

Human development begins at fertilization when a male gamete or sperm fuses with a female gamete or ovum to form a **zygote** (Gr. *zygotos*, yoked together). The zygote is the first cell of a new human being. By birth this one cell has given rise to millions of cells. Although a very large cell, *the zygote is just visible to the unaided eye.*

FERTILIZATION

Freshly ejaculated sperms are unable to fertilize secondary oocytes. They must undergo an *activation process* known as **capacitation** in the female genital tract during which *glycoproteins are removed from the surface of the acrosome.* Following capacitation the sperms show no morphological changes, but they are more active and are able to penetrate the corona radiata and zona pellucida surrounding the secondary oocyte. Usually sperms are capacitated in the uterus and uterine tubes by substances in the secretions of these parts of the female genital tract.

When a capacitated sperm contacts the corona radiata surrounding a secondary oocyte (Fig. 3–1A), the acrosome undergoes changes that result in the *development of perforations* in it (Fig. 3–1B). These changes, known as the **acrosome reaction,** are associated with the release of enzymes (e.g., hyaluronidase), which causes dissociation of the follicular cells of the corona radiata. Later other enzymes are released from the acrosome (e.g., acrosin), which produce a defect in the zona pellucida through which the sperm passes to the oocyte.

Fertilization is a sequence of events that begins with contact between a sperm and a secondary oocyte, and ends with the fusion of the nuclei of the sperm and ovum and the intermingling of maternal and paternal chromosomes at the metaphase of the first mitotic division of the zygote (Fig. 3–2D and E).

Fertilization usually occurs in the dilated portion of the uterine tube called the *ampulla* (see Fig. 2–2A). The fertilization process takes about 24 hours.

Fertilization may be summarized as follows (Figs. 3–1 and 3–2):

1. The sperm passes through the corona radiata. Dispersal of the corona radiata cells (Fig. 3–1) results from the action of enzymes released from the acrosome of the sperm.

2. The sperm penetrates the zona pellucida, following a pathway formed by other enzymes released from the acrosome.

3. The sperm head contacts the surface of the ovum.

4. The ovum reacts to sperm contact in two ways: (a) the zona pellucida and the ovum's plasma membrane change so that the entry of more sperms is prevented, and (b) *the secondary oocyte completes the second meiotic division* and expels the second polar body (Fig. 3–2B). The ovum is now mature and its nucleus is called the *female pronucleus.*

5. The sperm enters the cytoplasm of the ovum. Its head enlarges to form the rounded *male pronucleus* as the tail of the sperm degenerates (Fig. 3–2C).

6. The male and female pronuclei fuse and the maternal and paternal chromosomes intermingle (Fig.

25

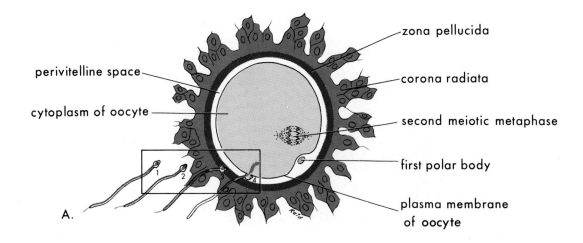

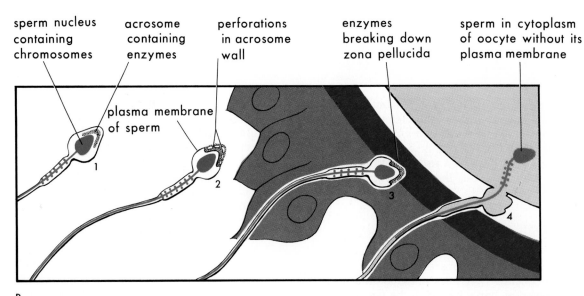

B.

Figure 3–1. Diagrams illustrating the early stages of fertilization. The acrosome reaction and penetration of a sperm into an ovum are shown. The details of the area outlined in *A* are given in *B*: (1) sperm during capacitation (a period of conditioning in the female reproductive tract during which a glycoprotein coat is removed), (2) sperm undergoing the acrosome reaction (perforations in the acrosome associated with the release of the enzymes), (3) sperm digesting a path for itself by the action of enzymes released from the acrosome, (4) sperm head fusing with ovum. Note that the sperm enters the oocyte but leaves its plasma membrane behind. (See Fig. 3–2 for the later stages of fertilization.)

3–2D and *E*). The new diploid cell is called a **zygote**. It is the primordium of a human being.

Results of Fertilization

1. Restoration of the Diploid Number of Chromosomes. Fusion of the two haploid gametes or germ cells (each with 23 chromosomes) produces a zygote, which is a diploid cell with 46 chromosomes, the normal number for the human species. One member of each of the 23 pairs of chromosomes is derived from each parent.

2. Species Variation. Because half the chromosomes in the zygote come from the mother and the other half from the father, the zygote contains a new combination of chromosomes that differs from that of either of the parents. Consequently, fertilization forms the basis of biparental inheritance and ensures variation of the human species.

Meiosis, or reduction division of the developing gametes, allows independent assortment of maternal

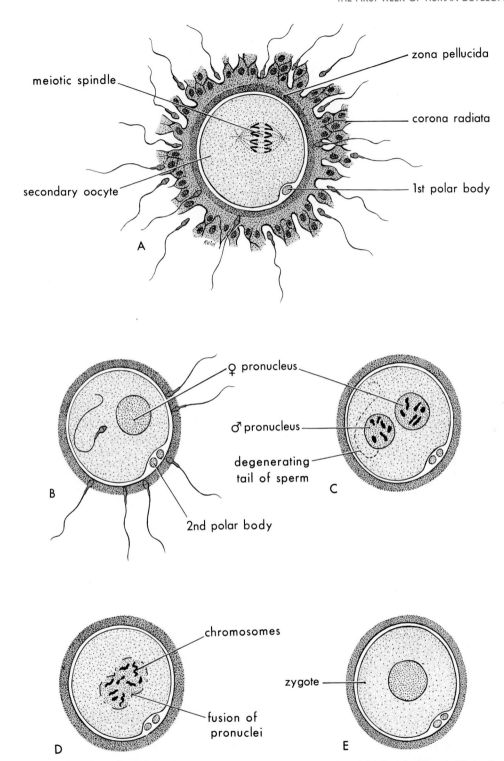

Figure 3–2. Diagrams illustrating fertilization. *A*, Secondary oocyte about to be fertilized. (Only four of the 23 chromosome pairs are shown.) *B*, The corona radiata has disappeared; a sperm has entered the ovum, and the second meiotic division has occurred. The nucleus of the ovum is now called the female pronucleus. *C*, The sperm head has enlarged to form the male pronucleus. *D*, The pronuclei are fusing. *E*, The zygote has formed and is preparing for the first cleavage division (see Fig. 3–3*A*). The polar bodies are small nonfunctional cells that soon degenerate.

and paternal chromosomes among the germ cells. Crossing over of chromosomes, resulting in the relocation of segments of the maternal and paternal chromosomes, "shuffles" the genes, thereby producing a recombination of genetic material.

3. Primary Sex Determination. The embryo's chromosomal sex is determined at fertilization by the kind of sperm that fertilizes the ovum. Fertilization by an X-bearing sperm produces an XX zygote, which normally develops into a female, whereas fertilization by a Y-bearing sperm produces an XY zygote, which normally develops into a male. Hence, *it is the father rather than the mother whose gamete determines the sex of the embryo.*

4. Initiation of Cleavage. Fertilization of the ovum by a sperm also initiates early human development by stimulating the zygote to undergo mitotic cell division or cleavage into two cells called blastomeres. Unfertilized ova degenerate within 24 hours of ovulation and are absorbed by the epithelium lining the uterine tubes.

In Vitro Fertilization and Embryo Transfer

Fertilization of ova or secondary oocytes *in vitro* (L. in glass) and transfer of the dividing zygotes (early embryos) into the uterus has provided an opportunity for many women who are sterile (e.g., owing to tubal occlusion) to bear children. The first of these so-called *test tube babies* was born in 1973. Since then several hundred pregnancies have occurred using this extracorporeal (outside the body) technique.

The steps involved in *in vitro* fertilization are as follows:

1. Ovarian follicles are stimulated to grow and mature by the administration of gonadotropins.

2. Several secondary oocytes are aspirated during *laparoscopy* (viewing the contents of the peritoneal cavity with a laparoscope) from the ovaries just prior to ovulation.

3. The ova are placed in a test tube or petri dish containing a special culture medium.

4. Sperms are added almost immediately.

5. Fertilization and cleavage are monitored microscopically until the 8-cell (blastomere) stage.

6. The "embryos" are inserted into the uterus via the cervical canal.

The probability of a successful pregnancy is enhanced by implanting two to four "embryos." Obviously the chance of multiple pregnancies is higher than when pregnancy results from normal ovulation and passage of the morula into the uterus via the uterine tube. The incidence of spontaneous abortion of transferred embryos is also higher than normal.

Early "embryos" (dividing zygotes) resulting from *in vitro* fertilization can be preserved for long periods by freezing them with liquid nitrogen (*cryopreservation*). Successful transfer of these human embryos to the uterus after thawing has been reported.

CLEAVAGE OF THE ZYGOTE

As the zygote passes down the uterine tube, it undergoes rapid cell division within its zona pellucida. Mitotic division of the zygote into two daughter cells, called *blastomeres* (Fig. 3–3A), begins shortly after fertilization. Subsequent divisions follow rapidly upon one another, forming progressively smaller blastomeres (Fig. 3–3B to D). Hence, there is a increase in cells without an increase in cytoplasmic mass. *The term cleavage is used to describe the mitotic divisions of the zygote.*

By the third day, a solid ball of 16 or so blastomeres has formed, which is called a **morula** (L. *morus*, mulberry). The morula, a mulberry-like cellular mass, enters the uterus and fluid passes into it from the uterine cavity and collects between its cells. As the fluid increases, it separates these cells into two parts: (1) an outer cell layer ("mass") called the *trophoblast*, and (2) a group of centrally located cells known as the *inner cell mass* or embryoblast. The inner cell mass or *embryoblast* subsequently differentiates into the *embryo*, whereas the trophoblast (Gr. *trophe*, nutrition) contributes to the formation of the placenta from which the embryo receives its nourishment.

By the fourth day after fertilization, the fluid-filled spaces fuse to form a single large space known as the *blastocyst cavity*. This converts the morula into a *blastocyst* (Fig. 3–3E). The inner cell mass (future embryo) projects into the blastocyst cavity and the trophoblast forms the wall of the blastocyst (Fig. 3–3F).

The blastocyst lies free in the uterine secretions for about two days. These secretions provide the nutritional requirements of the blastocyst (early embryo).

On about the fifth day after fertilization, the *zona pellucida* degenerates and disappears (Fig. 3–3E and F). The blastocyst attaches to the endometrial epithelium on about the sixth day, usually at the embryonic pole (Fig. 3–4A). The trophoblastic cells produce substances that destroy the adjacent endometrial epithelium (Fig. 3–4B).

As invasion of the trophoblast proceeds, two layers of trophoblasts form: (1) an inner *cytotrophoblast* (cellular trophoblast), and (2) an outer *syncytiotrophoblast* or syncytium. The syncytiotrophoblast is a *multinucleated mass* without recognizable cell boundaries. The finger-like processes of the syncytiotrophoblast produce substances that erode the maternal

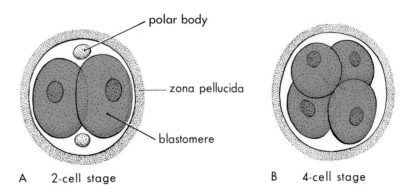

A 2-cell stage

B 4-cell stage

Figure 3–3. Drawings illustrating cleavage of the zygote and formation of the blastocyst. *E* and *F* are sections of blastocysts. Note that the zona pellucida has disappeared by the late blastocyst stage (about five days). The polar bodies shown in *A* are small, nonfunctional cells that soon degenerate. Cleavage of the zygote and formation of the morula occurs as the dividing zygote passes along the uterine tube. Blastocyst formation normally occurs in the uterus. Although cleavage increases the number of cells, called blastomeres, note that each of the daughter cells is smaller than the parent cells. As a result there is no increase in the size of the developing embryo until the zona pellucida degenerates. The blastocyst then enlarges considerably.

C 8-cell stage

D morula

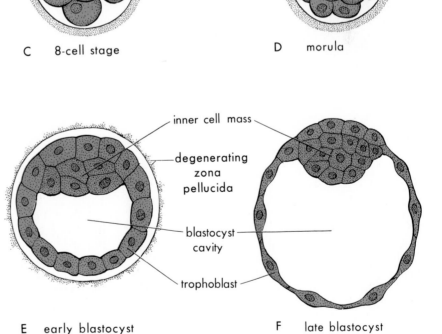

E early blastocyst

F late blastocyst

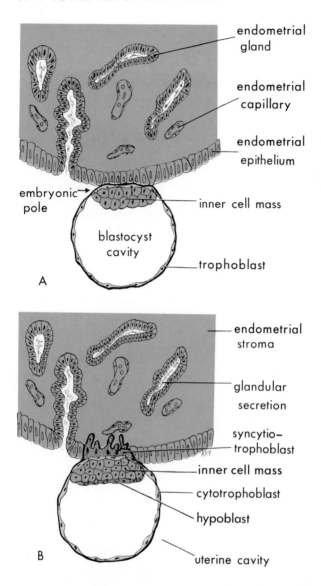

Figure 3—4. Drawings of sections illustrating the attachment of the blastocyst to the endometrial epithelium and the early stages of its implantation. *A,* Six days; the trophoblast is attached to the endometrial epithelium at the embryonic pole of the blastocyst. *B,* Seven days; the syncytiotrophoblast has formed from the trophoblast, has penetrated the endometrial epithelium, and has started to invade the endometrial stroma (framework of connective tissue).

tissues. This enables the blastocyst to penetrate the endometrial epithelium and invade the endometrial stroma. By the end of the first week, the blastocyst is superficially implanted in the endometrium of the uterus (Fig. 3—4B).

As the blastocyst implants, early differentiation of the inner cell mass occurs. A layer of cells, called the *hypoblast* (primitive embryonic endoderm), appears on the free surface of the inner cell mass (Fig. 3—4B). The hypoblast later forms the roof of the primary yolk sac (see Fig. 4—1C).

Abnormal Zygotes and Spontaneous Abortion. About 15 per cent of zygotes are aborted, but this estimate is undoubtedly low because the loss of zygotes during the first two weeks is thought to be high. *Implantation of the blastocyst is a critical period of development* that may fail to occur owing to the inadequate production of progesterone and estrogen by the corpus luteum (see Fig. 2—7).

The actual rate of early spontaneous abortion is unknown because the women are not certain that they are pregnant at this early stage. Clinicians occasionally have a patient who states that her last menstrual period was delayed by one or two weeks, and that her flow was then unusually profuse. Very likely, such a patient has had an early spontaneous abortion.

Early spontaneous abortion occurs for a variety of reasons, one being the presence of chromosomal abnormalities in the zygote. This early loss of embryos, once called *pregnancy wastage,* appears to be a means of disposing of abnormal embryos that could not have developed normally, i.e., in many cases *spontaneous abortion is a natural screening of embryos.*

SUMMARY

Fertilization of the ovum usually occurs in the ampulla of the uterine tube. The process is complete when the haploid male and female pronuclei of the sperm and ovum, respectively, fuse to form a *zygote* (Fig. 3–5). This diploid cell is the beginning of a new human being.

As it passes down the uterine tube, the zygote undergoes *cleavage* into a number of smaller cells called *blastomeres*. About three days after fertilization, a ball of 16 or so blastomeres, called a *morula*, enters the uterus. A fluid-filled cavity soon forms in the morula, converting it into a *blastocyst* consisting of the *inner cell mass* or embryoblast, the *trophoblast*, and the *blastocyst cavity*.

The zona pellucida disappears about five days after fertilization and the blastocyst contacts the epithelium of the uterus. Its syncytiotrophoblastic cells invade the endometrial epithelium and underlying endometrial stroma. By the end of the first week, the blastocyst is superficially implanted in the endometrium of the uterus.

The results of fertilization are: (1) restoration of the diploid number of chromosomes; (2) variation of the species; (3) primary determination of sex; and (4) initiation of cleavage of the zygote.

Commonly Asked Questions

1. Women do not commonly become pregnant after they are 50 years old, whereas men can impregnate women when they are very old. Why is this? Is there an increased risk of the Down syndrome or some other severe abnormality in the child when the father is over 50?
2. Why are there not contraceptive pills for men?
3. Is a polar body ever fertilized? If so, does the fertilized polar body give rise to a viable embryo?
4. I have heard that a woman could have dissimilar twins resulting from one ovum being fertilized by a sperm from one man and another one being fertilized by a sperm from another man. Is this possible?
5. Are there differences in meaning between the terms *impregnation, conception,* and *fertilization?*

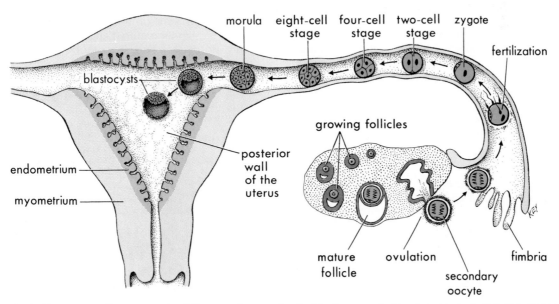

Figure 3–5. Diagrammatic summary of the ovarian cycle, fertilization, and development during the first week. *Development begins at fertilization.* The secondary oocyte is released from the ovary at ovulation and passes into the uterine tube where it is met and fertilized by a sperm. The zygote divides repeatedly as it passes down the uterine tube and becomes a morula. The morula enters the uterus, develops a cavity, and becomes a blastocyst. The blastocysts have been sectioned to show their structure. These stages are also illustrated in the timetable of development on page 2. The blastocyst then begins to invade the endometrium of the posterior wall of the uterus, as shown in Figure 3–4B.

6. Do the terms *cleavage* and *mitosis* of the zygote mean the same thing?
7. How is the dividing zygote (early embryo) nourished during the first week? Do the blastomeres contain any yolk?
8. Can one determine the sex of a dividing zygote (early embryo) developing *in vitro?* If so, are there medical reasons for doing so?

Answers

1. The ovarian and endometrial cycles cease between 47 and 55 years of age, the average being 48. This results from the gradual cessation of gonadotropin production by the pituitary gland, though it does not mean the ovaries have exhausted their supply of oocytes. This period is called the *menopause*. This can be perceived in a positive manner because it is known that there is an increased risk of the Down syndrome or some other trisomy in the children of women who are 35 years of age or older. *Spermatogenesis also decreases after the age of 45*, and the number of nonviable and abnormal sperms also increases with age. Nevertheless, sperm production continues until old age, and some very old men have fathered children. The risk of producing abnormal gametes is much less than in women, but *old men are more likely to have accumulated mutations* that the child might inherit. Mutations may produce congenital malformations.
2. Considerable research on new contraceptive methods is being conducted, including the development of *contraceptive pills for men*. This includes experimental work on nonhormonal prevention of spermatogenesis and the stimulation of immune responses to sperms. Arrest of the development of millions of sperms on a continuous basis is much more difficult than arresting the development of a single ovum monthly.
3. It is not known that polar bodies are ever fertilized, but it has been suggested that *dispermic chimeras* result from the fusion of a fertilized ovum with a fertilized polar body. Chimeras are rare individuals who are composed of a mixture of cells from two separate zygotes. More likely dispermic chimeras result from the fusion of dizygotic (fraternal) twin zygotes early in development. Dizygotic twins are derived from two zygotes (see Chapter 8). If a polar body was fertilized and remained separate from the normal zygote, it might form a small embryo, but it is doubtful that it would survive.
4. Yes, it is, but it is extremely rare. The term *superfecundation* designates the fertilization, by separate acts of coitus, of two or more ova that were ovulated at approximately the same time. In lower mammals that are characterized by multiple births and promiscuity (e.g., cats and dogs), superfecundity is known to occur. In such cases, litter mates are quite different and have characteristics of the different fathers. The possibility of this process occurring in humans cannot be discounted because evidence exists, from dizygotic (nonidentical) twins belonging to different blood groups, that cannot be accounted for in any other way.
5. Not too many. *Conception* means "to become pregnant." *Fertilization* occurs when a sperm fuses with an ovum, and when this occurs, conception takes place. *Impregnation* means "to make pregnant" (a male *impregnates* a female).
6. Essentially yes. *Mitosis* is the usual process of cell reproduction that results in the formation of daughter cells. *Cleavage* is the series of mitotic cell divisions occurring in the zygote immediately following its formation. This process results in the formation of daughter cells called blastomeres. The expressions "cleavage division" and "mitotic division" mean the same when referring to the dividing zygote. Hence, "cleavage" refers to the repeated mitotic divisions of the zygote.
7. The nutritional requirements of the dividing zygote are not great. They are nourished partly by the sparse yolk granules in the blastomeres, but the nutrients mainly come from the secretions of the uterine tubes and later from the secretions of the uterine glands.
8. Yes. One of the blastomeres could be removed and the Y chromosome could be identified by staining the cell with quinacrine mustard (see Fig. 7–12C). Blastomeres of a female embryo would lack a fluorescent body (Y chromosome). This technique could be available to couples with a family history of sex-linked genetic diseases (e.g., hemophilia or muscular dystrophy), or to women who have already given birth to a child with such a disease and are reluctant to have more children. In these cases, only female embryos developing *in vitro* would be transferred to the uterus.

4

The Second Week of Human Development

Implantation or *embedding of the blastocyst in the endometrium* ("lining") of the uterus is completed during the second week of development. Changes also occur in the inner cell mass which result in the formation of a thick, two-layered plate called the *embryonic disc* that will differentiate into the embryo.

The *amniotic cavity, yolk sac, connecting stalk,* and *chorion* also develop during the second week.

IMPLANTATION

The mucosa of the uterus is in the *secretory phase* (see Fig. 2–7) at the time of implantation. The erosive *syncytiotrophoblast* of the blastocyst continues to invade the endometrium containing connective tissue, capillaries, and glands. As a result, the blastocyst slowly embeds itself in the endometrium.

As more trophoblast contacts the endometrium, the trophoblast proliferates and differentiates into two layers (Fig. 4–1A). The *cytotrophoblast* is composed of cells (*cyto* means cell), whereas the *syncytiotrophoblast* consists of a thick multinucleated protoplasmic mass (i.e., a *syncytium*). The syncytiotrophoblast at the embryonic pole (adjacent to the embryo) soon forms a thick, multinucleated layer (Fig. 4–1B). *Syncytio* indicates the syncytium of trophoblast formed by the union of originally separate cells.

Isolated spaces, or *lacunae,* appear in the syncytiotrophoblast and soon become filled with a mixture of blood from ruptured maternal capillaries and secretions from eroded endometrial glands (Fig. 4–1C).

This nutritive fluid or *embryotroph* passes to the embryonic disc (early embryo) by diffusion.

As implantation progresses, a small space appears between the inner cell mass and the invading trophoblast. This space is the beginning of the *amniotic cavity* (Fig. 4–1A). As the amniotic cavity forms, changes occur in the inner cell mass, resulting in the formation of a flattened, essentially circular **embryonic disc.** It consists of two layers: (1) the *epiblast,* consisting of high columnar cells related to the amniotic cavity, and (2) the *hypoblast,* consisting of small cuboidal cells related to the blastocyst cavity.

As the amniotic cavity enlarges, a thin epithelial roof, the *amnion,* forms from cytotrophoblastic cells. The epiblast forms the floor of the amniotic cavity and is continuous peripherally with the amnion (Fig. 4–1C). Concurrently, other cells from the trophoblast form a thin *exocoelomic membrane* which encloses a cavity known as the *primary yolk sac* (primitive yolk sac). The human yolk sac contains no yolk, but it is an essential structure for the early formation of blood (see Fig. 5–7). Some trophoblastic cells give rise to a layer of loosely arranged mesenchymal tissue around the amnion and primary yolk sac, called *extraembryonic mesoderm.*

The 10-day conceptus (the embryo and its membranes) is completely embedded in the endometrium (Fig. 4–2). For a day or so, a small defect in the endometrial epithelium is indicated by a *closing plug* consisting of clotted blood and cellular debris (Figs. 4–2 and 4–3). By day 11 isolated spaces are visible within the extraembryonic mesoderm; these spaces

33

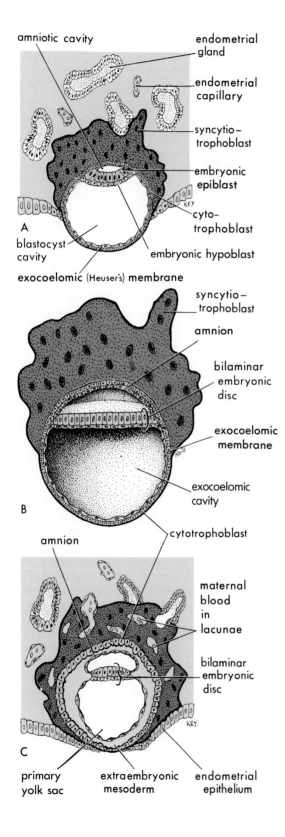

amniotic cavity

endometrial gland

endometrial capillary

syncytio-trophoblast

embryonic epiblast

cytotrophoblast

embryonic hypoblast

A

blastocyst cavity

exocoelomic (Heuser's) membrane

syncytio-trophoblast

amnion

bilaminar embryonic disc

exocoelomic membrane

exocoelomic cavity

cytotrophoblast

B

amnion

maternal blood in lacunae

bilaminar embryonic disc

C

primary yolk sac

extraembryonic mesoderm

endometrial epithelium

Figure 4–1. Drawings illustrating the implantation of a blastocyst into the endometrium. The actual size of the conceptus is about 0.1 mm. *A,* Drawing of a section through a blastocyst partially implanted in the endometrium (about 8 days). Note the slitlike amniotic cavity. *B,* An enlarged three-dimensional sketch of a slightly older blastocyst after removal from the endometrium. Note the extensive syncytiotrophoblast at the embryonic pole and the much larger amniotic cavity. *C,* Drawing of a section through a blastocyst of about 9 days implanted in the endometrium. (Based on Hertig and Rock, 1945.) Note the spaces or lacunae appearing in the syncytiotrophoblast. These lacunae soon communicate with the endometrial blood vessels. The type of implantation illustrated here, in which the blastocyst becomes completely embedded in the endometrium, is called *interstitial implantation.*

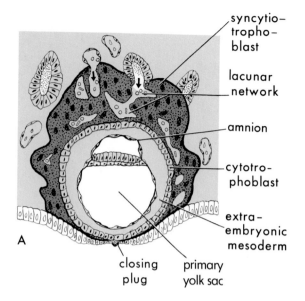

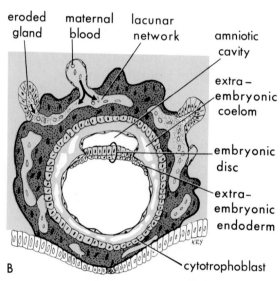

Figure 4–2. Drawings of sections through implanted blastocysts. *A,* 10 days; *B,* 12 days. (Based on Hertig and Rock, 1941.) This stage of development is characterized by the intercommunication of the lacunae filled with maternal blood. Note in *B* that large cavities have appeared in the extraembryonic mesoderm, forming the beginning of the extraembryonic coelom. Also note that extraembryonic endodermal cells have begun to form on the inside of the primary yolk sac.

rapidly fuse to form large isolated cavities of *extraembryonic coelom* (Figs. 4–2B and 4–3B).

By day 13 the endometrial epithelium covers over the blastocyst, producing a minute elevation or wart-like bulge on the endometrial surface (Fig. 4–4).

Meanwhile, adjacent syncytiotrophoblastic lacunae have fused to form intercommunicating *lacunar net-*

works (Fig. 4–2B), the primordia of the *intervillous spaces* of the placenta (see Fig. 5–9). The endometrial capillaries around the implanted embryo have also become dilated to form *sinusoids* and some have been eroded by the syncytiotrophoblast. Maternal blood now seeps into the lacunar networks and soon begins to flow slowly through the lacunar system, establishing a primitive *uteroplacental circulation.*

As maternal blood flows into the *syncytiotrophoblastic lacunae,* its nutritive substances become available to the embryo. As both arterial and venous branches of the maternal blood vessels come into communication with the syncytiotrophoblastic lacunae, blood circulation is established. Oxygenated blood and nutrients pass into the lacunae from the *spiral arteries,* and deoxygenated blood and waste products are removed from them via the veins of the uterus (see Fig. 2–2B). Hence, the maternal blood supplies a rich source of materials for *embryonic nutrition* and a disposal site for waste products.

By the end of the second week, *primary chorionic villi* (finger-like projections of the chorion) have also formed (Fig. 4–5). These villi will later differentiate into the chorionic villi of the placenta (see Fig. 5–9). The isolated coelomic spaces in the extraembryonic mesoderm have now fused to form a single large extraembryonic coelom or cavity (Fig. 4–4). This fluid-filled cavity surrounds the amnion and yolk sac, except where the amnion is attached to the chorion by the *connecting stalk.* As the extraembryonic coelom forms, the primitive yolk sac decreases in size, resulting in a smaller *secondary yolk sac.*

The extraembryonic coelom splits the extraembryonic mesoderm into two layers (see Fig. 4–4): the *extraembryonic somatic mesoderm* lines the trophoblast and covers the amnion, and the *extraembryonic splanchnic mesoderm* covers the yolk sac. The extraembryonic somatic mesoderm and the two layers of trophoblast constitute the *chorion* (Fig. 4–5B). The chorion forms *the chorionic sac,* within which the embryo and its attached amniotic and yolk sac are suspended by the connecting stalk.

The amniotic sac (with the embryonic epiblast forming its "floor") and the yolk sac (with the embryonic hypoblast forming its "roof") are analogous to two balloons pressed together to form the bilaminar embryonic disc and suspended by a cord (the connecting stalk) from the inside of a larger balloon (the chorionic sac).

IMPLANTATION SITES

Implantation of a blastocyst usually occurs in the uterus. Implantation of a blastocyst outside the uterus (*ectopic implantation*) gives rise to complications (see Fig. 4–7).

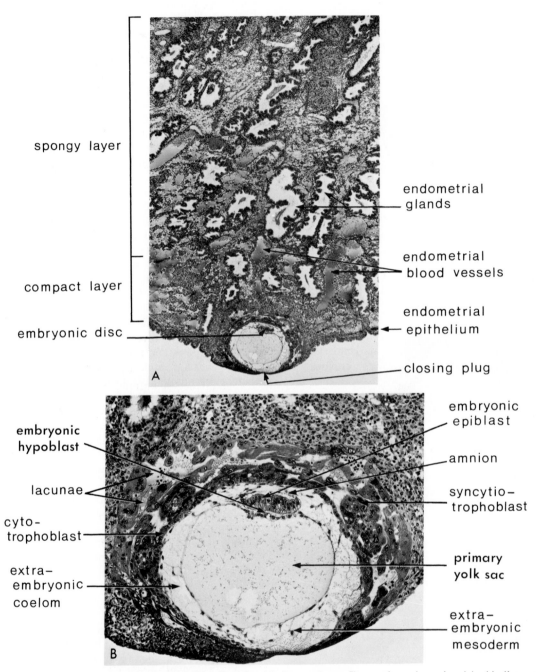

spongy layer

compact layer

embryonic disc

endometrial glands

endometrial blood vessels

endometrial epithelium

closing plug

A

embryonic hypoblast

lacunae

cyto-trophoblast

extra-embryonic coelom

B

embryonic epiblast

amnion

syncytio-trophoblast

primary yolk sac

extra-embryonic mesoderm

Figure 4–3. *A*, Section through the implantation site of a 12-day embryo. The embryo is embedded in the compact layer of the endometrium (× 30). *B*, Higher magnification of the conceptus and surrounding endometrium (× 100). (From Hertig, A. T., and Rock, J.: *Contr. Embryol. Carneg. Instn., Wash. 29*:127, 1941. Courtesy of the Carnegie Institution of Washington.)

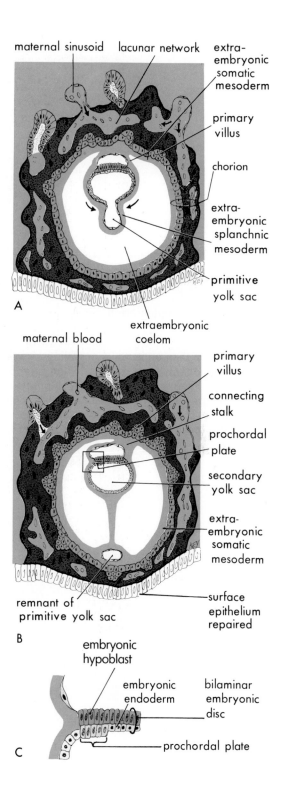

Figure 4–4. Drawings of sections through implanted human embryos. (Based mainly on Hertig et al., 1956.) In these drawings note that (1) the defect in the surface epithelium of the endometrium has disappeared; (2) a small secondary yolk sac has formed inside the primary yolk sac as it is "pinched off"; (3) a large cavity, the extraembryonic coelom, now surrounds the yolk sac and the amnion, except where the amnion is attached to the chorion by the connecting stalk; and (4) the extraembryonic coelom splits the extraembryonic mesoderm into two layers: extraembryonic somatic mesoderm lining the trophoblast and covering the amnion, and extraembryonic splanchnic mesoderm around the yolk sac. The trophoblast and extraembryonic somatic mesoderm together form the chorion, which eventually gives rise to the fetal part of the placenta. *A*, 13 days, illustrating the decrease in relative size of the primary yolk sac and the early appearance of primary chorionic villi at the embryonic pole. *B*, 14 days, showing the newly formed secondary yolk sac and the location of the prochordal plate (future site of mouth) in its roof. *C*, Detail of the prochordal plate area outlined in *B*.

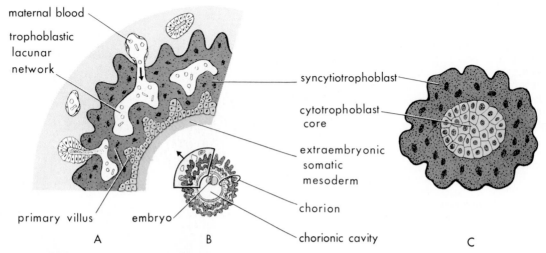

maternal blood

trophoblastic
lacunar
network

syncytiotrophoblast

cytotrophoblast
core

extraembryonic
somatic
mesoderm

chorion

primary villus

embryo

chorionic cavity

A

B

C

Figure 4–5. *A*, Detail of the section (outlined in *B*) of the wall of the chorionic sac. *B*, Sketch of a 14-day conceptus to illustrate the chorionic sac and the shaggy appearance created by the primary villi (× 6). *C*, Drawing of a transverse section through a primary chorionic villus (× 300).

Intrauterine Implantation Sites (Fig. 4–6). The blastocyst usually implants in the midportion of the body of the uterus, slightly more frequently on its posterior wall than on its anterior wall.

Implantation of the blastocyst in the inferior segment of the uterus, near the *internal ostium* (internal orifice of the cervix), results in *placenta previa*, a placenta that covers the internal ostium. This condition may cause bleeding during pregnancy and complications during delivery of the baby.

Extrauterine Implantation Sites (Figs. 4–6 to 4–8). Implantation often occurs *outside the cavity of the uterus.* These are called **ectopic pregnancies.**

More than 90 per cent of ectopic implantations occur in the uterine tube (Fig. 4–7). Most tubal pregnancies are in the ampulla or infundibulum of the uterine tube (Figs. 4–6 and 4–8). The incidence of tubal pregnancy varies from 1 in 80 to 1 in 250 pregnancies, depending on the socioeconomic level of the population studied.

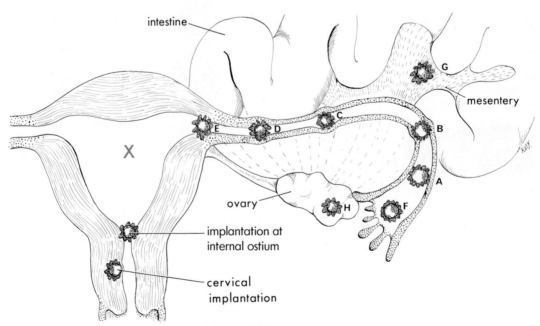

intestine

G

mesentery

E

D

C

B

A

X

ovary

implantation at
internal ostium

H

F

cervical
implantation

Figure 4–6. Drawing to illustrate various implantation sites; the usual site in the posterior wall is indicated by an X. The approximate order of frequency of ectopic implantations is indicated alphabetically. *A to F*, Tubal pregnancies. *G*, Abdominal pregnancy. *H*, Ovarian pregnancy.

Figure 4–7. Photograph showing the gross appearance of an unruptured ectopic pregnancy located in the ampulla of the uterine tube. When the chorionic sac distends the tube, partial separation of the placenta and rupture of the tube often occur. Spurts of blood escape from the ruptured tube and its infundibulum (shown at the left). Tubal rupture and the associated hemorrhage constitute a threat to the mother's life. (From Page, E. W., Villee, C. A., and Villee, D. B.: *Human Reproduction. Essentials of Reproductive and Perinatal Medicine*, 3rd ed. Philadelphia, W. B. Saunders Company, 1981.)

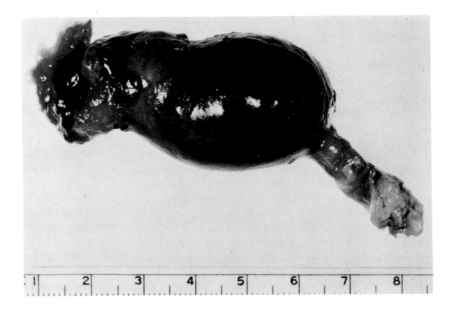

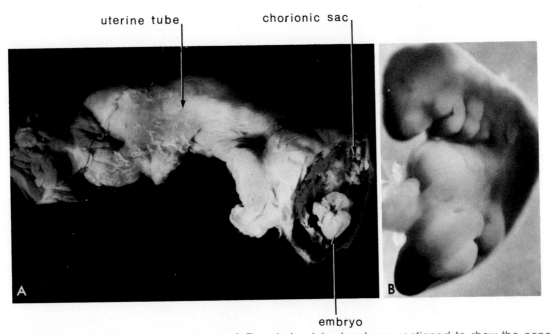

Figure 4–8. Photograph of a tubal pregnancy. *A*, The uterine tube has been sectioned to show the conceptus implanted in the mucous membrane (× 3). *B*, Enlarged photograph of the normal-appearing four-week embryo (× 13). Ectopic pregnancies occur most often in the ampulla of the uterine tube. This serious condition may be caused by a delay in the passage of the dividing zygote along the tube. Ectopic tubal pregnancy results in death of the embryo and usually sudden massive bleeding from the ruptured tube. (Photographed by Professor Jean Hay, Department of Anatomy, University of Manitoba.)

There are several causes of ectopic tubal pregnancy, but they are usually related to factors that delay or prevent transport of the dividing zygote to the uterus; for example, alterations resulting from *pelvic inflammatory disease.* In some cases, the blockage results from a previous tubal infection that has damaged the mucosa, causing adhesions between its folds.

Ectopic tubal pregnancies usually result in rupture of the uterine tube and hemorrhage into the peritoneal cavity during the first eight weeks, and in death of the embryo. Tubal rupture and hemorrhage constitute a threat to the mother's life and so are of major clinical importance. The affected tube and the conceptus are removed (Fig. 4–7).

Cervical implantations are uncommon (see Fig. 4–6). Some of these pregnancies are not recognized because the conceptus is expelled early in the gestation. In other cases, the placenta becomes firmly attached to the fibrous and muscular parts of the cervix, often resulting in bleeding and subsequent surgical intervention, e.g., *hysterectomy* (excision of the uterus).

Blastocysts expelled from the uterine tube ("early abortions") may implant in the ovary (see Fig. 4–6H) or in the abdominal cavity (see Fig. 4–6G), but *ovarian and abdominal pregnancies are extremely rare.* In exceptional cases, an abdominal pregnancy may progress to full term and the fetus may be delivered alive. Usually an abdominal pregnancy creates a serious condition because the placenta often attaches to vital structures and causes considerable bleeding.

Inhibition of Implantation. The administration of relatively large doses of estrogen ("morning-after" pills) for several days after sexual intercourse will interrupt pregnancy by preventing implantation of the blastocyst that develops. Normally, the endometrium progresses to the secretory phase of the menstrual cycle as the zygote forms, undergoes cleavage, and the blastocyst enters the uterus. The large amount of estrogen, usually administered as the synthetic estrogen *diethylstilbestrol (DES)*, disturbs the normal balance between estrogen and progesterone that is necessary for preparation of the endometrium for implantation of the blastocyst (see Fig. 2–7). When the secretory phase does not develop normally, implantation cannot take place and the blastocyst soon dies.

This hormone treatment results in the death of the blastocyst rather than in prevention of its formation; therefore, use of this method is largely *restricted to special cases* in which impregnation is not desired (e.g., after a rape). Another reason this method is not used routinely for birth control is that the treatment is associated with a relatively high frequency of nausea, vomiting, and other adverse effects. Consequently, *contraception is preferable to contraimplantation.*

Various types of *intrauterine devices* (IUD) also prevent implantation of the blastocyst, presumably by inducing a foreign-body response in the endometrium that inhibits implantation.

SPONTANEOUS ABORTIONS

Abortion is defined as the termination of a pregnancy before 20 weeks' gestation, i.e., *before the period of viability of the embryo or fetus.* Almost all abortions that occur during the first three weeks occur spontaneously, that is, they are not induced.

The frequency of early abortions is difficult to establish because they often occur before the woman

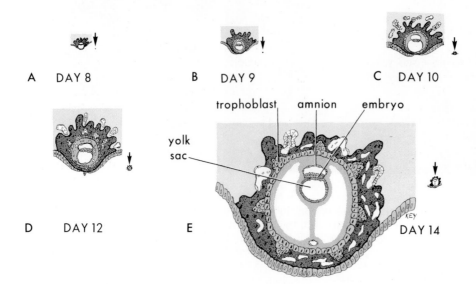

A   DAY 8   B   DAY 9   C   DAY 10

D   DAY 12   E

trophoblast   amnion   embryo

yolk
sac

DAY 14

Figure 4–9. Drawings of sections of human blastocysts during the second week, illustrating the rapid expansion of the trophoblast and the relatively minute size of the embryos (× 25); the sketches indicated by the arrows show the actual size of the blastocysts. Obviously, an aborted conceptus (embryo and its membranes) would be difficult to detect in the menstrual fluid.

is aware she is pregnant. An abortion that occurs a few days after the first missed period is very likely to be mistaken for a delayed menstruation. Detection of the conceptus in the menstrual blood is very difficult owing to its small size (Fig. 4–9).

A study of 34 early embryos recovered from women of known fertility revealed that 10 of them were so abnormal that they probably would have aborted by the end of the second week. The incidence of chromosome abnormalities in early spontaneous abortions is high.

Summarizing the data of several studies, *it has been* *estimated that about 50 per cent of all known spon-* *taneous abortions result from chromosomal abnor-* *malities.* The higher incidence of early abortions in older women probably results from the increasing frequency of nondisjunction during oogenesis (*see* Chapter 2).

It has been estimated that from one third to one half of all zygotes never become blastocysts and implant. Failure of blastocysts to implant may result from a poorly developed endometrium, but in many cases there are probably lethal chromosomal abnormalities in the zygote.

SUMMARY

Rapid proliferation of the trophoblast occurs *during the second week* (Fig. 4–9). The trophoblast consists of an internal cellular layer, known as the *cytotrophoblast,* and an external syncytial layer, known as the *syncytiotrophoblast.*

Lacunae develop in the syncytiotrophoblast that soon fuse to form *lacunar networks.* The syncytiotrophoblast erodes maternal blood vessels and blood seeps into the networks, forming a primitive *uteroplacental circulation.*

Primary *chorionic villi* form on the external surface of the chorionic sac. Implantation is complete when the conceptus is completely embedded in the endometrium and the surface epithelium has grown over the embedded blastocyst.

Concurrently, *extraembryonic mesoderm* arises from the cytotrophoblast. This reduces the relative size of the blastocyst cavity and forms a *primary yolk sac.* As the *extraembryonic coelom* forms from spaces in the extraembryonic mesoderm, the primary yolk sac becomes smaller and is called the *secondary yolk sac.* The *amniotic cavity* appears as a slitlike space between the trophoblast and the inner cell mass, and the *amnion* forms from cells that arise from the cytotrophoblast.

Early in the second week, the inner cell mass differentiates into a *bilaminar embryonic disc* consisting of a layer of embryonic *epiblast* and a layer of embryonic *hypoblast.* At the end of the second week, a localized thickening of the hypoblast, called the *prochordal plate,* indicates the site of the future mouth.

Commonly Asked Questions

1. What is meant by the term "*implantation bleeding*"?
2. Can drugs taken during the first two weeks of pregnancy cause congenital malformations of the embryo?
3. Recently I heard the term "*interception*" in reference to birth control. What does it mean?
4. Can an ectopic pregnancy occur in a woman who has an intrauterine device (IUD)?
5. Can a blastocyst that implants in the abdomen (*abdominal pregnancy*) develop into a full-term fetus?

Answers

1. "*Implantation bleeding*" refers to the loss of small amounts of blood from the implantation site of blastocyst that may occur at the expected time of menstruation. Persons unfamiliar with this possible occurrence may interpret the bleeding as a light menstrual flow. In such cases they would give the wrong date for their last menstrual period (LMP).
2. *Drugs or other agents do not cause congenital* *malformations if taken during the first two weeks* *of development.* A teratogenic drug either damages all the embryonic cells, killing the embryo, or it injures only a few cells and the embryo recovers to develop normally. Despite this, it is unwise to give teratogenic drugs to a female during her reproductive years. If she has a malignant tumor and needs chemotherapy, contraceptive techniques would be used because many chemotherapeutic drugs are teratogenic.
3. The term "*interception*" is sometimes used in reference to *postcoital contraception.* Interceptive pills (e.g., composed of ethinyl estradiol and norgestrel) may be given after a rape to prevent the

sperms from fertilizing an ovum. The risk of pregnancy from unprotected midcycle intercourse is up to 30 per cent.

4. The insertion of an *intrauterine device* (e.g., a coil) usually prevents implantation of a blastocyst in the uterus, but it does not prevent sperms from entering the uterine tubes and fertilizing an oocyte, if one is present. As the endometrium is hostile to implantation, a blastocyst could develop and implant in the uterine tube.

5. *Abdominal pregnancies are very uncommon.* Although the pregnancy can result from a primary implantation of a blastocyst in the abdomen, most of them are believed to result from the implantation of a blastocyst that spontaneously aborted from the uterine tube. The risk of severe maternal bleeding and fetal mortality is high in cases of abdominal pregnancy, but if the diagnosis is made late in pregnancy and the patient (mother) is free of symptoms, the pregnancy may be allowed to continue until the viability of the fetus is ensured. It would then be delivered by the technique of *cesarean section.*

The Third Week of Human Development

The third week is the beginning of a period of rapid development of the embryo from the embryonic disc that formed during the second week. It follows the first missed menstrual period (see the *Timetable of Human Prenatal Development,* Fig. 1–1). Cessation of menstruation is usually the first sign that a woman may be pregnant.

Relatively simple and rapid tests are now available for detecting pregnancy as early as the second week. These tests depend on the presence of *human chorionic gonadotropin* (hCG), a hormone produced by the syncytiotrophoblast that enters the mother's blood and is excreted in her urine (see Chapter 8).

Bleeding at the expected time of menstruation does not rule out pregnancy because there may be light bleeding from the implantation site of the blastocyst in some cases. This *implantation bleeding* results from leakage of blood into the uterine cavity from disrupted blood vessels around the implanted blastocyst. When such bleeding is interpreted as menstruation, an error occurs in determining the expected delivery date of the baby.

The third week is important because three germ layers develop and three important structures form (the primitive streak, the notochord, and the neural tube).

GASTRULATION

The process by which the inner cell mass (see Fig. 3–3) is converted into a trilaminar embryonic disc is called gastrulation. The process begins at the end of the first week with the formation of the *hypoblast* (see Fig. 3–4). It continues during the second week with the formation of the *epiblast* (see Figs. 4–1 and 4–4), and is completed during the third week with the formation of the three *primary germ layers:* ectoderm, mesoderm, and endoderm (Fig. 5–1). As development proceeds these layers give rise to the tissues and organs of the embryo (see Fig. 6–2).

The Primitive Streak

At the beginning of the third week, a thick linear band of embryonic epiblast, known as the *primitive streak,* appears caudally in the midline of the dorsal aspect of the embryonic disc (Figs. 5–1 and 5–2). The primitive streak results from the "heaping up" of cells of the epiblast that proliferate and migrate to the center of the embryonic disc.

As the primitive streak elongates by addition of cells to its caudal end (Fig. 5–3), its cranial end enlarges to form a *primitive knot.* The primitive streak gives rise to mesenchymal cells which form loose embryonic connective tissue, called *mesoblast* (see Fig. 5–2). The mesoblast spreads laterally and cranially from the primitive streak and some of it aggregates to form a layer between the epiblast and the hypoblast known as the *intraembryonic mesoderm* (Fig. 5–1B). Some mesoblastic cells invade the hypoblast and displace most, if not all, of the hypoblastic cells laterally. This newly formed germ layer is known as the intraem-

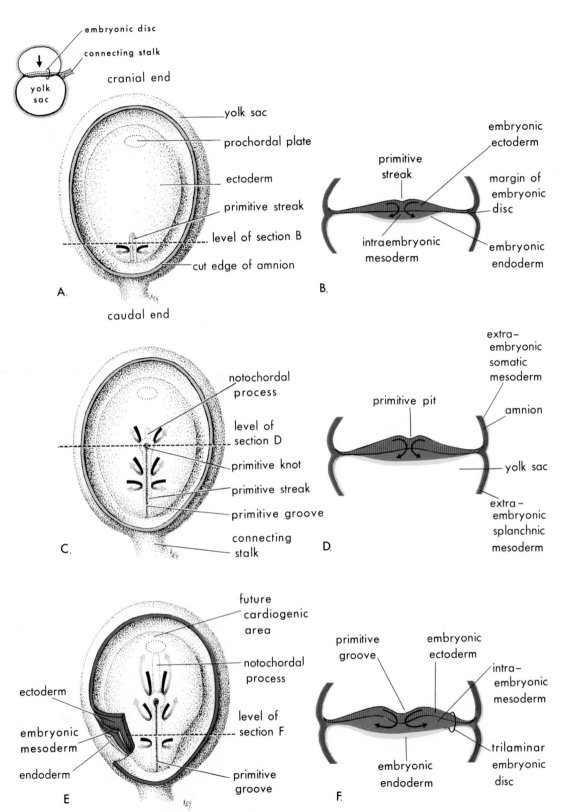

embryonic disc

connecting stalk

yolk sac

cranial end

yolk sac

prochordal plate

ectoderm

primitive streak

level of section B

cut edge of amnion

A.

caudal end

primitive streak

embryonic ectoderm

margin of embryonic disc

intraembryonic mesoderm

embryonic endoderm

B.

notochordal process

level of section D

primitive knot

primitive streak

primitive groove

connecting stalk

C.

primitive pit

extra-embryonic somatic mesoderm

amnion

yolk sac

extra-embryonic splanchnic mesoderm

D.

future cardiogenic area

notochordal process

level of section F

primitive groove

ectoderm

embryonic mesoderm

endoderm

E.

primitive groove

embryonic ectoderm

intra-embryonic mesoderm

embryonic endoderm

trilaminar embryonic disc

F.

Figure 5–1 *See legend on opposite page*

Figure 5–2. Drawing of the cranial half of the embryonic disc during the third week. The disc has been cut transversely to show the migration of mesenchymal cells from the primitive streak. This illustration also indicates that most of the definitive embryonic endoderm may also arise from the epiblast. Presumably most of the hypoblastic cells are displaced to extraembryonic regions.

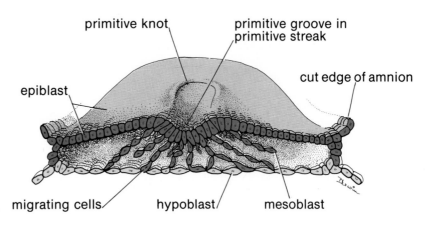

primitive knot

primitive groove in primitive streak

cut edge of amnion

epiblast

migrating cells

hypoblast

mesoblast

bryonic or *embryonic endoderm*. The cells that remain in the epiblast form the layer called the intraembryonic or *embryonic ectoderm*.

Formation of the intraembryonic mesoderm converts the bilaminar embryonic disc into a trilaminar, or three-layered, embryonic disc (Fig. 5–1E and F). The *embryonic ectoderm* gives rise to the epidermis and the nervous system (see Fig. 6–2). The *embryonic endoderm* forms the linings of the digestive and respiratory tracts. The *embryonic mesoderm* gives rise to muscle, connective tissues, bone, and blood vessels.

The Notochordal Process. Cells migrate cranially from the primitive knot of the primitive streak and form a midline cellular cord known as the *notochordal process* (Figs. 5–1C and D and 5–3B). This cord grows cranially between the ectoderm and endoderm until it reaches the *prochordal plate*, which indicates the future site of the *mouth*. The notochordal process can extend no further because the prochordal plate is firmly attached to the overlying ectoderm, forming the *oropharyngeal membrane* (Figs. 5–3C and 5–4C).

Caudal to the primitive streak there is a circular area that is known as the *cloacal membrane*. The embryonic disc remains bilaminar here also because the ectoderm and endoderm are fused (Figs. 5–3C and 5–4E). The cloacal membrane indicates the future site of the *anus*.

Fate of the Primitive Streak. The primitive streak continues to form mesenchyme until about the end of the fourth week; thereafter, mesenchyme production from this source slows down. The primitive streak diminishes in relative size and becomes an insignificant structure in the sacrococcygeal region of the embryo (Fig. 5–3D). Normally it undergoes degenerative changes and disappears, but primitive streak remnants may persist and give rise to a tumor known as a *sacrococcygeal teratoma*. As primitive streak cells are pleuripotent, teratomas often contain various types of tissue.

The Notochord

The notochord is a cellular rod that develops from the *notochordal process* (Fig. 5–4). The notochord defines the *primitive axis of the embryo* and gives it some rigidity. In the lower chordate, *Amphioxus*, the notochord forms the skeleton of the adult animal. This cellular rod forms the mesenchymal axial skeleton in the human embryo and the basis of the adult bony axial skeleton (vertebral column, ribs, sternum, and skull).

The notochord is the structure around which the vertebral column forms (see Chapter 16). It degenerates and disappears where it is surrounded by the

Figure 5–1. Drawings illustrating formation of the trilaminar embryonic disc (three-layered embryo). The small sketch at the upper left is for orientation; the arrow indicates the dorsal aspect of the embryonic disc as shown in A. The arrows in all other drawings indicate migration of mesenchymal cells between the ectoderm and endoderm. A, C, and E, Dorsal views of the embryonic disc early in the third week, exposed by removal of the amnion. B, D, and F, Transverse sections through the embryonic disc at the levels indicated. *The intraembryonic mesoderm forms as follows:* Cells of the epiblast move medially to the primitive streak and enter the primitive groove. These cells lose their attachment to the epiblast and migrate between the epiblast and the hypoblast. These *mesoblastic cells* pass laterally and form a network of cells called the *mesoblast* (see Fig. 5–2). Some mesoblastic cells become organized into a layer called the *intraembryonic mesoderm*.

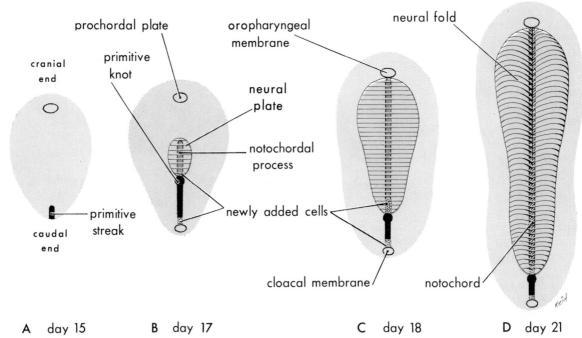

Figure 5–3. Sketches of dorsal views of the embryonic disc showing how it lengthens and changes shape during the third week. The primitive streak lengthens by addition of cells to its caudal end; the notochordal process lengthens by migration of cells from the primitive knot. The notochordal process and adjacent mesoderm induce the overlying embryonic ectoderm to form the neural plate, the primordium of the central nervous system. Observe that as the notochordal process elongates, the primitive streak shortens. At the end of the third week the notochordal process is transformed into the notochord (see Figs. 4–5 and 4–6). Note that the embryonic disc is originally egg-shaped, but soon becomes pear-shaped and then slipper-like as the notochordal process and notochord develop.

vertebral bodies, but it persists as the *nucleus pulposus* of each intervertebral disc.

The developing notochord induces the overlying ectoderm to form the neural plate, the primordium of the central nervous system (the brain and spinal cord). By the end of the third week, the notochord is almost completely formed and extends from the oropharyngeal membrane cranially to the primitive knot caudally.

NEURULATION

The process of formation of the *neural plate,* the *neural folds,* and their closure to form the *neural tube* is called neurulation (Figs. 5–3 to 5–6). This process is completed by the end of the fourth week.

The Neural Plate

As the notochord develops, the embryonic ectoderm over it thickens to form the *neural plate* (Figs. 5–3, 5–4, and 5–6A).

The neural plate gives rise to the *central nervous system* (see Chapter 17). It first appears close to the primitive knot, but as the notochordal process elongates, the neural plate broadens cranially and eventually extends as far as the *oropharyngeal membrane* (Fig. 5–3C).

On about the 18th day, the neural plate invaginates along its central axis to form a *neural groove* with neural folds on each side (Figs. 5–3D, 5–5, and 5–6).

The Neural Tube

By the end of the third week, the *neural folds* near the middle of the embryo have moved together and fused, converting the neural plate into a *neural tube* (Figs. 5–5F and 5–6). Formation of this tube begins in the middle of the embryo and progresses toward the cranial and caudal ends. Progression of closure is more rapid toward the cranial end. Closure of the ends of the neural tube occurs by the end of the fourth week (see Chapter 6).

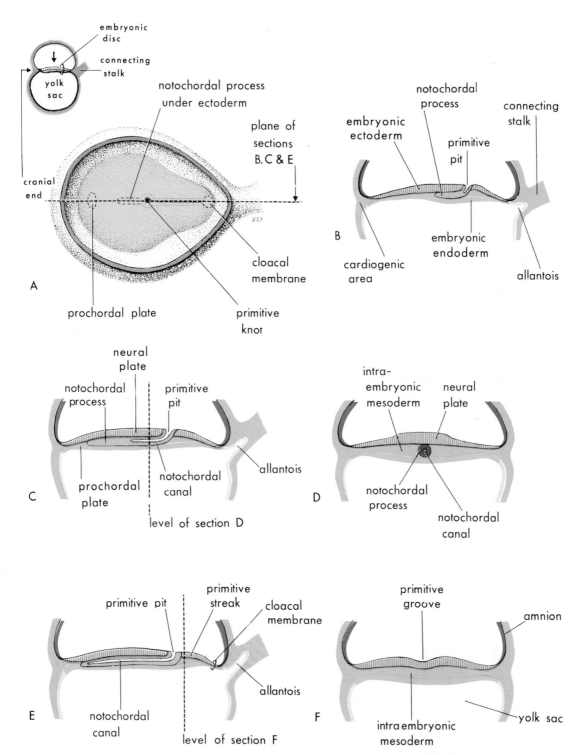

Figure 5–4. Drawings illustrating early stages of notochord development. The small sketch at the upper left is for orientation; the short arrow indicates the dorsal aspect of the embryonic disc. *A,* Dorsal view of the embryonic disc (about 16 days), exposed by removal of the amnion. The notochordal process is shown as if it were visible through the embryonic ectoderm. *B, C,* and *E,* Sagittal sections at the plane shown in *A,* illustrating successive stages in the development of the notochordal process and canal. Stages shown in *C* and *E* occur at about 18 days. *D* and *F,* Transverse sections through the embryonic disc at the levels shown.

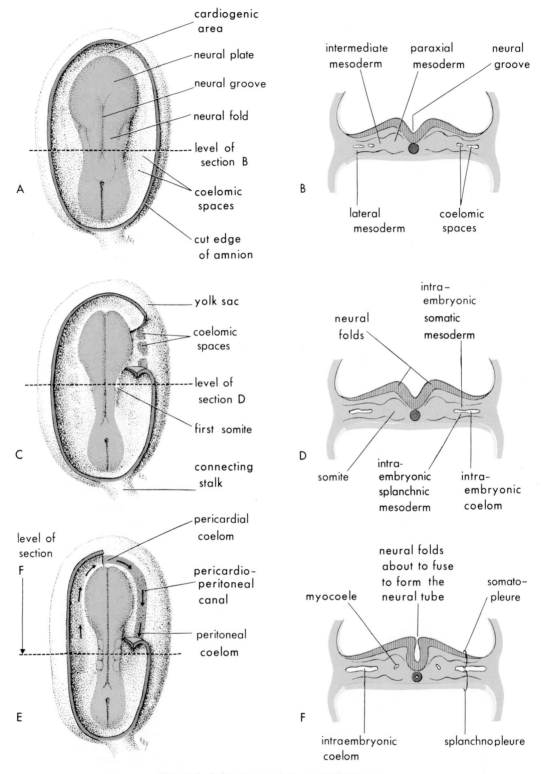

cardiogenic area

neural plate

neural groove

neural fold

level of section B

coelomic spaces

cut edge of amnion

A

intermediate mesoderm **paraxial mesoderm** **neural groove**

lateral mesoderm **coelomic spaces**

B

yolk sac

coelomic spaces

level of section D

first somite

connecting stalk

C

intra-embryonic somatic mesoderm

neural folds

somite intra-embryonic splanchnic mesoderm intra-embryonic coelom

D

level of section F

pericardial coelom

pericardio-peritoneal canal

peritoneal coelom

E

neural folds about to fuse to form the neural tube

myocoele somato-pleure

intraembryonic coelom **splanchnopleure**

F

Figure 5–5 *See legend on opposite page*

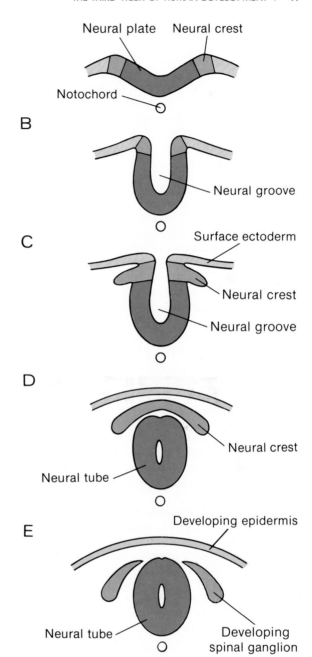

Neural plate   Neural crest

Notochord

B

Neural groove

C

Surface ectoderm

Neural crest

Neural groove

D

Neural crest

Neural tube

E

Developing epidermis

Neural tube

Developing
spinal ganglion

Figure 5–6. Diagrammatic horizontal sections through progressively older embryos, illustrating formation of the neural groove, the neural tube, and the neural crest up to the end of the fourth week.

Figure 5–5. Drawings of embryos of 19 to 21 days, illustrating development of somites and the intraembryonic coelom. *A, C,* and *E,* Dorsal views of the embryonic disc exposed by removal of the amnion. *B, D,* and *F,* Transverse sections through the embryonic disc at the levels shown. Note the notochord in *F,* the cellular structure around which the vertebral column subsequently forms (see Chapter 16). *A,* Presomite embryo of about 19 days. *C,* An embryo of about 20 days showing the first pair of somites. A portion of the ectoderm and mesoderm on the right side has been removed to show the coelomic spaces in the lateral mesoderm. *E,* A three-somite embryo of about 21 days showing the horseshoe-shaped intraembryonic coelom, exposed on the right by removal of the ectoderm and mesoderm of the embryo. The myocoele is an unimportant transitory cavity in the somite.

The Neural Crest

As the neural folds fuse to form the neural tube, some neuroectodermal cells lying along the crest of each neural fold lose their epithelial affinities and attachments to the neighboring cells. As the neural tube separates from the surface ectoderm (Fig. 5–6C), these neuroectodermal cells, called *neural crest cells*, migrate to the sides of the neural tube. Initially these cells form an irregular flattened mass, called the *neural crest* (Fig. 5–6D), between the neural tube and the overlying surface ectoderm. The neural crest soon separates into right and left parts that migrate to the dorsolateral aspects of the neural tube, where they give rise to the *sensory ganglia* of the spinal and cranial nerves. Many neural crest cells begin to migrate in lateral and ventral directions and disperse. Although these cells are difficult to identify, special tracer techniques have revealed that they disseminate widely and have important derivatives, as illustrated in Figure 17–8.

Neural crest cells give rise to the spinal ganglia (dorsal root ganglia) and the ganglia of the autonomic nervous system. The ganglia of cranial nerves V, VII, IX, and X are also partly derived from the neural crest. In addition to forming ganglion cells, neural crest cells form the sheaths of nerves (Schwann cells) and the meningeal covering of the brain and the spinal cord (at least the pia mater and arachnoid). They also contribute to the formation of pigment cells, the suprarenal (adrenal) medulla, and several skeletal and muscular components in the head (see Fig. 6–2 and Chapter 11).

Congenital Malformations of the Central Nervous System Resulting From Abnormal Neurulation. Because the primordium of the central nervous system (neural plate) appears during the third week and gives rise to the neural folds and the beginning of the neural tube, disturbance of neurulation may result in *severe abnormalities of the brain and spinal cord* (see Chapter 17).

Available evidence suggests that the primary disturbance (e.g., a teratogenic drug) affects the neuroectoderm, which results in *failure of closure of the neural tube* in the brain and/or spinal cord regions. Extroversion (a turning outward) of the neural tissue then occurs and the exposed tissue degenerates. In *meroanencephaly*, the brain is represented by a mass of degenerated neural tissue exposed on the surface of the head (see Fig. 16–8).

THE ALLANTOIS

The allantois (Gr. *allas*, sausage) appears early in the third week as a relatively small, finger-like outpouching or diverticulum from the caudal wall of the yolk sac (see Fig. 5–4B). The allantois remains very small in human embryos, but it is involved with early blood and blood vessel formation and is associated with development of the urinary bladder (see Fig. 14–7). As the bladder enlarges, the allantois becomes the *urachus.*

DEVELOPMENT OF SOMITES

At the end of the third week, as the notochord and neural tube form, the mesoderm beside them forms longitudinal columns called *paraxial mesoderm* (Fig. 5–5B). These columns soon begin to divide into paired cuboidal bodies called *somites* (Fig. 5–5C and D). The first pair of somites (Gr. *soma*, body) develops a short distance caudal to the cranial end of the notochord, and subsequent pairs form in a craniocaudal sequence. About 38 pairs of somites form during the so-called *somite period of development* (days 20 to 30); eventually 42 to 44 pairs develop. During the somite period the somites are used as one of the criteria for determining the embryo's age (see Table 6–1).

The somites form distinct surface elevations on the embryo (Fig. 5–5E) and are somewhat triangular in transverse section. The somites give rise to most of the axial skeleton (vertebral column, ribs, sternum, and skull) and associated musculature, as well as the adjacent dermis of the skin (see Chapters 16 and 19).

DEVELOPMENT OF THE INTRAEMBRYONIC COELOM

The intraembryonic coelom (embryonic body cavity) first appears as isolated *coelomic spaces* in the lateral mesoderm and the mesoderm that will form the heart, called the *cardiogenic mesoderm* (see Fig. 5–5A and B). These spaces soon coalesce to form a horseshoe-shaped cavity called the *intraembryonic coelom* (see Fig. 5–5E).

The intraembryonic coelom divides the lateral mesoderm into two layers (see Fig. 5–5D): a *somatic or parietal layer* continuous with the extraembryonic mesoderm covering the amnion, and a *splanchnic or visceral layer* continuous with the extraembryonic mesoderm covering the yolk sac. The somatic mesoderm and the overlying embryonic ectoderm form the body wall called the *somatopleure* (see Fig. 5–5F), whereas the splanchnic mesoderm and the embryonic endoderm form the gut wall called the *splanchnopleure* (see Fig. 6–1).

During the second month, the intraembryonic coelom is divided into three body cavities: (1) the *peri-*

cardial cavity containing the heart, (2) the *pleural cavities* containing the lungs, and (3) the *peritoneal cavity* containing the abdominal and pelvic viscera (see Chapter 10).

DEVELOPMENT OF THE PRIMITIVE CARDIOVASCULAR SYSTEM

Blood and blood vessel formation (*angiogenesis*) starts at the beginning of the third week in the extraembryonic mesoderm of the yolk sac, connecting stalk, and chorion (Fig. 5–7). Embryonic blood vessels begin to develop about two days later.

The early formation of the cardiovascular system is correlated with the absence of a significant amount of yolk in the ovum and yolk sac. At the end of the second week, embryonic nutrition is obtained from the maternal blood by diffusion across the extraembryonic coelom and yolk sac. As the embryo develops in the third week, there is a need for vessels to bring nourishment and oxygen to the embryo from the maternal circulation (Fig. 5–8).

Blood and blood vessel formation during the third

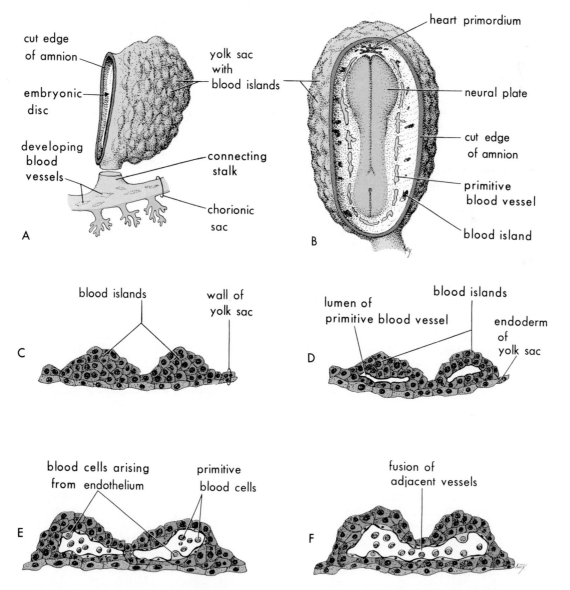

Figure 5–7. Successive stages in the development of blood and blood vessels. *A,* The yolk sac and a portion of the chorionic sac at about 18 days. *B,* Dorsal view of an embryo of about 19 days, exposed by removing the amnion. *C,* to *F,* Sections of blood islands showing progressive stages of development of blood and blood vessels.

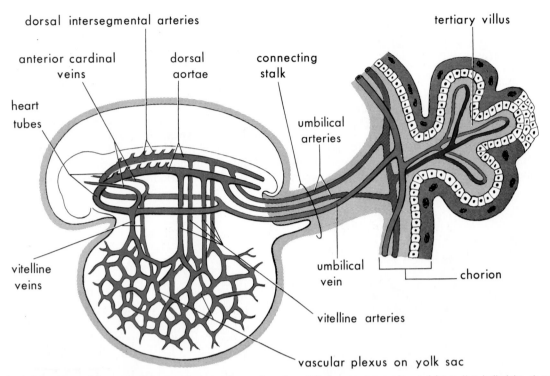

Figure 5–8. Diagram of the primitive cardiovascular system in a 20-day embryo viewed from the left side, showing the transitory stage of paired symmetrical vessels. Each heart tube continues dorsally into a *dorsal aorta* which passes caudally. Branches of the aortae are (1) *umbilical arteries,* establishing connections with vessels in the chorion, (2) *vitelline arteries* to the yolk sac, and (3) *dorsal intersegmental arteries* to the body of the embryo. An *umbilical vein* returns blood from the chorion and divides into right and left umbilical veins within the embryo. Vessels on the yolk sac form a *vascular plexus* which is connected to the heart tubes by *vitelline veins.* The *anterior cardinal veins* return blood from the head region. The umbilical vein is shown in red to indicate that it carries oxygenated blood and nutrients from the chorion (embryonic part of the placenta) to the embryo.

week may be summarized as follows (Fig. 5–7): (1) mesenchymal cells, known as *angioblasts,* aggregate to form isolated masses and cords known as *blood islands;* (2) cavities appear within these islands; (3) cells arrange themselves around each cavity to form a primitive *endothelium;* (4) the vessels fuse to form networks of endothelial channels; and (5) vessels extend into adjacent areas by fusing with other vessels, which have formed independently.

Primitive plasma and blood cells develop from the endothelial cells of the vessels in the walls of the yolk sac and allantois (Fig. 5–7E). *Blood formation does not begin in the embryo until the fifth week.* It first occurs in the liver and later in the spleen, bone marrow, and lymph nodes. The mesenchymal cells surrounding the primitive endothelial blood vessels differentiate into the muscular and connective tissue elements of the vessels.

The *primitive heart* forms in a similar manner from mesenchymal cells in the *cardiogenic area* (Fig. 5–7B). Paired *endocardial heart tubes* develop before the end of the third week and begin to fuse into a primitive heart tube (see Fig. 15–2).

By the end of the third week, the heart tubes have linked up with blood vessels in the embryo, connecting stalk, chorion, and yolk sac to form a primitive cardiovascular system (Fig. 5–8). The circulation of blood starts by the end of the third week when the heart begins to beat. Hence *the cardiovascular system is the first organ system to reach a functional state.*

DEVELOPMENT OF CHORIONIC VILLI

Shortly after the primary chorionic villi appear at the end of the second week (see Figs. 4–4 and 4–5), they begin to branch. Early in the third week mesenchyme begins to grow into the primary chorionic villi, forming a core of loose connective tissue. The villi at this stage, called *secondary chorionic villi,* cover the entire surface of the chorion (Fig. 5–9A and B). Soon mesenchymal cells in the villi begin to differentiate into blood capillaries, which soon form *arteriocapillary venous networks* (about 15 to 20 days). After blood vessels have developed in the villi, they are called *tertiary chorionic villi* (Fig. 5–9D). Vessels in these mature villi soon become connected with the embryonic heart via vessels that differentiate in the mesenchyme of the chorion and in the connecting stalk (Fig. 5–8). By the end of the third week, embryonic blood begins to circulate through the capillaries of the chorionic villi. *Oxygen and nutrients* in the maternal blood in the intervillous spaces diffuse through the walls of the villi and enter the fetal capillaries. *Carbon dioxide and waste products* diffuse from blood in the fetal capillaries through the walls of the villi into the maternal blood.

Concurrently, cytotrophoblast cells of the chorionic villi proliferate and extend through the syncytiotrophoblastic layer and join to form a *cytotrophoblastic shell* (Fig. 5–9), which attaches the chorionic sac to the endometrium. Chorionic villi that are attached to the maternal tissues via the cytotrophoblastic shell are called *stem villi* or *anchoring villi*. The villi that grow from the sides of the stem villi are called *branch villi*, and it is through them that the main exchange of material between the blood of the mother and the embryo takes place.

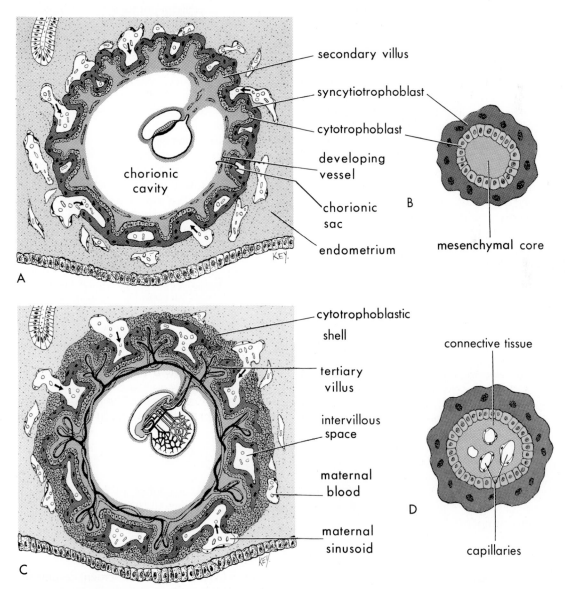

Figure 5–9. Diagrams illustrating further development of the chorionic villi and placenta. *A,* Sagittal section of an embryo (about 16 days). *B,* Section of a secondary chorionic villus. *C,* Section of an implanted embryo (about 21 days). *D,* Section of a tertiary chorionic villus. The fetal blood in the capillaries is separated from the maternal blood surrounding the villus by the placental membrane, composed of the endothelium of the capillary, mesenchyme, cytotrophoblast, and syncytiotrophoblast.

SUMMARY

Rapid development of the embryo begins during the third week. This important period of development coincides with the week following the first missed menstrual period. As the primitive streak forms intraembryonic mesoderm, *the bilaminar embryonic disc is converted into a trilaminar embryo composed of three primary germ layers* (ectoderm, mesoderm, and endoderm). These layers will later give rise to all tissues and organs in the embryo (see Fig. 6–2).

The primitive streak appears at the beginning of the third week as a midline thickening of the embryonic *epiblast*. It gives rise to mesenchymal cells which migrate laterally and cranially between the epiblast and hypoblast. As soon as the primitive streak begins to produce these mesenchymal cells, the epiblast layer is known as the *embryonic ectoderm*, and the hypoblast is known as the *embryonic endoderm*. The cells produced by the primitive streak soon organize into a *third germ layer*, the *intraembryonic mesoderm*. Cells from the primitive knot give rise to the *notochordal process*. This cellular cord soon becomes hollowed out to form a notochordal canal. When fully developed the notochordal process extends from the primitive knot to the prochordal plate.

The *notochord* develops from the notochordal process and forms the primitive skeletal support of the embryo around which the adult axial skeleton later forms.

The *neural plate* appears as a midline thickening of the embryonic ectoderm, cranial to the primitive knot. Formation of the neural plate is induced to form by the developing notochord and the mesenchyme adjacent to it.

A longitudinal *neural groove* develops in the neural plate which is flanked by *neural folds*. These folds meet and fuse to form the *neural tube*. As this process occurs, some cells migrate ventrolaterally to form the *neural crest*.

Neural crest cells give rise to spinal and autonomic ganglia, pigment cells, the suprarenal medulla, the meninges of the brain and spinal cord, and skeletal components of the head.

The mesoderm on each side of the notochord thickens to form longitudinal columns of *paraxial mesoderm*. Division of these paraxial mesodermal columns into pairs of *somites* begins cranially by the end of the third week. The somites give rise to the vertebral column, ribs, and associated back muscles.

The intraembryonic coelom arises as isolated spaces in the *lateral mesoderm* and *cardiogenic mesoderm*. These coelomic spaces subsequently coalesce to form a single, horseshoe-shaped cavity which eventually gives rise to the body cavities (e.g., the peritoneal cavity).

Blood vessels first appear on the yolk sac, around the allantois, and in the chorion. They develop within the embryo shortly thereafter. Blood and blood vessels develop as follows. Spaces appear within aggregations of mesenchyme (*blood islands*) which soon become lined with endothelium derived from the mesenchymal cells. These primitive vessels unite with other vessels to form a *primitive cardiovascular system*.

At the end of the third week, the heart is represented by paired *heart tubes* which are connected to blood vessels in the extraembryonic membranes (yolk sac, umbilical cord, and chorionic sac).

The primitive blood cells are derived mainly from the endothelial cells of blood vessels in the walls of the yolk sac and allantois. Blood begins to form in the embryo about two weeks later.

Primary chorionic villi become *secondary chorionic villi* as they acquire mesenchymal cores. Before the end of the third week, capillaries develop in the villi, transforming them into *tertiary chorionic villi*. Cytotrophoblastic extensions from the chorionic villi mushroom out and join to form a *cytotrophoblastic shell* that anchors the stem villi and the chorionic sac to the endometrium. The rapid development of chorionic villi during the third week greatly increases the surface area of the chorion for the exchange of nutrients and other substances between the maternal and embryonic circulations.

Commonly Asked Questions

1. Do women who have been taking contraceptive pills for many years have more early spontaneous abortions than women who have used other contraceptive techniques?

2. Is the third week of development considered to be part of the embryonic period?

3. What is meant by the term "menstrual extraction"?

4. Can drugs and other agents cause congenital malformations of the embryo if they are present in the mother's blood during the third week?

5. Are there increased risks associated with women over 40 having children?

Answers

1. Yes, if they become pregnant soon after they stop taking the pills. *It takes at least three months for normal menstrual cycles to occur.* If pregnancy occurs before this time, spontaneous abortions often occur a week or so after the first missed menstrual period. Most of the embryos have been found to have severe chromosomal abnormalities. For this reason, most physicians recommend that other contraceptive techniques be used for a few months after cessation of birth control pills, in order to allow normal menstrual cycles to occur.

2. Now it is. Traditionally the fourth to eighth weeks were considered to constitute the embryonic period, but the third week is now included because fundamental embryonic stages of development occur during the third week (e.g., early development of the nervous and cardiovascular systems).

3. *"Menstrual extraction"* refers to suction or *vacuum curettage* of the uterus in the first few weeks after a missed menstrual period. It is the most widely used method of early abortion in North America. The conceptus is evacuated utilizing an electrically powered vacuum source.

4. Yes, certain ones. *Antineoplastic agents (antitumor drugs) can produce severe skeletal and neural tube defects in the embryo* (e.g., meroanencephaly or partial absence of the brain) if administered during the third week.

5. Yes, to the mother and her embryo. *Increased maternal age is a predisposing factor to certain medical conditions* (e.g., kidney disorders and hypertension). *Toxemia,* for example, occurs more frequently in older pregnant women than in younger ones. Advanced maternal age also produces a significantly increased risk to the embryo/fetus. Most common are birth defects associated with chromosomal abnormalities (e.g., the *Down syndrome;* see Chapter 9).

The Fourth to Eighth Weeks of Human Development

These five weeks constitute a critical period of development when all the organs and systems of the body are established. Although the fourth to eighth weeks are commonly referred to as the **embryonic period,** it is important to realize that this period begins in the third week when the nervous and cardiovascular systems begin to form.

The embryonic period is a very important period of human development because the beginnings of all major external and internal structures develop during this time. As the organs develop, the shape of the embryo gradually changes. By the end of the eighth week after fertilization, *the embryo has a remarkably human appearance.*

Because the beginnings of all major external and internal structures develop during the embryonic period, exposure of an embryo to certain agents (drugs, viruses, and so on) during this *critical period of development* may cause major congenital malformations (see Chapter 9).

FOLDING OF THE EMBRYO

The significant event in the establishment of general body form is the folding of the flat trilaminar embryonic disc into a somewhat cylindrical embryo (Fig. 6–1).

During the fourth week, the embryo grows rapidly, tripling its size, and its shape changes significantly as the result of folding. The gradual establishment of body form results from folding of the embryonic disc and the development of the organs (e.g., the heart).

The infolding in both median and horizontal planes is mainly caused by rapid growth of the neural tube. The formation of these folds is a simultaneous process of constriction at the junction of the embryo and yolk sac and is not a separate sequence of events.

Folding in the median plane produces head and tail folds that result in the cranial and caudal regions "swinging" ventrally as if on a hinge (Fig. 6–1A_2 to D_2). During folding, part of the yolk sac is incorporated into the embryo.

The Head Fold (Fig. 6–1A_2 to D_2). The developing brain grows cranially beyond the oropharyngeal membrane and soon overhangs the primitive heart. As the head folds, the heart and oropharyngeal membrane move to the ventral surface. After folding, the mass of mesoderm cranial to the pericardial coelom, called the *septum transversum,* lies caudal to the heart. Subsequently, this septum develops into a major part of the diaphragm (see Chapter 10).

During folding of the head region, part of the yolk sac is incorporated into the embryo as the *foregut;* it lies between the brain and the heart and ends blindly at the *oropharyngeal membrane.* This membrane separates the foregut from the *stomodeum,* or primitive mouth cavity.

The Tail Fold (Fig. 6–1B_2 to D_2). Folding of the caudal end of the embryo occurs a little later than that of the cranial end. As the embryo grows, the tail region projects over the *cloacal membrane.*

During folding of the tail region, part of the yolk sac is incorporated into the embryo as the *hindgut.* After folding, the *connecting stalk* is attached to the ventral surface of the embryo as the *umbilical cord* forms (Fig. 6–1D_2).

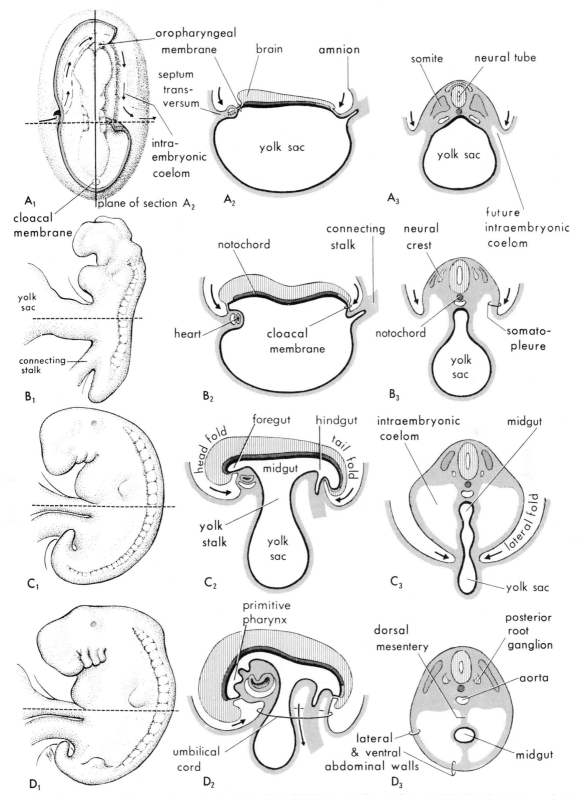

Figure 6–1. Drawings of four-week embryos illustrating folding in both median and horizontal planes. A_1, Dorsal view of a 22-day embryo. The continuity of the intraembryonic coelom and extraembryonic coelom is illustrated on the right side by removal of a portion of the embryonic ectoderm and mesoderm. B_1, C_1, and D_1, Lateral views of embryos of about 24, 26, and 28 days, respectively. A_2 to D_2, Longitudinal sections at the plane shown in A_1, A_3 to D_3, Transverse sections at the levels indicated in A_1 to D_1.

The Lateral Folds (Fig. 6–1A_3 to D_3). Folding of the embryo in the horizontal plane produces right and left *lateral folds*. Each lateral body wall folds toward the median plane, rolling the edges of the embryonic disc ventrally and forming a roughly cylindrical embryo.

As the lateral and ventral body walls form, part of the yolk sac is incorporated into the embryo as the *midgut*. Concurrently, the connection of the midgut with the yolk sac is reduced to a narrow *yolk stalk*. After folding, the region of the attachment of the amnion to the embryo is reduced to a relatively narrow region where the umbilical cord attaches to the ventral surface.

As the midgut separates from the yolk sac, it becomes attached to the dorsal abdominal wall by a thin *dorsal mesentery* (Fig. 6–1D_3).

GERM LAYER DERIVATIVES

The three germ layers (embryonic ectoderm, mesoderm, and endoderm), formed from the inner cell mass during the third week, give rise to all the tissues and organs of the embryo (Fig. 6–2). The cells of each germ layer divide, migrate, aggregate, and differentiate in rather precise patterns as they form the various organ systems. Tissues that develop from the different germ layers are commonly associated in the formation of an organ *(organogenesis)*. The main germ layer derivatives are as follows:

Ectoderm. This layer gives rise to the central nervous system (brain and spinal cord), the peripheral nervous system, the sensory epithelia of the eye, ear, and nose, the epidermis and its appendages (hair and nails), the mammary glands, the hypophysis cerebri (pituitary gland), the subcutaneous glands, and the enamel of teeth.

Neural crest cells, derived from neuroectoderm, give rise to the cells of the *spinal, cranial,* and *autonomic ganglia;* ensheathing cells of the peripheral nervous sytem; *pigment cells* of the dermis; muscle, connective tissues, and *bone of branchial arch origin* (see Chapter 11); the *suprarenal medulla* (adrenal medulla), and the membranes covering the brain and spinal cord (meninges).

Mesoderm. This layer gives rise to cartilage, bone, and connective tissue, striated and smooth muscles, the heart, blood and lymph vessels and cells, the kidneys, the gonads (ovaries and testes), and the genital ducts, the serous membranes lining the body cavities (pericardial, pleural, and peritoneal), the spleen, and the cortex of the suprarenal gland.

Endoderm. This layer gives rise to the epithelial lining of the gastrointestinal and respiratory tracts, the parenchyma of the tonsils, the thyroid gland, the parathyroid glands, the thymus, the liver, and the pancreas, the epithelial lining of the urinary bladder and the urethra, and the epithelial lining of the tympanic cavity, the tympanic antrum, and the auditory tube.

CONTROL OF DEVELOPMENT

Development results from genetic plans contained in the chromosomes. The individuality of each person is largely determined at fertilization by the genes contained in the chromosomes of the sperm and the ovum. These genes control the processes by which the body develops before and after birth.

Most developmental processes depend upon a precisely coordinated interaction of genetic and environmental factors. There are control mechanisms that guide differentiation and ensure synchronized development, e.g., tissue interactions, regulated migrations of cells and cell colonies, controlled proliferations, and cell death. Each system of the body has its own developmental pattern, but most processes of morphogenesis are similar.

Defective genetic plans (abnormal number of chromosomes, gene mutations, and so forth) result in maldevelopment. Abnormal development may also be caused by environmental factors (discussed in Chapter 9). Most developmental processes depend upon a precisely coordinated interaction of genetic and environmental factors.

Induction

For a limited time during early development, certain embryonic tissues markedly influence the development of adjacent tissues. The tissues producing these influences or effects are called *inductors* or organizers. In order to induce, an inductor must be close to but not necessarily in contact with the tissue to be induced. For example, during the development of the eye, the optic vesicle is believed to induce the development of the lens from the surface ectoderm covering the head. In the absence of the optic vesicle, the lens fails to develop. Moreover, if the optic vesicle is removed and placed in association with surface ectoderm which is not usually involved in lens development, lens formation can be induced. Clearly then, development of a lens is dependent on the ectoderm acquiring an association with a second tissue.

Once the basic embryonic plan has been established by primary organizers, a chain of *secondary inductions* occurs. The nature of the inductive agents is not clearly understood, but it is generally accepted that some signal passes from the inducing tissue to

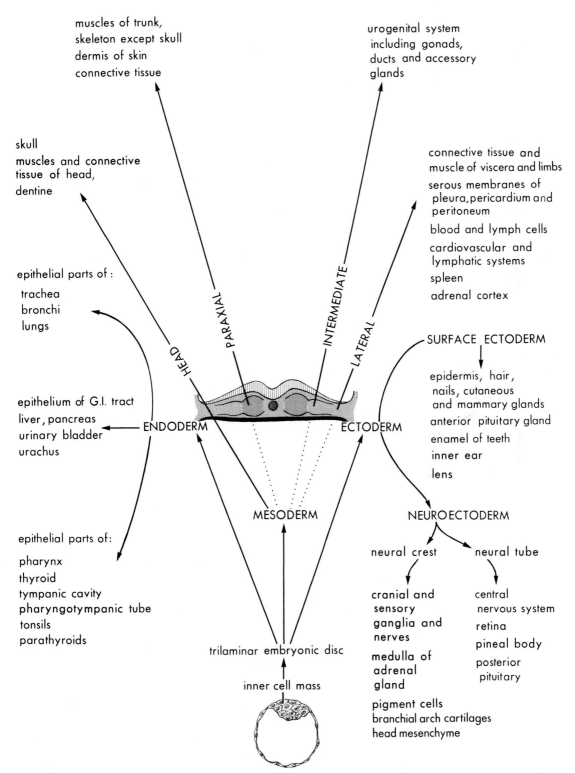

muscles of trunk,
skeleton except skull
dermis of skin
connective tissue

urogenital system
including gonads,
ducts and accessory
glands

skull
muscles and connective
tissue of head,
dentine

connective tissue and
muscle of viscera and limbs

serous membranes of
pleura, pericardium and
peritoneum

blood and lymph cells

cardiovascular and
lymphatic systems

spleen

adrenal cortex

epithelial parts of :
trachea
bronchi
lungs

PARAXIAL

INTERMEDIATE

LATERAL

HEAD

SURFACE ECTODERM

epidermis, hair,
nails, cutaneous
and mammary glands

anterior pituitary gland

enamel of teeth

inner ear

lens

epithelium of G.I. tract
liver, pancreas
urinary bladder
urachus

ENDODERM

ECTODERM

epithelial parts of:

pharynx
thyroid
tympanic cavity
pharyngotympanic tube
tonsils
parathyroids

MESODERM

NEUROECTODERM

neural crest

neural tube

cranial and
sensory
ganglia and
nerves

medulla of
adrenal
gland

pigment cells
branchial arch cartilages
head mesenchyme

central
nervous system

retina

pineal body

posterior
pituitary

trilaminar embryonic disc

inner cell mass

Figure 6–2. Scheme illustrating the origin and derivatives of the three germ layers ectoderm, endoderm, and mesoderm. Cells from these layers make contributions to the formation of the different tissues and organs, e.g., the endoderm forms the epithelial lining of the gastrointestinal tract and the mesoderm gives rise to its connective tissues and muscles.

the induced tissue. The precise nature of the signal is not known; however, the mechanism of the signal transfer appears to vary with the specific tissues involved. In some cases, the signal appears to take the form of a diffusible molecule that passes from the inductor to the reacting tissue. In others, the message is mediated through a nondiffusible extracellular matrix, secreted by the inductor, with which the reacting tissue comes in contact. In still others, the signal appears to require that physical contacts occur between the inducing and the responding tissues.

HIGHLIGHTS OF THE FOURTH TO EIGHTH WEEKS

The following descriptions summarize the main developmental events and changes in external form that occur during this period. The details of organ formation are given with discussions of the various systems (Chapters 12 to 19). Useful criteria for estimating developmental stages in human embryos are listed in Table 6–1.

The Fourth Week (Figs. 6–3 to 6–7). Initially the embryo is almost straight and the *somites* (representing the beginnings of muscles and vertebrae) produce conspicuous surface elevations. The *neural tube* is formed opposite the somites, but it is widely open at rostral and caudal openings called *neuropores*.

By 24 days the first or *mandibular arch* and the second or *hyoid branchial arch* are visible (Fig. 6–3C). The major portion of the first branchial arch, called the mandibular prominence (process), forms the mandible or lower jaw, and an extension of it, the maxillary prominence (process), contributes to the maxilla or upper jaw (see Chapter 11).

Table 6–1. Criteria for Estimating Developmental Stages in Human Embryos

Age (Days)	Carnegie Stage	No. of Somites	Length (mm)	Main Characteristics
20–21	9	1–3	1.5–3.0	*Deep neural groove and first somites present.* Head fold evident.
22–23	10	4–12	2.0–3.5	*Embryo straight or slightly curved.* Neural tube forming or formed opposite somites, but widely open at rostral and caudal neuropores. First and second pairs of branchial arches visible.
24–25	11	13–20	2.5–4.5	*Embryo curved owing to head and tail folds.* Rostral neuropore closing. Otic placodes present. Optic vesicles formed.
26–27	12	21–29	3.0–5.0	*Upper limb buds appear.* Rostral neuropore closed. Caudal neuropore closing. Three pairs of branchial arches visible. Heart prominence distinct. Otic pits present.
28–30	13	30–35	4.0–6.0	*Embryo has C-shaped curve.* Caudal neuropore closed. *Upper limb buds are flipper-like.* Four pairs of branchial arches visible. Lower limb buds appear. *Otic vesicles* present. Lens placodes distinct. Attenuated *tail* present.
31–32	14	*	5.0–7.0	*Upper limbs are paddle-shaped.* Lens pits and nasal pits visible. Optic cups present.
33–36	15		7.0–9.0	*Hand plates formed.* Lens vesicles present. Nasal pits prominent. *Lower limbs are paddle-shaped.* Cervical sinuses visible.
37–40	16		8.0–11.0	*Foot plates formed.* Pigment visible in retina. Auricular hillocks developing.
41–43	17		11.0–14.0	*Digital rays appear in hand plates.* Auricular hillocks outline future auricle of external ear. Trunk beginning to straighten. Cerebral vesicles prominent.
44–46	18		13.0–17.0	*Digital rays appear in foot plates.* Elbow region visible. Eyelids forming. Notches between digital rays in the hands. Nipples visible.
47–48	19		16.0–18.0	*Limbs extend ventrally.* Trunk elongating and straightening. Midgut herniation prominent.
49–51	20		18.0–22.0	*Upper limbs longer and bent at elbows. Fingers and thumb distinct but webbed.* Notches between digital rays in the feet. Scalp vascular plexus appears.
52–53	21		22.0–24.0	*Hands and feet approach each other. Fingers are free and longer.* Toes *distinct* but webbed. Stubby tail present.
54–55	22		23.0–28.0	*Toes free and longer.* Eyelids and auricles of external ears are more developed.
56	23		27.0–31.0	*Head more rounded and shows human characteristics.* External genitalia still have sexless appearance. Distinct bulge still present in umbilical cord; caused by herniation of intestines. *Tail has disappeared.*

*At this and subsequent stages, the number of somites is difficult to determine and so is not a useful criterion.

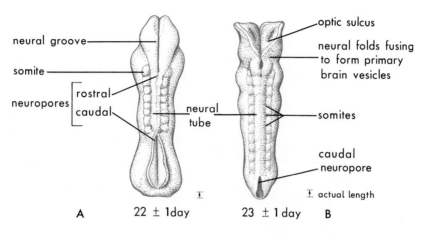

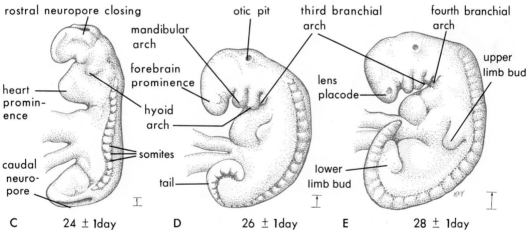

Figure 6–3. Drawings of four-week embryos. *A* and *B,* Dorsal views of embryos early in the fourth week with 8 and 12 somites, respectively. *C, D,* and *E,* Lateral views of older embryos with 16, 27, and 33 somites, respectively. The rostral neuropore is normally closed by 26 to 27 days and the caudal neuropore is usually closed by the end of the fourth week.

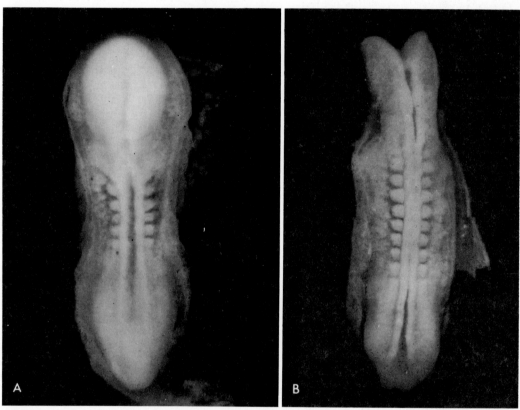

Figure 6–4. Photographs of embryos early in the fourth week. In *A*, the embryo is essentially straight, whereas the embryo in *B* is slightly curved. In *A*, the neural groove is deep and is open throughout its entire extent. In *B*, the neural tube has formed opposite the somites but is widely open at the rostral and caudal neuropores. Compare with Figure 6–3*A*. The neural tube is the primordium of the central nervous system (brain and spinal cord). (Courtesy of Professor Hideo Nishimura, Kyoto University, Kyoto, Japan.)

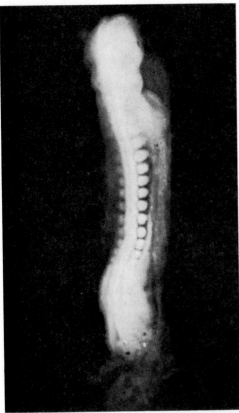

Figure 6–5. Photograph of an embryo during the fourth week (24 to 25 days). Ten of the 13 pairs of somites are easily recognized. The embryo is curved owing to folding of the cranial and caudal ends. Observe the ventral prominence produced by the primitive heart (see Fig. 6–3C). The rostral neuropore is almost closed and the caudal neuropore is closing. (Courtesy of Professor Hideo Nishimura, Kyoto University, Kyoto, Japan.)

A slight curve is produced in the embryo by the head and tail folds (see Fig. 6–1), and the heart produces a large ventral prominence.

Three branchial arches are visible by 26 days (Figs. 6–3D and 6–6), and the forebrain produces a prominent swelling on the head. Continued longitudinal folding has given the embryo a characteristic C-shaped curvature.

The *upper limb buds* become recognizable as small swellings on the lateral body walls (Figs. 6–3D and 6–7). The *otic pits*, the primordia of the internal ears, are also clearly visible. The *lower limb buds* appear as small swellings on the lateral body walls by 28 days (Fig. 6–3E). Lens placodes, ectodermal thickenings indicating the future lenses, are visible on the sides of the head. The fourth pair of branchial arches is also visible by the end of the fourth week.

The Fifth Week (Fig. 6–8A). Changes in body form are minor compared with the fourth week. Extensive head growth is caused mainly by rapid development of the brain. The *upper limbs become paddle-shaped* and the lens and nasal pits become visible.

By the end of the fifth week the *hand plates* have formed and the lower limbs have become paddle-shaped. Note that development of the lower limb occurs somewhat later than that of the upper limb.

The Sixth Week (Figs. 6–8B and C and 6–9). The head is now much larger relative to the trunk and is further bent over the *heart prominence*. This head position results from bending of the brain in the cervical region.

The limbs now show considerable regional differentiation, especially the upper limbs. The elbow and wrist regions become identifiable and the paddle-shaped hand plates develop ridges, called *digital rays* (finger rays), indicating the future *digits* (fingers and thumb). Note that development of the lower limb still occurs somewhat later than that of the upper limb.

Several small swellings develop around the branchial groove between the first two branchial arches (Fig. 6–8C). This groove becomes the *external acoustic meatus* and the swellings eventually fuse to form the auricle of the external ear. Largely because retinal pigment begins to appear, the eye becomes more obvious. The somites are visible in the lumbosacral region until the middle of the week but are not useful criteria for estimating age at this time. By the end of the sixth week, the trunk and neck have begun to straighten.

The Seventh Week (Figs. 6–10 and 6–11A). The communication between the primitive gut and the yolk sac has been reduced to a relatively small duct, the *yolk stalk*. The intestines have entered the extraembryonic coelom in the proximal portion of the umbilical cord; this is called the *umbilical herniation*.

The limbs undergo considerable change during the seventh week. Notches appear between the digital rays in the hand plates, indicating the future digits (fingers and thumb).

The Eighth Week (Figs. 6–11B, 6–12, and 6–13). At the beginning of the final week of the embryonic period, the digits of the hand are short and noticeably webbed (Fig. 6–11B). Notches are visible between the digital rays (toe rays) in the foot plates, and the tail is still visible, but it is stubby (Fig. 6–13A).

By the end of the eighth week, the regions of the limbs are apparent, the fingers have lengthened, and the toes are distinct. All evidence of the tail disappears by the end of the eighth week (Figs. 6–13B and 6–14).

Text continued on page 69

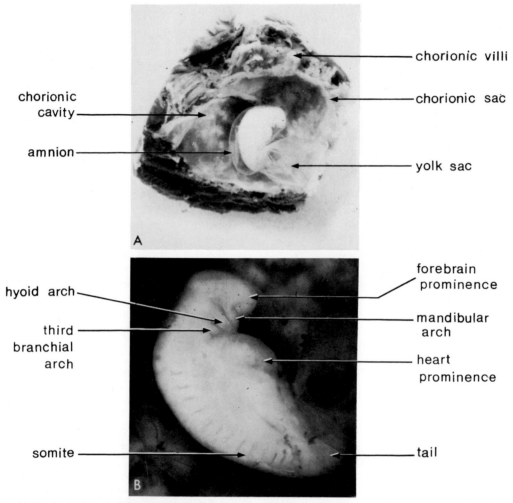

Figure 6–6. *A,* Photograph of a four-week embryo in its amniotic sac, exposed by opening the chorionic sac (×5). *B,* Higher magnification of the embryo of 26 to 27 days (×18). For a discussion of the branchial arches and other parts of the branchial apparatus, see Chapter 11. Although present, the upper limb bud is not visible in this photograph. (Photographed by Professor Jean Hay, Department of Anatomy, University of Manitoba.)

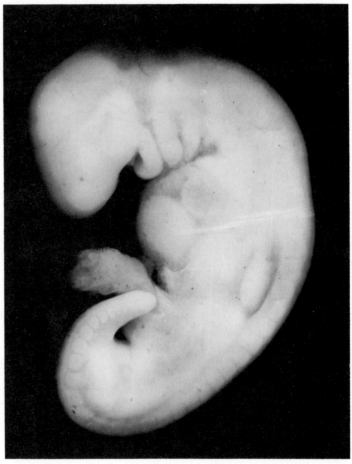

Figure 6–7. Photograph of an embryo 28 days old. The embryo has a characteristic C-shaped curvature, four branchial arches, and upper and lower limb buds. The lower limb bud is not recognizable in this photograph. The heart prominence is easily recognized. The ventrally curled attenuated tail, with its somites, is a characteristic feature of this stage. Compare with Figure 6–3E. (Courtesy of Professor Hideo Nishimura, Kyoto University, Kyoto, Japan.)

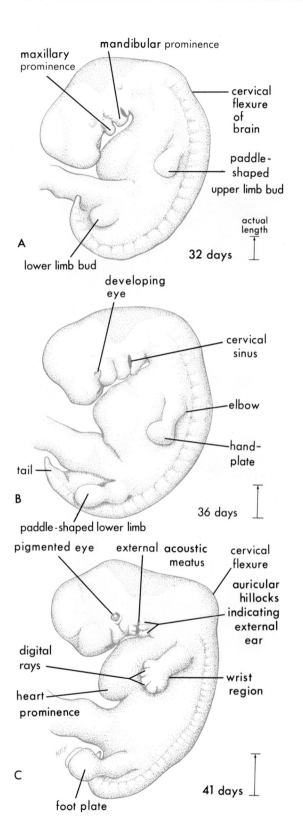

maxillary prominence

mandibular prominence

cervical flexure of brain

paddle-shaped upper limb bud

actual length

A

lower limb bud

32 days

developing eye

cervical sinus

elbow

hand-plate

tail

B

paddle-shaped lower limb

36 days

pigmented eye

external acoustic meatus

cervical flexure

auricular hillocks indicating external ear

digital rays

wrist region

heart prominence

C

foot plate

41 days

Figure 6–8. Drawings of lateral views of embryos during the fifth and sixth weeks.

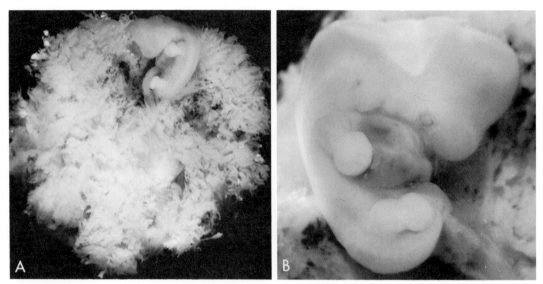

Figure 6–9. *A*, Photograph of a six-week embryo in its amniotic sac, exposed by opening the chorionic sac (×2). *B*, Higher magnification of the embryo of about 41 days (×6). Compare with Figure 6–8*C*. Note the large size of the head compared with the rest of the body, and the prominence of the cerebral vesicles, the primordia of the cerebral hemispheres of the brain. (Photographed by Professor Jean Hay, Department of Anatomy, University of Manitoba.)

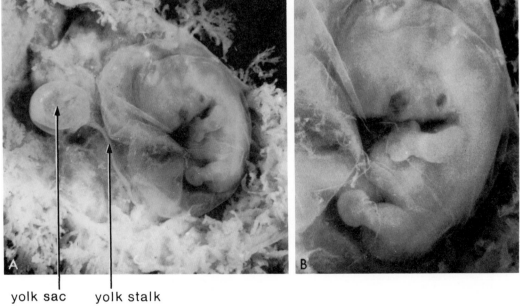

yolk sac   yolk stalk

Figure 6–10. *A* Photograph of a seven-week embryo in its amniotic sac. It has been exposed by opening the chorionic sac (×2.8). *B*, Higher magnification of the embryo of 44 to 46 days (×5). Note the low position of its ear at this stage and the notches between the digital rays of its hand.

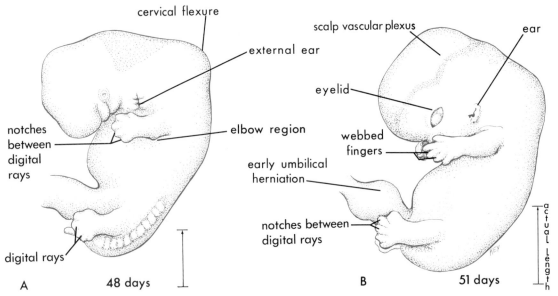

Figure 6–11. Drawings of lateral views of embryos at the end of the seventh and the beginning of the eighth weeks.

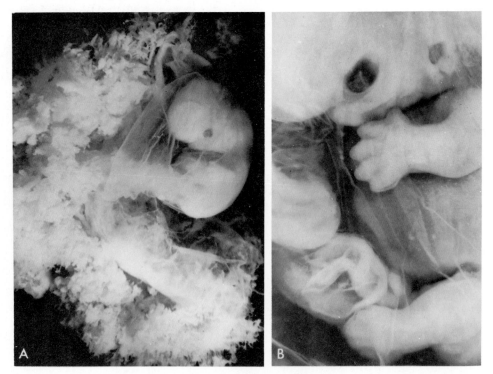

Figure 6–12. *A,* Photograph of an embryo in its amniotic sac, exposed by opening the chorionic sac (×2). *B,* Higher magnification of this embryo of about 51 days (×7). Note the webbed fingers and the notches between the digital rays of the foot. (Photographed by Professor Jean Hay, Department of Anatomy, University of Manitoba.)

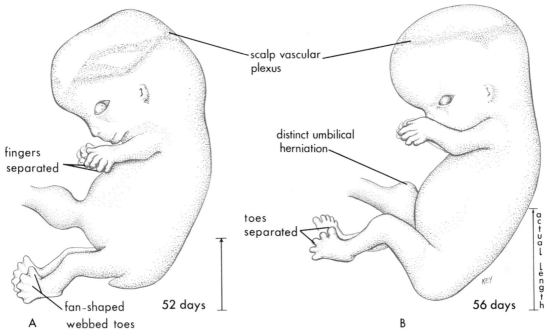

scalp vascular plexus

fingers separated

distinct umbilical herniation

toes separated

fan-shaped webbed toes

52 days

56 days

actual length

A

B

Figure 6–13. Drawings of lateral views of embryos during the eighth week.

The embryo now has unquestionably human characteristics. The head is more round and erect, but is still disproportionately large, constituting almost half of the embryo. The neck region has become established and the eyelids are more obvious.

The abdomen is less protuberant; however, the intestines are still in the proximal portion of the umbilical cord (Figs. 6–13 and 6–14).

During the eighth week, the eyes are usually open, but toward the end of the week, the eyelids may meet and become united by epithelial fusion. The auricles of the external ears begin to assume their final shape, but they are still low-set on the head. Although sex differences exist in the appearance of the external genitalia, they are not distinct enough to permit accurate sexual identification to be made by lay persons.

ESTIMATION OF EMBRYONIC AGE

Information about the starting date of pregnancies may be unreliable, partly because it depends on the mother's memory. Two reference points are commonly used for estimating age: the onset of the *last menstrual period (LMP),* and the time of *fertilization* (see Fig. 1–1).

The probability of error in establishing the last normal menses is highest in women who become pregnant after discontinuing oral contraceptives. This is because the interval between stopping the hormones and ovulation is variable. In addition, uterine

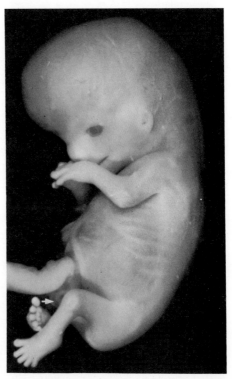

Figure 6–14. Photograph of an embryo of about 56 days (×2). The intestines are still in the umbilical cord (arrow). The digits (fingers and toes) are clearly defined. Note the relatively large head and that the tail has disappeared. (Photographed by Professor Jean Hay, Department of Anatomy, University of Manitoba.)

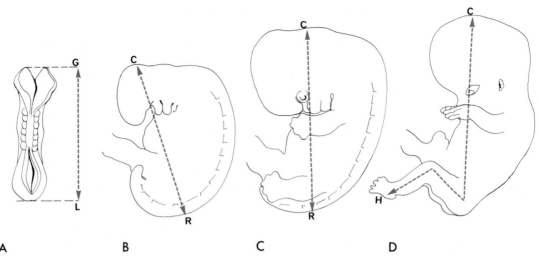

A	B	C	D

Figure 6–15. Sketches showing methods of measuring the length of embryos. *A,* Greatest length. *B* and *C,* Crown-rump length. *D,* Crown-heel length.

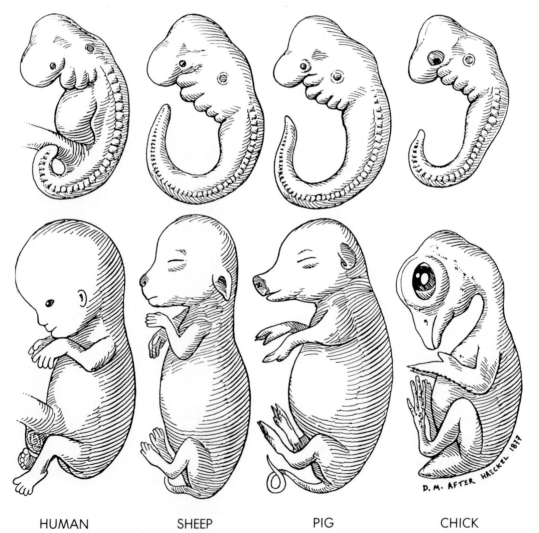

HUMAN	SHEEP	PIG	CHICK

Figure 6–16. Drawings of embryos of four species showing how their early characteristics are similar. By the eighth week, human embryos have distinctive characteristics.

bleeding or "spotting" sometimes occurs after implantation of the blastocyst that may be incorrectly regarded as menstruation by the woman.

It must be emphasized that the zygote does not form until about two weeks after the onset of the last menstrual period (see Fig. 1–1). Consequently, 14 ± 2 days must be deducted from the "menstrual age" to obtain the actual or *fertilization age* of an embryo. The day fertilization occurs is the most accurate reference point for estimating age. This is commonly calculated from the estimated time of ovulation because the ovum is usually fertilized within 12 hours after ovulation.

Because it may be important to know the fertilization age of an embryo, e.g., for determining its sensitivity to drugs (Chapter 9), all statements about age should indicate the reference point used, i.e., weeks after LMP or the estimated time of fertilization.

Estimates of the age of recovered embryos (e.g.,

after abortion) are determined from external characteristics and measurements of length (Table 6–1). The changing appearance of the developing limbs is a very useful criterion. Size alone may be an unreliable criterion because some embryos probably undergo a progressively slower rate of growth prior to death.

Methods of Measurement (Fig. 6–15). Because embryos early in the fourth week are nearly straight, measurements indicate their *greatest length* (GL). The sitting height or *crown-rump length* (CR) is most frequently used for older embryos, but standing height or *crown-heel length* (CH) is sometimes used.

The size of the embryo in a pregnant woman can also be estimated using ultrasound measurements. At four weeks (six weeks after LMP), the embryo, amnion, and yolk sac form a structure about 5 mm long that is detectable with careful scanning. After the fifth week (seven weeks after LMP), discrete embryonic structures can be visualized, and "crown-rump" measurements can be made.

SUMMARY

Early in the embryonic period, *longitudinal and transverse folding* converts the flat trilaminar embryonic disc into a C-shaped, cylindrical embryo. The dorsal part of the yolk sac is incorporated into the embryo during this folding and gives rise to the *primitive gut*. The gut becomes pinched off from the yolk sac, but remains attached to it by the narrow *yolk stalk*.

The head fold results in the heart coming to lie ventrally and the brain becoming the most cranial part of the embryo. The tail fold causes the connecting stalk (future umbilical cord) to move to the ventral surface of the embryo.

The three germ layers differentiate into various tissues and organs, so that by the end of the embryonic period, the beginnings of all the main organ systems have been established. The external appearance of the embryo is greatly affected by

the formation of the brain, heart, liver, somites, limbs, ears, nose, and eyes. As these structures develop, they produce characteristics that mark the embryo as unquestionably human.

Because the beginnings of all essential external and internal structures are formed during the embryonic period, *the fourth to eighth weeks constitute the most critical period of development.* Developmental disturbances during this period may give rise to major congenital malformations.

Reasonable estimates of the age of embryos can be determined from (1) the day of onset of the last normal menstrual period, (2) the estimated time of fertilization, (3) measurements of length, and (4) external characteristics. The age of an embryo can also be estimated by using ultrasound measurements.

Commonly Asked Questions

1. I have heard that the human embryo could be confused with the offspring of many other species, e.g., a pig, mouse, or chick. Is this true?
2. I cannot see any difference between an eight-week-old embryo and a nine-week-old fetus. Why do embryologists give them different names?
3. When does the embryo become human?
4. Can sex be determined by ultrasound techniques during the embryonic period?

5. What is the difference between the terms *primigravida* and *primipara*? I have also heard a woman referred to as a "primip." What does this mean?

Answers

1. Until the fifth week, human embryos resemble the embryos of several other species because of common characteristics (e.g., large head, branchial arches, and tail), but thereafter embryos acquire

characteristics that are distinctly human (e.g., loss of the tail and the human appearance of the face and limbs, Fig. 6–16).

2. Embryos early in the eighth week look different from nine-week-old fetuses because of their webbed toes and stubby tails, but by the end of the eighth week embryos and young fetuses look similar. The name change is made to indicate that a new phase of development (growth and differentiation) has begun. Similarly, a full-term fetus is indistinguishable from a newborn infant, but the name change signifies that a new phase of development has begun, as it is no longer attached to its mother by the umbilical cord.

3. This is a difficult question to answer because one's views are affected by one's religion and the views of one's peers. The scientific answer is that the embryo *always* had human potential, and no *other,* from the time of fertilization because of its human chromosome constitution. Two things are definite: (1) human development begins at fertilization and (2) the zygote and early embryo are living organisms. My personal view is that the embryo becomes a human being during the eighth week when it acquires distinctive human characteristics, but you will have to decide for yourself after wide consultation.

4. No. During the embryonic period there are more similarities than differences in the external genitalia. It would be impossible to know whether the primitive sexual organ (*genital tubercle* at five weeks and *phallus* at seven weeks) will become a penis or a clitoris. Sexual differences are not clear until the 10th to 12th weeks.

5. *Primigravida* is a woman who is pregnant for the first time (L. *primus,* first, + *gravida,* a pregnant woman). *Primipara* is a woman who has given birth for the first time to an infant or infants, alive or dead, weighing 500 gm or more, or having a gestation of 20 weeks or more. Hence, a mother who had previously had a spontaneous abortion at six weeks would be referred to as a *multigravida* because she has been pregnant more than once. *"Primip"* is an abbreviation for the term *primipara,* a woman who has given birth to her first child.

The Ninth to Thirty-eighth Weeks of Human Development

The fetal period lasts from the beginning of the **ninth week** after fertilization until **full term** (usually 38 weeks). *This is primarily a period of increase in size.*

At nine weeks the human embryo is referred to as a *fetus* (L. offspring), signifying that it has developed into a recognizable human being. In addition, the fetus is far less vulnerable than the embryo to the deforming effects of drugs, viruses, and radiation (see Chapter 9).

The transition from embryo to fetus is not abrupt, but the name change is intended to signify the change from embryonic to fetal development.

Development during the fetal period is primarily concerned with growth and differentiation of tissues and organs that appeared during the embryonic period. Very few new structures appear during the fetal period.

The rate of body growth during the fetal period is remarkable, especially between the 9th and 16th weeks (Figs. 7–1 and 7–4), and weight gain is phenomenal during the terminal months (see Table 7–2 and Fig. 7–10).

Fetuses weighing less than 500 gm at birth usually do not survive. The term *abortion* is applied to all pregnancies that terminate before the period of viability, i.e., before 22 weeks (see Table 7–2). If given expert postnatal care, fetuses weighing 500 to 1000 gm may survive if born prematurely. They are referred to as *immature infants.* Fetuses weighing between 1000 and 2500 gm are called *premature infants.* Most of them survive; however, *prematurity is one of the most common causes of perinatal death.*

During a pregnant woman's first visit to a doctor, the age of the embryo or fetus is estimated. The date of the *last mentrual period (LMP)* is a time-honored guide to establishing *gestational age,* and it is reliable in most cases. To determine the actual age, or *fertilization age of the embryo,* two weeks must be deducted from the gestational age because development does not begin until about two weeks after LMP (see Fig. 1–1).

ESTIMATION OF FETAL AGE

A pregnancy or gestational period may be divided into days, weeks, or months (Table 7–1). Confusion arises if it is not stated whether a given time is calculated from the onset of the last menstrual period (LMP), or from the estimated day of fertilization of the ovum. More uncertainty arises when months are used, particularly when it is not stated whether *calendar months* (28 to 31 days) or *lunar months* (28 days) are meant. Unless otherwise stated, *developmental age in this book is calculated from the estimated time of fertilization,* and months refer to calendar months.

It is best to express the age of a fetus in weeks and to state whether the beginning or the end of a week is meant.

Clinically, gestation in humans is commonly divided into three parts, or trimesters, each lasting three calendar months. By the end of the first trimester, all major systems are developed and the crown-rump length of the fetus is about the width of one's palm (see Fig. 7–6).

Table 7–1. Comparison of Gestational Time Units

Reference Point	Days	Weeks	Calendar Months	Lunar Months
Fertilization*	266	38	8¾	9½
Last menstrual period	280	40	9	10

*The date of birth is calculated as about 266 days after fertilization, or 280 days after the onset of the last normal menstrual period. From fertilization to the end of the embryonic period, age is best expressed in days; thereafter age is commonly given in weeks. Because ovulation and fertilization are usually separated by not more than 12 hours, these events are more or less interchangeable in expressing prenatal age.

At the end of the second trimester, the fetus is usually too immature to survive, if born prematurely, even though its length is now equal to about the span of one's hand (see Fig. 7–8).

Various measurements and external characteristics are useful in *estimating fetal age* (Table 7–2). *Foot length* correlates well with CR length and is particularly useful for estimating the age of incomplete or macerated fetuses. *Fetal weight* is often a useful criterion, but there may be a discrepancy between the fertilization age and the weight of a fetus, particularly when the mother has had metabolic disturbances during pregnancy; e.g., diabetes mellitus. In these cases, fetal weight often exceeds values considered normal for the length.

The fetal dimensions obtained from measurements of fetuses using *ultrasound* closely approximate the crown-rump measurements obtained from aborted fetuses (Table 7–2). In addition, the *diameter of the head* and the dimension of the trunk may be obtained. At 9 to 10 weeks, the head is still slightly larger than the trunk. Ultrasound crown-rump measurements of the fetus are predictive of fetal age with an accuracy of ± one to four days. Assessment of fetal size and age is enhanced when head and trunk dimensions are considered along with crown-rump measurements.

Determination of the size of the fetus, especially of its head, is of great value to the obstetrician for the management of patients (e.g., those women with small

Table 7–2. Criteria for Estimating Fertilization Age During the Fetal Period

Age (weeks)	CR Length (mm)*	Foot Length (mm)*	Fetal Weight (gm)†	Main External Characteristics
PREVIABLE FETUSES				
9	50	7	8	Eyes closing or closed. Head more rounded. External genitalia still not distinguishable as male or female. Intestines in umbilical cord.
10	61	9	14	Intestine in abdomen. Early fingernail development.
12	87	14	45	Sex distinguishable externally. Well-defined neck.
14	120	20	110	Head erect. Lower limbs well developed. Early toenail development.
16	140	27	200	Ears stand out from head.
18	160	33	320	Vernix caseosa present.
20	190	39	460	Head and body hair (lanugo) visible.
VIABLE FETUSES‡				
22	210	45	630	Skin wrinkled and red.
24	230	50	820	Fingernails present. Lean body.
26	250	55	1000	Eyes partially open. Eyelashes present.
28	270	59	1300	Eyes open. Good head of hair. Skin slightly wrinkled.
30	280	63	1700	Toenails present. Body filling out. Testes descending.
32	300	68	2100	Fingernails reach finger tips. Skin pink and smooth.
36	340	79	2900	Body usually plump. Lanugo hairs almost absent. Toenails reach toe tips. Flexed limbs; firm grasp.
38	360	83	3400	Prominent chest; breasts protrude. Testes in scrotum or palpable in inguinal canals. Fingernails extend beyond finger tips.

*These measurements are averages and so may not apply to specific cases; dimensional variations increase with age. The method for taking CR (crown-rump) measurements is illustrated in Figure 6–15.

†These weights refer to fetuses that have been fixed for about two weeks in 10 per cent formalin. Fresh specimens usually weigh about 5 per cent less.

‡There is no sharp limit of development, age, or weight at which a fetus automatically becomes viable or beyond which survival is ensured, but experience has shown that it is uncommon for a baby to survive whose weight is less than 500 gm or whose fertilization age is less than 22 weeks. Even fetuses born during the 26- to 28-week period have difficulty surviving, mainly because the respiratory and central nervous systems are not completely differentiated. The term *abortion* refers to all pregnancies that terminate before the period of viability.

pelves and/or those fetuses with *intrauterine growth retardation*).

HIGHLIGHTS OF THE FETAL PERIOD

No formal system of staging is used for the fetal period, but it is useful to consider the changes that occur in four- to five-week periods.

Nine to Twelve Weeks (Figs. 7–1 to 7–5). At the beginning of the ninth week, the *head constitutes half the crown-rump length of the fetus*. Thereafter, growth in body length accelerates rapidly so that by the end of 12 weeks, fetal length has more than doubled (Table 7–2). Growth of the head slows down considerably, however, compared with that of the rest of the body. The face is broad, the eyes widely separated, and the ears low-set. The eyes are usually closed during the ninth week.

At the beginning of the ninth week, the legs are short and the thighs are relatively small (Fig. 7–3). At the end of 12 weeks, the upper limbs have almost reached their final relative lengths, but the lower limbs are still not so well developed and are slightly shorter than their final relative length (Fig. 7–2).

The external genitalia of males and females appear somewhat similar until the end of the ninth week.

Their mature form is not established until the twelfth week (see Chapter 14). Intestinal coils are visible within the proximal end of the umbilical cord (Fig. 7–3B) until the middle of the tenth week. By the eleventh week, the intestines have usually returned to the abdomen.

At the beginning of the ninth week, the liver is the major site of *erythropoiesis*. By the end of the twelfth week, this activity has decreased in the liver and has begun in the spleen.

Urine starts to form between the ninth and twelfth weeks and is excreted into the amniotic fluid. It reabsorbs some of this after swallowing it. Waste products then pass into the maternal circulation by passage across the placenta (see Fig. 8–6).

The fetus begins to move during the nine- to twelve-week period, but these movements cannot be detected by the mother.

Thirteen to Sixteen Weeks (Figs. 7–4 and 7–6). *Growth is very rapid during this period* (Table 7–2). At the end of this period, the head is relatively small compared with that of the 12-week fetus, and the lower limbs have lengthened. The skeleton shows clearly on x-ray films toward the end of this period.

At 16 weeks the appearance of the fetus is even more human because the eyes are facing anteriorly rather than laterally. In addition, the external ears are

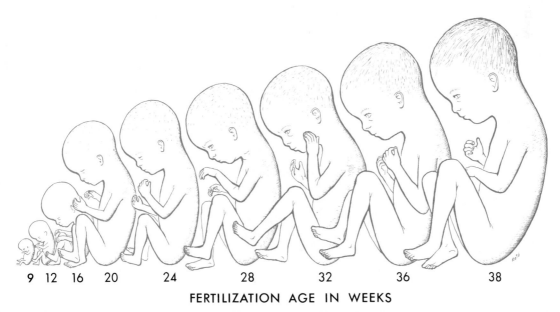

FERTILIZATION AGE IN WEEKS

9   12   16   20   24   28   32   36   38

Figure 7–1. Drawings of fetuses, about *one-fifth actual size*. Head hair begins to appear at about 20 weeks. Eyebrows and eyelashes are usually recognizable by 24 weeks, and the eyes are open by 26 weeks. Fetuses born prematurely (22 weeks or more) may survive, but intensive care is required. The mean duration of pregnancy is 266 days (38 weeks) from fertilization, with a standard deviation of 12 days. *In clinical practice,* it is customary to refer to full term as 40 weeks from the first day of the last menstrual period (LMP). Thus when a doctor refers to a pregnancy of 20 weeks, the true duration or actual age of the fetus is 18 weeks. The fetus begins to move by the twelfth week, but the mother does not usually feel the fetus move before the sixteenth week.

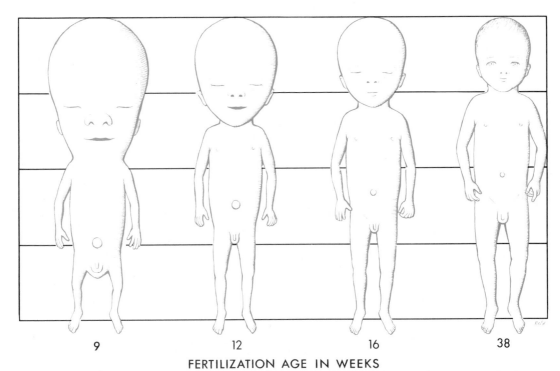

FERTILIZATION AGE IN WEEKS

9   12   16   38

Figure 7–2. Diagram illustrating the changing proportions of the body during the fetal period. By 36 weeks, the circumferences of the head and the abdomen are approximately equal. After this, the circumference of the abdomen may be greater. All stages are drawn to the same total height.

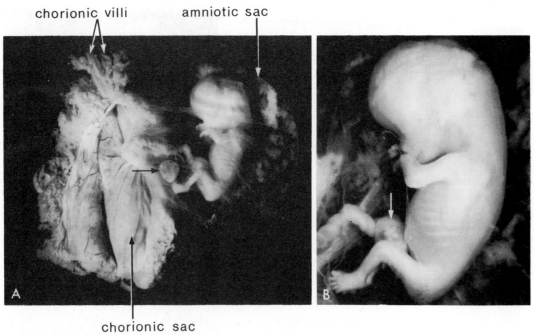

chorionic villi   amniotic sac

chorionic sac

Figure 7–3. Photographs of a nine-week fetus in its amniotic sac which has been exposed by removal from its chorionic sac. *A, Actual size.* The remnant of the yolk sac is indicated by an arrow. *B, Enlarged* photograph of the fetus (×2). Note the following features: (1) large head, (2) cartilaginous ribs, and (3) intestines in the umbilical cord (arrow). Ultrasound crown-rump measurements of the fetus can ascertain fetal age with an accuracy of ± one to four days. Determination of fetal size, especially of the head, allows the obstetrician to improve the management of patients (e.g., women whose fetuses may have congenital malformations such as hydrocephalus; see Chapter 17). (Photographed by Professor Jean Hay, Department of Anatomy, University of Manitoba.)

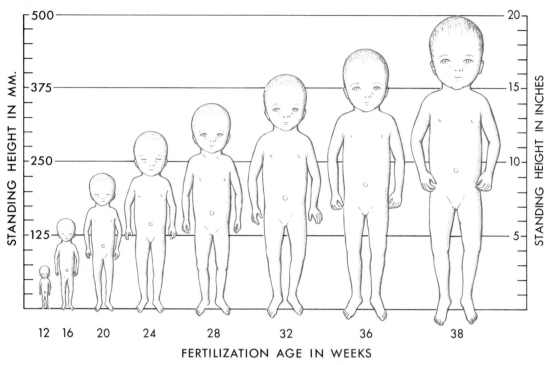

Figure 7–4. Diagram illustrating the changes in size of the human fetus when drawn to scale.

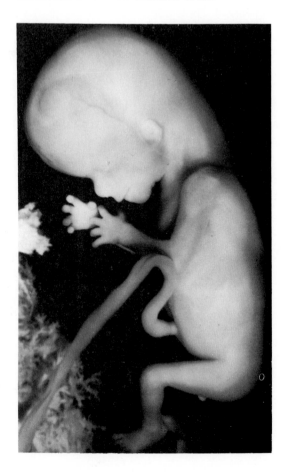

Figure 7–5. Photograph of an 11-week fetus exposed by removal from its chorionic and amniotic sacs (×1.5). Note the relatively large head and that the intestine is no longer in the umbilical cord. Note that its head is still disproportionately large. (Photographed by Professor Jean Hay, Department of Anatomy, University of Manitoba.)

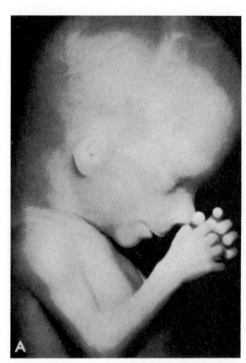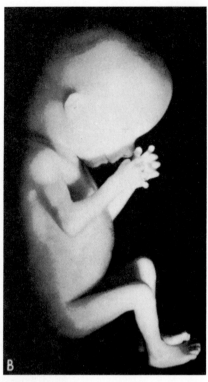

Figure 7–6. Photographs of a 13-week fetus. *A, Enlarged* photograph of the head and shoulders of this fetus (× 2). Note that its eyes are closed at this stage. *B, Actual size.* Note that its crown-rump length is about the same as the width of your palm. (Photographed by Professor Jean Hay, Department of Anatomy, University of Manitoba.)

close to their definitive positions on the sides of the head.

Seventeen to Twenty Weeks (Fig. 7–7). Growth slows down during this period (Table 7–2). Fetal movements, known as *quickening,* are commonly recognized by the mother.

The skin is covered with a greasy cheeselike material known as *vernix caseosa.* It consists of a mixture of a fatty secretion from the fetal sebaceous glands and dead skin (see Chapter 19). The vernix caseosa protects the fetus' delicate skin from abrasions, chapping, and hardening as a result of being bathed in amniotic fluid.

The bodies of 20-week fetuses are usually completely covered with fine downy hair called *lanugo;* this may help hold the vernix on the skin. Eyebrows and head hair are also visible at the end of this period.

Brown fat forms during this time and is the site of heat production, particularly in the newborn infant. This specialized adipose tissue produces heat by oxidizing fatty acids. Brown fat is chiefly found (1) on the floor of the anterior triangle of the neck surrounding the subclavian and carotid vessels, (2) posterior to the sternum, and (3) in the perirenal area. Brown

fat has a high content of mitochondria, giving it a definite brown hue.

Twenty-one to Twenty-five Weeks (Fig. 7–8). There is a substantial weight gain during this period. Although the body is still somewhat lean, it is better proportioned. The skin is usually wrinkled and is pink to red because blood in the capillaries is now visible.

By 24 weeks, alveolar cells of the lung have begun to make surfactant, a surface-active lipid that maintains alveolar patency. Although all organs are rather well developed, a 22- to 25-week fetus may die if born prematurely, mainly because its respiratory system is still immature.

Twenty-six to Twenty-nine Weeks. A fetus may now survive if born prematurely (Table 7–2), because *the lungs are capable of breathing air,* and because the lungs and pulmonary vasculature have developed sufficiently to provide gas exchange. In addition, the central nervous system has matured to the stage at which it can direct rhythmic breathing movements and control body temperature.

The eyes reopen during this period, and head and lanugo hair are well developed. Considerable subcutaneous fat has now formed under the skin, smoothing

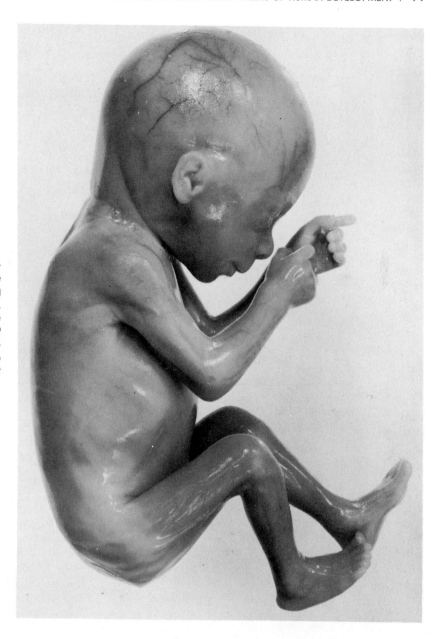

Figure 7–7. Photograph of a 17-week fetus. *Actual size.* Because the skin is very thin, the underlying scalp vessels are clearly visible. Movements of the fetus should be felt by the mother at this time (19 weeks after LMP). Fetuses born prematurely at this age are unable to survive because their lungs are not well developed.

out many of the wrinkles. During this period, the quantity of white fat in the body increases to about 3.5 per cent of body weight. *Erythropoiesis in the spleen ends by 28 weeks.* The bone marrow now becomes the major site of this process.

The fetus usually assumes an upside-down position as the time of birth approaches; this positioning results partly from the shape of the uterus and partly because the head is heavier than the feet.

Thirty to Thirty-four Weeks. *The pupillary light reflex is present by 30 weeks.* Usually by the end of this period, the skin is pink and smooth, and the upper and lower limbs often have a chubby appear-

ance. At this stage, the quantity of white fat in the body is about 7 to 8 per cent of body weight. Fetuses 32 weeks and older usually survive if born prematurely.

Thirty-five to Thirty-eight Weeks (Fig. 7–9). Fetuses at 35 weeks have a firm grasp and exhibit a spontaneous orientation to light. Most fetuses during this "finishing period" are plump.

At 36 weeks, the circumference of the head and the abdomen are approximately equal. After this, the circumference of the abdomen is greater than that of the head.

There is a slowing of growth as the time of birth

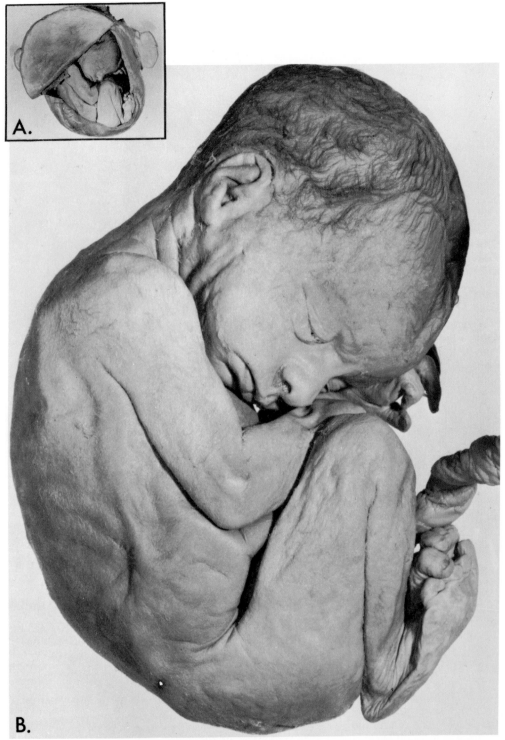

Figure 7–8. Photographs of a 25-week fetus. *A*, in the uterus. *B Actual size.* Note the wrinkled skin and rather lean body caused by the scarcity of subcutaneous fat. Observe that the eyes are beginning to open. A fetus of this size might survive if born prematurely; hence it is considered a viable fetus. Termination of pregnancy after the period of viability is uncommon (see Table 7–2). The mother of this fetus was killed in an automobile accident, and the fetus died before it could be removed by cesarean section.

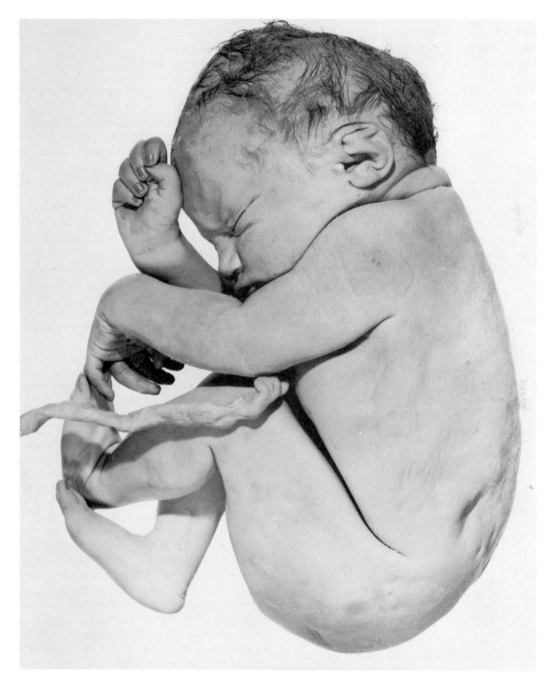

Figure 7–9. Photograph of a 36-week fetus. *Half actual size*. Fetuses at this size and age usually survive. Note the plump body resulting from the deposition of subcutaneous fat. This fetus' mother was killed in an automobile accident, and the fetus died before it could be delivered by cesarean section.

approaches (Fig. 7–10). Fetuses usually reach a CR length of 360 mm and weigh about 3400 gm. By full term, the amount of white fat in the body is about 16 per cent of body weight. A fetus lays down about 14 gm of fat a day during the last few weeks of gestation. In general, male fetuses grow faster than females and male infants generally weigh more than female infants at birth.

By *full term* (38 weeks after fertilization, or 40 weeks after LMP), the skin is usually white or bluish-pink in color. The chest is prominent and the breasts protrude in both sexes.

The testes are usually in the scrotum in full-term male infants; descent begins at about 28 to 32 weeks. Thus, premature male infants commonly have undescended testes. Usually the testes in these babies descend during early infancy.

The Expected Time of Birth. The expected date of confinement (often indicated as EDC) for the birth of a baby is roughly calculated as 266 days or 38 weeks after fertilization, or 280 days or 40 weeks from the onset of the last menstrual period (see Table 7–1). Most fetuses are born within 10 to 15 days of this time.

The common way of setting the expected date of delivery is to count back three calendar months from the first day of the last menstrual period and then add a year and one week.

FACTORS INFLUENCING FETAL GROWTH

Glucose is the primary source of energy for fetal metabolism and growth, but amino acids are also required. These substances are derived from the mother via the placenta (see Chapter 8). The insulin required for the metabolism of glucose is secreted mainly by the fetal pancreas.

Maternal Malnutrition. Severe maternal malnutrition resulting from a poor-quality diet is known to cause reduced fetal growth (Fig. 7–10). Poor nutrition and faulty food habits are common and they are not restricted to mothers belonging to poverty groups.

Smoking. The growth rate of fetuses of mothers who smoke cigarettes is less than normal during the last six to eight weeks of pregnancy (Fig. 7–10). The effect is greater on fetuses whose mothers also eat a poor-quality diet.

Multiple Pregnancy. Individuals of twins, triplets, and other multiple births usually weigh considerably less than infants resulting from a single pregnancy. It is evident that the total requirements of twins (Fig. 7–10) exceed the nutritional supply available from the placenta during the third trimester.

Drugs. Infants born to alcoholic mothers often exhibit intrauterine growth retardation (IUGR) as part of the *fetal alcohol syndrome* (see Chapter 9). Similarly, narcotic addiction can cause IUGR and other obstetrical complications.

Impaired Uteroplacental Blood Flow. Maternal placental circulation may be reduced by a variety of conditions which decrease uterine blood flow (e.g., severe hypotension and renal disease). Chronic reduction of uterine blood flow can cause fetal starvation and result in fetal growth retardation.

Placental Insufficiency. Placental defects can also cause intrauterine fetal growth retardation. These placental changes reduce the total surface area available for exchange of nutrients between the fetal and maternal blood streams (Chapter 8).

Genetic Factors and Chromosomal Aberrations. It is well established that genetic factors can cause retarded fetal growth. In recent years structural and numerical chromosomal aberrations (Chapter 9) have also been associated with cases of retarded fetal growth. Intrauterine growth retardation is pronounced in the Down syndrome and is very characteristic of

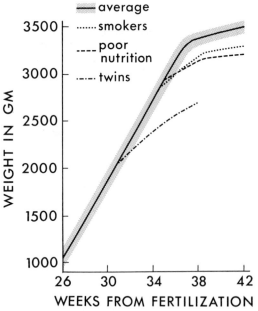

Figure 7–10. Graph showing the rate of fetal growth during the last trimester. Average refers to babies born in the United States. After 36 weeks the growth rate deviates from the straight line. The decline, particularly after full term (38 weeks), probably reflects inadequate fetal nutrition caused by placental changes. Note the adverse effect on fetal weight created by mothers who smoke heavily or eat a poor-quality diet. (Adapted from Gruenwald, P.: Growth of the human fetus. I. Normal growth and its variation. *Am. J. Obstet. Gynecol.* 94:1112, 1966.)

persons with the trisomy 18 syndrome (*see* Chapter 9).

PERINATOLOGY

Perinatology is the branch of medicine that is primarily concerned with the health of the fetus and newborn infant, generally covering the *perinatal period* from about 26 weeks after fertilization to about four weeks after birth. The subspecialty known as *perinatal medicine* combines certain aspects of obstetrics and pediatrics.

The older fetus is now commonly regarded as an unborn patient on whom diagnostic and therapeutic procedures may be performed. Several techniques are now available for assessing the status of the human fetus and for providing prenatal treatment.

Amniocentesis (Fig. 7–11A). Amniotic fluid is sampled by inserting a hollow needle through the mother's abdominal wall into the amniotic cavity. A syringe is then attached and amniotic fluid withdrawn. Because there is relatively little amniotic fluid, amniocentesis is difficult to perform prior to the thirteenth week.

Amniocentesis is relatively devoid of risk, especially when the procedure is performed by an experienced obstetrician who is guided by ultrasonography for placental localization. Amniocentesis is the most common technique for detecting genetic disorders and is usually performed 13 to 14 weeks after the estimated time of fertilization.

Sex Chromatin Patterns. Fetal sex can be diagnosed by noting the presence or absence of sex chromatin in cells recovered from amniotic fluid (Fig. 7–12). Knowledge of fetal sex can be useful in diagnosing the presence of severe sex-linked hereditary diseases such as hemophilia or muscular dystrophy. *These tests are not done to diagnose fetal sex for curious parents.*

Cell Cultures. Fetal sex can also be determined by studying the sex chromosomes of cultured amniotic cells. These studies are commonly done when an autosomal abnormality is suspected, such as occurs in the Down syndrome (discussed in Chapter 9).

Inborn errors of metabolism and enzyme deficiencies in fetuses can also be detected by studying cell cultures. Cell cultures permit prenatal diagnosis of severe diseases for which there is no effective treatment and afford the opportunity to interrupt the pregnancy.

Chorionic Villi Sampling (Fig. 7–11B). Pieces of chorionic villi may be obtained by inserting a needle, guided by ultrasonography, through the mother's abdominal and uterine walls into the uterine cavity.

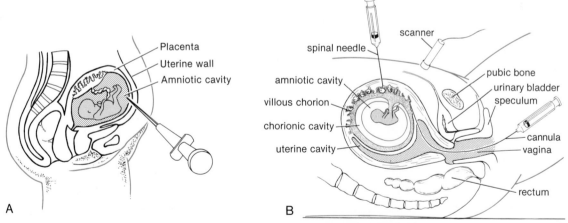

Figure 7–11. *A,* Drawing illustrating the technique of amniocentesis. A needle is inserted through the lower abdominal wall and the uterine wall into the amniotic cavity. A syringe is attached, and amniotic fluid is withdrawn for diagnostic purposes (e.g., for cell cultures or protein studies). Amniocentesis is relatively devoid of risk because it is combined with ultrasonography for placental localization. For the same reason, the risk of injuring the fetus with the needle is highly unlikely. Amniocentesis is usually performed 13 to 14 weeks after fertilization. Prior to this stage of development, there is relatively little amniotic fluid, and the difficulties in obtaining it without endangering the mother or the fetus are consequently greater. *B,* A drawing illustrating chorionic villus sampling (CVS). Two sampling approaches are illustrated: via the maternal anterior abdominal wall with a spinal needle, and via the vagina and cervical canal using a malleable cannula. Success and safety in both approaches depend upon use of a scanner (ultrasound imaging). This technique is usually performed 7 to 9 weeks after fertilization.

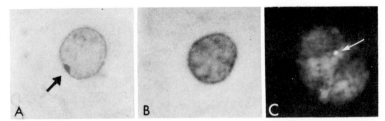

Figure 7–12. Nuclei of cells in amniotic fluid obtained by amniocentesis. *A,* Chromatin-positive nucleus indicating the presence of a female fetus; the sex chromatin is indicated by an arrow. *B,* Chromatin-negative nucleus indicating the presence of a male fetus. No sex chromatin is visible. Cresylecht violet stain (× 1000). *C,* Y-chromatin-positive nucleus indicating the presence of a male fetus. The arrow indicates the Y-chromatin as an intensely fluorescent body obtained after staining the cell in quinacrine mustard. *(A* and *B* from Riis, M., and Fuchs, F.: Sex chromatin and antenatal sex diagnosis; *in* K. L. Moore [Ed.]: *The Sex Chromatin.* Philadelphia, W. B. Saunders Company, 1966. *C* courtesy of Dr. M. Ray, Department of Human Genetics and Department of Anatomy, University of Manitoba and Health Sciences Centre, Winnipeg, Canada.)

To understand how such a biopsy is obtained, see Figure 7–11*B.* Chorionic villi sampling can also be performed transcervically using ultrasound guidance.

Biopsy of chorionic villi is used for detecting chromosomal abnormalities, inborn errors of metabolism, and X-linked disorders. This technique can be performed between 9 and 11 weeks of gestation (7 to 9 weeks fertilization age).

Fetoprotein Measurements. Chemical components are known to leak from fetuses with neural tube defects into the amniotic fluid (*see* Chapter 17). The concentration of α-*fetoprotein (AFP)* in the amniotic fluid surrounding fetuses with spina bifida cystica and meroanencephaly is very high. Thus, it is possible to detect the presence of these severe abnormalities by measuring the concentration of α-fetoprotein in amniotic fluid.

Detection of an increased concentration of α-fetoprotein in amniotic fluid is likely to be a useful diagnostic tool for detecting the presence or absence of *open neural tube defects,* e.g., meroanencephaly (partial absence of the brain) and other severe types

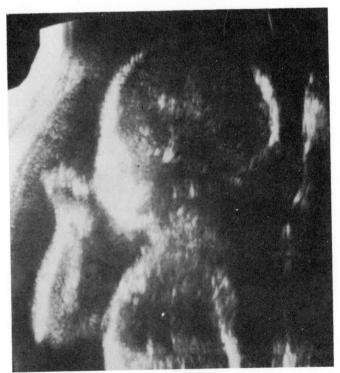

Figure 7–13. Ultrasound scan of a 30-week fetus that is sucking its thumb. Observe that its forearm bones are visible. The biparietal diameter of the head can be determined and compared with the abdominal diameter. Determination of these measurements facilitates estimation of the age and weight of the fetus. (From Thompson, J. S., and Thompson, M. W.: *Genetics in Medicine,* 3rd ed. Philadelphia, W. B. Saunders Company, 1980. Courtesy of Stuart Campbell.)

of spina bifida in fetuses of mothers who have already had a child with a neural tube defect (see Fig. 17–10). The findings would help to decide whether the pregnancy should be terminated.

Intrauterine Fetal Transfusion. Fetuses can be given intrauterine blood transfusions (e.g., for the treatment of erythroblastosis fetalis). The blood is injected through a needle inserted into the fetal peritoneal cavity. Over a period of five to six days, most of the cells pass into the fetal circulation via the lymphatics of the diaphragm.

Fetoscopy. Using fiberoptic lighting instruments, one may directly visualize parts of the fetal body. It is possible to scan the entire fetus, looking for congenital malformations such as cleft lip. The fetoscope is usually introduced through the anterior abdominal wall and the uterine wall into the amniotic cavity, similar to the way the needle is inserted during amniocentesis (see Fig. 7–11). One can not only see the fetus but can also take skin biopsies or blood samples.

Ultrasonography (Fig. 7–13). Chorionic sacs may be visualized during the embryonic period by using ultrasound techniques; placental and fetal size, multiple births, and abnormal presentations can also be determined.

Ultrasonic scans give accurate measurements of the biparietal diameter of the fetal skull, from which close estimates of fetal length can be made. Thus "small for date" fetuses can be detected. In most cases, the male genitalia can be visualized by ultrasound.

Recent advances in ultrasonography have made this technique a major tool for prenatal diagnosis of fetal abnormalities such as meroanencephaly, hydrocephaly, microcephaly, fetal ascites, and renal agenesis. Because of the cost, ultrasonography for estimation of gestational age and for the determination of congenital malformations is not routine. It is indicated in *high-risk obstetrical patients* (e.g., when there is a medical indication for induction of labor).

SUMMARY

The fetal period begins nine weeks after fertilization and ends at birth. It is *characterized by rapid body growth and differentiation of organ systems.* An obvious change is the relative slowing of head growth compared with that of the rest of the body.

Lanugo and head hair appear, and the skin is coated with *vernix caseosa* by the beginning of the twentieth week. The eyelids are closed during much of the fetal period, but reopen at about 26 weeks. Until this time the fetus is usually incapable of extrauterine existence, mainly because of the immaturity of its respiratory system. *Fetuses born prematurely during the 26- to 36-week period usually survive,* but full-term fetuses have the best chance of survival.

Until about 30 weeks the fetus appears reddish and wizened because of the thinness of its skin and the relative absence of subcutaneous fat. Fat usu-ally develops rapidly during the last six to eight weeks, making the fetus smooth and plump. This terminal period is devoted mainly to building up of tissues and preparation of systems involved in the transition from intrauterine to extrauterine environments.

Changes occurring during the fetal period are not so dramatic as those in the embryonic period, but they are very important. The fetus is far less vulnerable to the teratogenic or deforming effects of drugs, viruses, and radiation, but these agents may interfere with normal functional development, especially of the brain and eyes (see Fig. 9–12).

Various techniques are available for assessing the status of the fetus and for diagnosing certain diseases and developmental abnormalities before birth.

Commonly Asked Questions

1. I have heard that the fetus begins to move its limbs during the early fetal period. Can the mother feel her baby kick at this time?
2. Some women have *"morning sickness"* during early pregnancy. What type of illness is it?
3. I have heard that the baby can cause cavities in the mother's teeth. Is this true?
4. I read in the paper that vitamin supplementation will prevent neural tube defects such as spina bifida. Is there scientific proof for this statement?

5. Can the fetus be injured during amniocentesis? Is there a risk of inducing a miscarriage or causing maternal or fetal infection?

Answers

1. No. Although the fetus begins to move in the early fetal period, the mother cannot usually feel her baby move until the seventeenth to twentieth week. Women who have borne several children usually detect this movement, called *"quickening,"*

sooner than a woman who is pregnant for the first time.

2. About half of all pregnant women experience *nausea,* and some of them vomit a little every day. Although the urge to vomit usually occurs in the morning, it may occur anytime. Usually eating dry crackers and restricting water intake during meals dispels the nauseated feeling.

3. No. Although the fetus is competing with the mother for the nutrients and calcium in her blood, *the fetus cannot take calcium from the mother's teeth* and produce caries (cavities). The fetus needs calcium for its growing skeleton; therefore, the mother's intake of calcium should be sufficient for herself and the fetus.

4. At present it is too early to state that vitamin supplementation is effective in reducing the incidence of neural tube defects, but preliminary studies are encouraging. They have shown that the risk of a mother having a child with a neural tube defect is significantly lowered when vitamin supplementation is received.

5. *There is no risk of damaging the fetus during amniocentesis,* because ultrasonography is used to locate the position of the fetus. As a result, the needle is not going to injure it. There is a slight risk of inducing an abortion (about 1 in 200). Maternal or fetal infection is an unlikely complication when the technique is performed by a trained person.

The Placenta and Fetal Membranes

The placenta is a fetomaternal organ, that is, it consists of fetal and maternal portions (Fig. 8–1E). It functions primarily as an organ that *permits the exchange of materials* carried in the bloodstreams of the mother and the embryo or fetus (see Fig. 8–5). It allows food materials and respiratory gases to reach the embryo and it also provides a route for the disposal of waste products.

The *chorion, amnion, yolk sac,* and *allantois* constitute the fetal membranes. These membranes develop from the zygote but they do not form embryonic structures, except for portions of the yolk sac and allantois.

Before birth, the placenta and fetal membranes perform the following functions and activities: *protection, nutrition, respiration, excretion,* and *hormone production.* At birth, the placenta and fetal membranes separate from the fetus. Shortly after birth the placenta and fetal membranes are expelled from the uterus as the *afterbirth* (see Fig. 8–9F).

THE DECIDUA

The term *decidua*[1] is applied to the functional layer of the gravid or pregnant endometrium (see Fig. 2–2B), to indicate that it is shed or "cast off" at *parturition* (birth).

For descriptive purposes, *three regions of the decidua* are designated according to their relation to the

implantation site (Fig. 8–1): (1) the part underlying the conceptus and forming the maternal component of the placenta is the *decidua basalis;* (2) the superficial portion overlying the conceptus is the *decidua capsularis;* and (3) all the remaining uterine mucosa of the uterine wall is the *decidua parietalis* (L. *paries,* wall).

As the conceptus enlarges, the decidua capsularis bulges into the uterine cavity and eventually fuses with the decidua parietalis, thus obliterating the uterine cavity (Fig. 8–1F). By about 22 weeks, the decidua capsularis degenerates and disappears.

DEVELOPMENT OF THE PLACENTA

The rapid proliferation of the trophoblast and development of the chorionic sac were described in Chapters 4 and 5. By the fourth week, the essential arrangements necessary for physiological exchanges between the mother and embryo are established (see Figs. 5–9 and 8–1C).

Chorionic villi cover the entire surface of the chorionic sac until about the eighth week (Figs. 8–1C and 8–2A). As the sac grows, the chorionic villi associated with the decidua capsularis become compressed and their blood supply is reduced. Subsequently, these chorionic villi degenerate, producing a bare area known as the chorion laeve (L. *levis,* smooth) or *smooth chorion* (Figs. 8–1D and 8–2B). As this occurs, the chorionic villi associated with the decidua basalis rapidly increase in number, branch profusely, and enlarge. This portion of the chorionic

---

[1]From Latin *deciduus,* a falling-off, as the leaves of deciduous trees in the autumn.

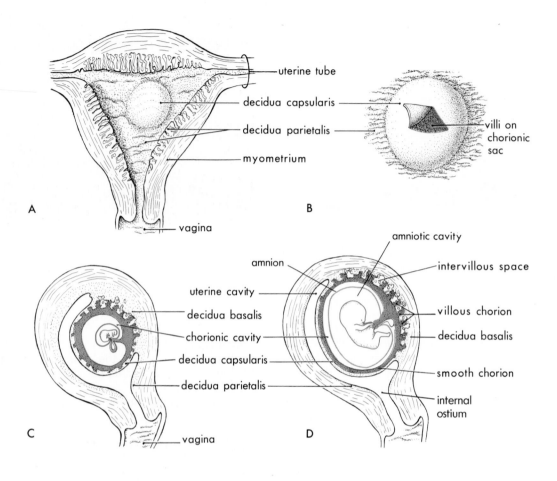

A

uterine tube
decidua capsularis
decidua parietalis
myometrium
vagina

B

villi on chorionic sac

C

uterine cavity
decidua basalis
chorionic cavity
decidua capsularis
decidua parietalis
vagina

D

amniotic cavity
amnion
intervillous space
villous chorion
decidua basalis
smooth chorion
internal ostium

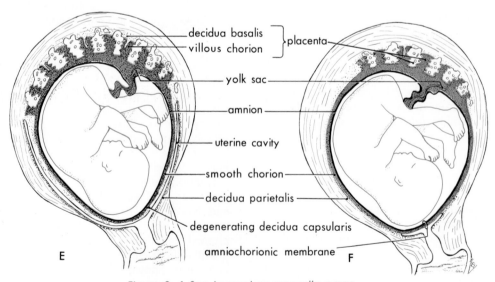

E

decidua basalis
villous chorion
placenta
yolk sac
amnion
uterine cavity
smooth chorion
decidua parietalis
degenerating decidua capsularis
amniochorionic membrane

F

Figure 8–1 *See legend on opposite page*

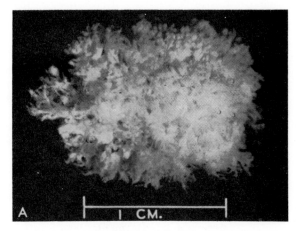

Figure 8–2. Photographs of human chorionic sacs that have been removed from the uterus. *A*, 21 days. The entire sac is covered with chorionic villi (×4). *B*, Eight weeks. *Actual size.* Note that some villi have degenerated, leaving the chorion smooth. The remaining villous chorion forms the fetal contribution to the placenta. (Reproduced with permission from Potter, E. L.: *Pathology of the Fetus and Infant*, 2nd ed. Copyright © 1961 by Year Book Medical Publishers, Inc., Chicago.)

smooth chorion   villous chorion

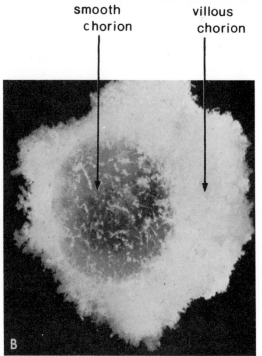

Figure 8–1. *A*, Drawing of a frontal section of the uterus showing the elevation of the decidua capsularis caused by the expanding chorionic sac of an implanted four-week embryo. *B*, Enlarged drawing of the implantation site shown in *A*; the chorionic villi have been exposed by cutting an opening in the decidua capsularis. *C* to *F*, Drawings of sagittal sections of the gravid uterus from the fourth to twenty-second weeks, showing the changing relations of the fetal membranes to the decidua. In *F*, the amnion and chorion are fused with each other and the decidua parietalis, thus obliterating the uterine cavity. Note that the chorionic villi persist only where the chorion is associated with the decidua basalis; here they form the villous chorion. Initially the placenta is larger than the fetus, but during the last half of pregnancy the fetus grows faster than the placenta.

sac, known as the chorion frondosum (L. *frondosus*, leafy) or *villous chorion*, forms the fetal component of the placenta (Figs. 8–1F and 8–3).

The fetal component of the placenta is formed by the wall of the chorion, often called the *chorionic plate* (Fig. 8–4), and the chorionic villi that arise from it and project into the intervillous spaces containing maternal blood (Figs. 8–1 and 8–5).

The maternal component of the placenta is formed by the decidua basalis (Figs. 8–1 and 8–4). This constitutes all the endometrium that is deep to the fetal component of the placenta.

The final shape of the placenta is determined by the form of the persistent area of chorionic villi; usually this is circular, giving the placenta a discoid shape (see Figs. 8–3 and 8–11). As the villi erode the decidua basalis, they leave several wedge-shaped areas of decidual tissue called *placental septa* (Fig. 8–5). These septa divide the fetal part of the placenta into 10 to 38 irregular areas called *cotyledons* (see Fig. 8–11A). Each cotyledon consists of two or more main stem villi and their many branches.

The fetal portion of the placenta (or villous chorion) is anchored to the maternal portion of the placenta (decidua basalis) by *anchoring villi* (Fig. 8–5).

The Intervillous Space (see Figs. 8–1D and 8–4). The blood-filled intervillous spaces are derived mainly from the lacunae which developed in the syncytiotrophoblast during the second week. As the chorionic villi enlarge, these spaces enlarge. Collectively, the spaces form a large blood sinus, the *intervillous space,* which is bounded by the *chorionic plate* and decidua basalis (Figs. 8–4 and 8–5).

The intervillous space is divided into compartments by the placental septa. Because the septa do not reach the *chorionic plate,* there is communication between the intervillous spaces of different compartments. The intervillous space is drained by *endometrial veins,* which open over the entire surface of the decidua basalis (Fig. 8–5).

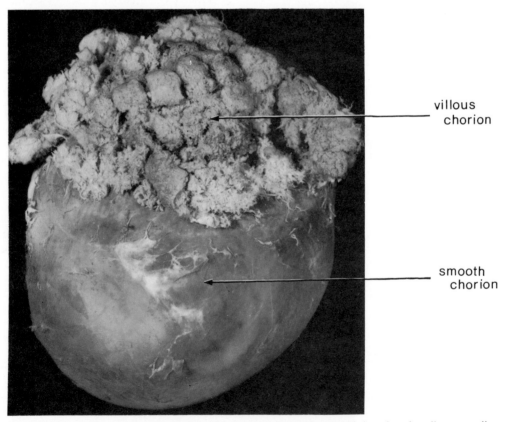

villous chorion

smooth chorion

Figure 8–3. Photograph of a human chorionic sac containing a 13-week fetus showing the smooth and villous areas of the chorion. *Actual size.* To visualize how this chorionic sac was situated in the uterus prior to its spontaneous abortion, see Figures 8–1E and 8–4.

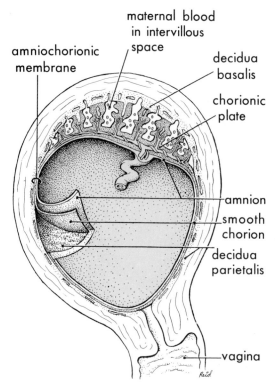

amniochorionic
membrane

maternal blood
in intervillous
space

decidua
basalis

chorionic
plate

amnion

smooth
chorion

decidua
parietalis

vagina

Figure 8–4. Drawing of a sagittal section of the gravid uterus at 22 weeks showing the relations of the fetal membranes to each other and to the decidua. The fetus has been removed, and the amnion and smooth chorion have been cut and reflected. The fetal component of the placenta consists of the chorionic plate and the chorionic villi that arise from it and project into the intervillous spaces containing maternal blood. The maternal component of the placenta is formed by the decidua basalis. This comprises all the endometrium related to the fetal component of the placenta.

Maternal blood circulates through the intervillous spaces, bringing food materials, respiratory gases, and other substances necessary for embryonic and fetal development, and taking away the waste products of fetal metabolism.

PLACENTAL CIRCULATION

The placenta provides a large area where materials may be exchanged across the *placental membrane* interposed between the fetal and maternal circulations (see Fig. 8–7). From the maternal blood the fetal blood acquires nutrients and oxygen. Waste products formed within the embryo are carried to the placenta and transferred to the maternal blood. Within the

placenta, the maternal and fetal bloodstreams flow close to each other, but they do not normally mix.

The Placental Membrane (Figs. 8–6 and 8–7). This membrane consists of the fetal tissues separating the maternal and fetal blood. Until about 20 weeks, it consists of four layers (Fig. 8–6*B*): (1) the syncytiotrophoblast, (2) the cytotrophoblast, (3) the connective tissue core of the villus, and (4) the endothelium of the fetal capillary.

The placental membrane is often called the placental "barrier," but this term is inappropriate because there are few compounds, endogenous or exogenous, that are unable to cross the placental membrane in detectable amounts. The placental membrane acts as a true barrier only when the molecule has a certain size, configuration, and charge (e.g., heparin).

As pregnancy advances, the placental membrane becomes progressively thinner and many capillaries come to lie very close to the syncytiotrophoblast (Fig. 8–6*C*). Most drugs and other substances present in the maternal plasma will also be found in the fetal plasma.

At some sites the syncytiotrophoblastic nuclei form nuclear aggregations or *syncytial knots.* Toward the end of pregnancy, *fibrinoid material* forms on the surfaces of villi; it consists of fibrin and other substances. These changes result from placental aging.

Fetal Placental Circulation (see Fig. 8–5). Deoxygenated blood leaves the fetus and passes in the umbilical arteries to the placenta. The blood vessels form an extensive *arterio-capillary-venous system* within the chorionic villus (see Fig. 8–6*A*), bringing the fetal blood very close to the maternal blood. The oxygenated fetal blood passes into thin-walled veins which converge to form the umbilical vein. This large vessel carries the oxygenated blood to the fetus.

Maternal Placental Circulation (see Fig. 8–5). The blood in the intervillous space is temporarily outside the maternal circulatory system. It enters the intervillous space through 80 to 100 *spiral arteries* or endometrial arteries (see Fig. 2–2*B*). The blood is propelled in jetlike streams by the maternal blood pressure and spurts toward the chorionic plate or "roof" of the intervillous space. The blood slowly flows around and over the surface of the villi, allowing an exchange of metabolic and gaseous products with the fetal blood. The maternal blood eventually reaches the floor of the intervillous space, where it enters the endometrial veins (see Fig. 8–5).

The welfare of the embryo and fetus depends more on the adequate bathing of the chorionic villi by maternal blood than on any other factor. Acute reductions of uteroplacental circulation result in *fetal hypoxia* (e.g., from prolapse of the umbilical cord).

Chronic reductions of uteroplacental circulation re-

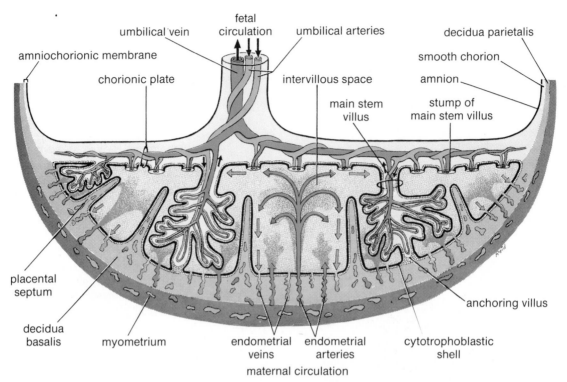

Figure 8–5. Schematic drawing of a section through a full-term placenta, showing (1) the relation of the villous chorion (fetal placenta) to the decidua basalis (maternal placenta), (2) the fetal placental circulation, and (3) the maternal placental circulation. Maternal blood flows into the intervillous spaces in funnel-shaped spurts, and exchanges occur with the fetal blood as the maternal blood flows around the villi. The inflowing arterial blood pushes venous blood out into the endometrial veins, which are scattered over the entire surface of the decidua basalis. *Note that the umbilical arteries carry deoxygenated fetal blood* (shown in blue) to the placenta and that the umbilical vein carries oxygenated blood (shown in red) to the fetus. Note that the cotyledons are separated from each other by decidual septa of the maternal portion of the placenta. Each cotyledon consists of two or more main stem villi and their many branches. In this drawing only one main stem villus is shown in each cotyledon, but the stumps of those that have been removed are indicated.

sult in disturbances of growth and development that constitute a syndrome known as *intrauterine growth retardation.*

PLACENTAL ACTIVITIES

The placenta has three main activities: (1) *metabolism,* (2) *transfer,* and (3) *endocrine secretion* that are essential for maintaining pregnancy and promoting normal embryonic development.

Placental Transfer

Gases. Oxygen, carbon dioxide, and carbon monoxide cross the placental membrane by *simple diffu-*sion. The interruption of oxygen transport for even a few minutes will endanger embryonic/fetal survival.

Nutrients. Water is rapidly and freely exchanged between mother and fetus, and in increasing amounts as pregnancy advances. There is little or no transfer of maternal cholesterol, triglycerides, or phospholipids. There is transport of free fatty acids, but the amount transferred is probably relatively small. Vitamins cross the placenta and are essential for normal development. Water-soluble vitamins cross the placental membrane more quickly than fat-soluble ones. Glucose is quickly transferred.

Hormones. Protein hormones do not reach the fetus in significant amounts, except for a slow transfer of thyroxine and triiodothyronine. Unconjugated steroid hormones pass the placental membrane rather freely, unless they are firmly bound to proteins. Tes-

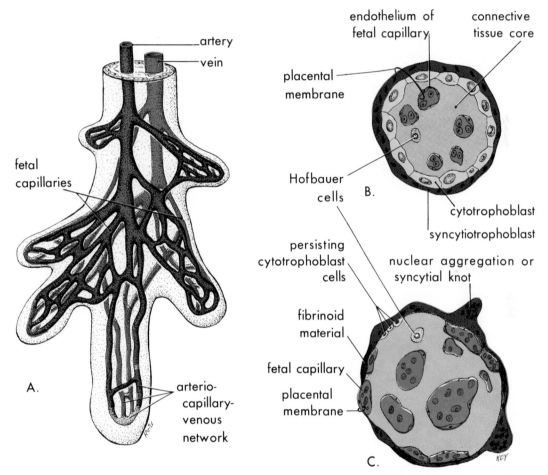

Figure 8–6. *A,* Drawing of a chorionic villus showing the arterio-capillary-venous system carrying fetal blood. The artery carries deoxygenated blood and waste products from the fetus, whereas the vein carries oxygenated blood and nutrients to the fetus. *B* and *C,* Drawings of sections through a chorionic villus at 10 weeks and at full term, respectively. The villi are bathed externally in maternal blood. The placental membrane, composed of fetal tissues, separates the maternal blood from the fetal blood. Hofbauer cells have the general qualities of macrophages (scavenger cells).

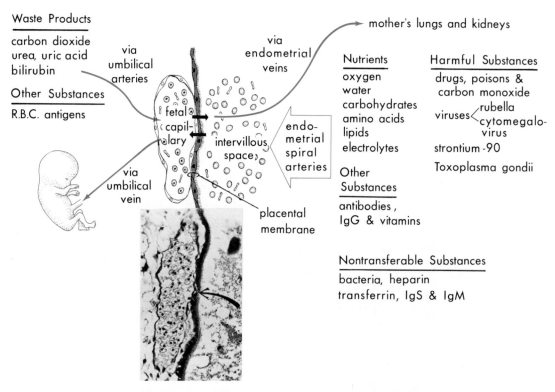

Waste Products

carbon dioxide
urea, uric acid
bilirubin

via umbilical arteries

via endometrial veins

mother's lungs and kidneys

Other Substances

R.B.C. antigens

fetal capil-lary

intervillous space

endo-metrial spiral arteries

via umbilical vein

placental membrane

Nutrients

oxygen
water
carbohydrates
amino acids
lipids
electrolytes

Other Substances

antibodies,
IgG & vitamins

Harmful Substances

drugs, poisons &
carbon monoxide

viruses ⎰rubella
       ⎱cytomegalo-
         virus

strontium-90

Toxoplasma gondii

Nontransferable Substances

bacteria, heparin
transferrin, IgS & IgM

Figure 8–7. Diagrammatic illustration of transfer across the placental membrane. Note that the intervillous space contains maternal blood and that the placental membrane is composed of fetal tissues. (Inset photomicrograph from Javert, C. T.: *Spontaneous and Habitual Abortion,* Copyright © 1957 by McGraw-Hill, Inc. Used by permission of McGraw-Hill Book Company.)

tosterone and certain synthetic progestins cross the placenta and may cause external masculinization of female fetuses (see Chapter 9).

Electrolytes. These are freely exchanged across the placenta in significant quantities, each at its own rate.

When a mother receives intravenous fluids, they also pass to the fetus and affect its water and electrolyte status.

Antibodies. Some passive immunity is conferred upon the fetus by transplacental transfer of maternal antibodies. The alpha and beta globulins reach the fetus in very small quantities, but many of the gamma globulins, notably the IgG (7S) class, are readily transported to the fetus.

Maternal antibodies confer immunity on the fetus to such diseases as diphtheria, smallpox, and measles, but no immunity is acquired to pertussis (whooping cough) or chickenpox. The fetus has a poor capacity to produce antibodies until well after birth.

Although the placental membrane separates the maternal and fetal circulations, small amounts of blood may pass from the fetus to the mother. If the fetus is Rh-positive and the mother Rh-negative, the fetal cells

may stimulate the formation of anti-Rh antibody by the mother. This passes to the fetal bloodstream and causes hemolysis of fetal Rh-positive blood cells and anemia in the fetus.

Some fetuses with this condition, known as *hemolytic disease of the newborn (HDN),* or erythroblastosis fetalis, fail to make a satisfactory intrauterine adjustment and may die unless delivered early or given intrauterine blood transfusions (discussed in Chapter 7).

Exchange transfusions of blood are also performed after birth, using the umbilical vein. Most of the infant's blood is replaced with Rh-negative donor blood. This technique prevents death of erythroblastotic babies who are very anemic. It also avoids brain damage by preventing or controlling hyperbilirubinemia.

When the placenta separates at birth (see Fig. 8–9F), the mother often receives a small transfusion of fetal blood into her circulation from ruptured fetal chorionic vessels. If she is Rh-negative and the infant Rh-positive, the fetal red cells can stimulate a permanent antibody response in the mother. These fetal red blood cells can be destroyed rapidly by giving the mother high-titer anti-Rh antibody. In this way, she does not become sensitized.

Wastes. The major waste product, carbon dioxide, diffuses across the placenta even more rapidly than oxygen. Urea and uric acid pass the placental membrane by simple diffusion.

Drugs. Almost all drugs cross the placenta freely; some cause congenital malformations (see Chapter 9). *Fetal drug addiction* may occur following maternal use of drugs such as heroin, resulting in withdrawal symptoms. Except for the muscle relaxants, such as succinylcholine and curare, most agents used for the management of labor readily cross the placenta. These drugs may cause respiratory depression of the newborn infant. All sedatives and analgesics affect the fetus to some degree.

Infectious Agents. Rubella, cytomegalovirus, and coxsackie viruses and those associated with variola, varicella, measles, encephalitis, and poliomyelitis may pass through the placental membrane and cause fetal infection. In some cases (e.g., *rubella virus*), congenital malformations may be produced (see Chapter 9).

Placental Endocrine Secretion

The *syncytiotrophoblast* synthesizes the following hormones:

Protein Hormones. The two well-documented protein products of the placenta are: (1) *human chorionic gonadotropin* (hCG) and (2) human chorionic soma-tomammotropin (hCS) or human placental lactogen (hPL). *Human chorionic gonadotropin maintains the corpus luteum* in the ovary and therefore prevents the onset of menstruation (see Chapter 2).

Steroid Hormones. Estrogens and progesterones are the only steroid hormones known to be secreted by the placenta.

UTERINE GROWTH DURING PREGNANCY

The uterus normally lies entirely in the pelvis (Fig. 8–8A). During pregnancy the uterus expands as the fetus grows, and rises out of the pelvic cavity to the level of the mother's umbilicus (navel) by about 20 weeks (Fig. 8–8B). By 28 to 30 weeks, the uterus in the pregnant female occupies a large part of the abdominopelvic cavity and reaches the epigastric region (Fig. 8–8C).

PARTURITION OR LABOR

The *birth process* by which the fetus, placenta, and fetal membranes are expelled from the mother's reproductive tract (Figs. 8–9 and 8–10) is called *parturition* (labor, or childbirth). The onset of labor (L. toil, suffering) is caused mainly by hormonal influences (e.g., oxytocin). Although occurring in a continuous sequence, labor is divided into three stages for convenience of description.

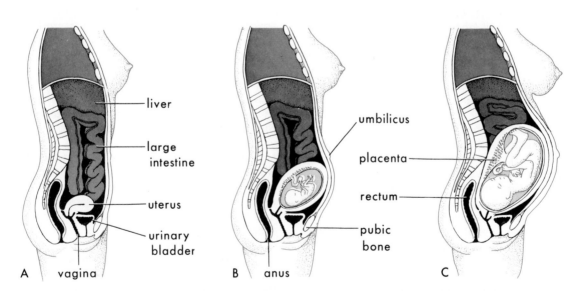

Figure 8–8. Drawings of sagittal sections of a woman. *A,* Not pregnant. *B,* 20 weeks pregnant. *C,* 30 weeks pregnant. Note that as the fetus enlarges, the uterus increases in size and its superior part rises out of the pelvic cavity to accommodate the rapidly growing fetus. The mother's intestines are displaced by the growth of the fetus and uterus and her abdominal skin and muscles are greatly stretched.

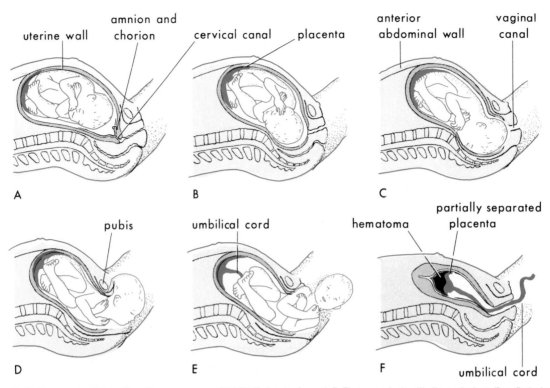

Figure 8–9. Drawings illustrating the process of birth (labor). *A* and *B,* The cervix is dilating during the first stage of labor, partly as the result of the amnion and chorion being forced into the cervical canal. *C* to *E,* The fetus passes through the cervix and vagina during the second stage of labor. *F,* As the uterus contracts during the third stage of labor, the placenta folds and pulls away from the uterine wall. Separation of the placenta results in bleeding, forming a large hematoma. Later the placenta and its associated membranes are expelled from the uterus (not shown) by further uterine contractions.

The *first stage of labor* is the dilatation stage. The amnion and chorion are forced into the cervical canal by contractions of the uterus (Fig. 8–9*A*). The cervix dilates slowly, and when it is fully dilated, or even before, the amniotic and chorionic sacs rupture, allowing the fluid to escape.

During the *second stage of labor,* the expulsion stage, the contractions of the uterus become stronger and are aided by voluntary contractions of the maternal abdominal muscles. The baby is forced through the cervical canal and the vagina (Fig. 8–9*B* to *E*).

The *third stage of labor* is the interval from birth to the expulsion of the placenta and membranes, which are now referred to as the "afterbirth."

The placenta separates through the spongy layer of the decidua basalis (see Fig. 2–2*B*). After delivery of the baby, the uterus continues to contract. As a result, a hematoma forms behind the placenta (Fig. 8–9*F*) and separates it from the decidua basalis. After delivery of the placenta, the uterine contractions constrict the spiral arteries that formerly supplied the intervillous spaces. These persistent contractions prevent excessive bleeding from the placental site.

THE FULL-TERM PLACENTA

The placenta (Gr. *plakous,* a flat cake) commonly has the form of a flat circular or oval disc (Fig. 8–11) with a diameter of 15 to 20 cm and a thickness of 2 to 3 cm. The placenta weighs 500 to 600 gm, and it is usually about one-sixth the weight of the fetus. The margins of the placenta are continuous with the ruptured amniotic and chorionic sacs (see Figs. 8–5 and 8–11*A* and *C*). Several variations in placental shape occur.

Maternal Surface (Fig. 8–11*A*). The characteristic cobblestone appearance of this surface is caused by the cotyledons. The surface of the cotyledons is usually covered by thin grayish shreds of decidua basalis. Most of the decidua is temporarily retained in the uterus and shed with subsequent uterine bleeding.

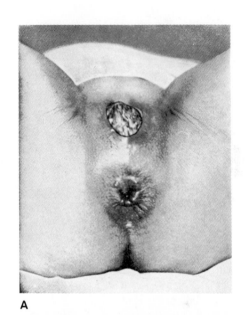

Figure 8–10. Photographs illustrating delivery of the baby's head during the second stage of labor. *A,* The head distends the mother's perineum, and part of the scalp becomes visible; this is called "crowning." *B,* The perineum slips back over the face. *C,* The head is delivered; subsequently the body of the fetus is expelled. (From Greenhill, J. B., and Friedman, E. A.: *Biological Principles and Modern Practice of Obstetrics.* Philadelphia, W. B. Saunders Company, 1974.)

A

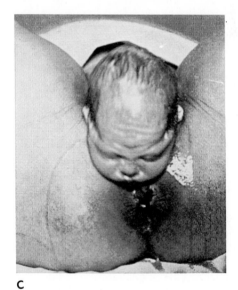

B   C

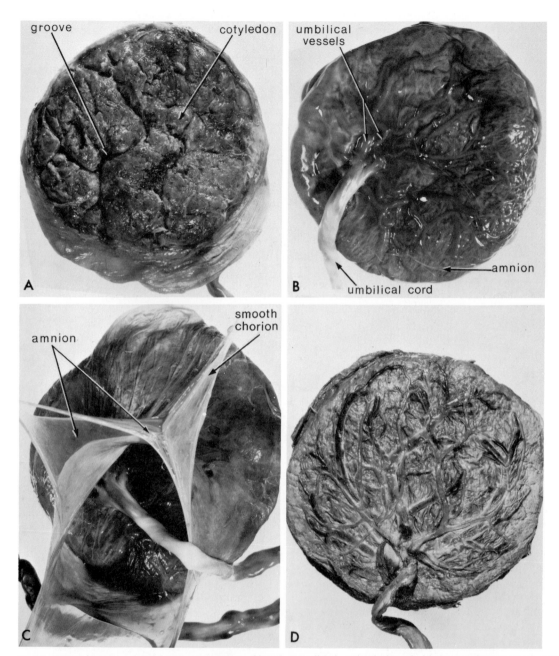

Figure 8–11. Photographs of full-term placentas. *About one third actual size. A,* Maternal (or uterine) surface, showing cotyledons and grooves. *B,* Fetal (or amniotic) surface, showing the blood vessels running under the amnion and converging to form the umbilical vessels at the attachment of the umbilical cord. *C,* The amnion and smooth chorion are arranged to show that they are (1) fused and (2) continuous with the margins of the placenta. *D,* Placenta with a marginal attachment of the cord, often called a battledore placenta because of its resemblance to the bat used in the medieval game of battledore and shuttlecock.

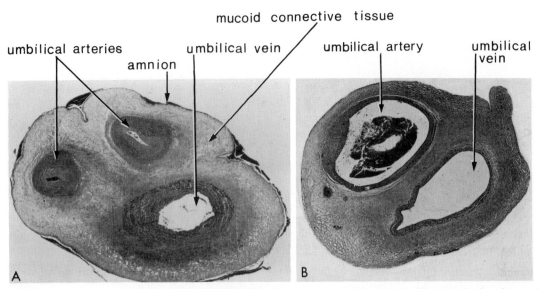

Figure 8–12. Transverse sections through full-term umbilical cords. *A*, Normal. *B*, Abnormal, showing only one artery. About 15 per cent of fetuses that have only one umbilical artery have cardiovascular malformations. (×3.) (From Javert, C. T.: *Spontaneous and Habitual Abortion.* Copyright © 1957 by McGraw-Hill, Inc. Used by permission of McGraw-Hill Book Company.)

Fetal Surface (Fig. 8–11*B*). The umbilical cord attaches to this surface, and its amniotic covering is continuous with the amnion adherent to this surface of the placenta (see Fig. 8–15). The vessels radiating from the umbilical cord are clearly visible through the smooth, transparent amnion.

The Umbilical Cord

The umbilical cord is a *vascular cable* that connects the embryo or fetus to the placenta (see Fig. 8–15). The attachment of the umbilical cord is usually near the center of the placenta (Fig. 8–11*B*), but it may be located anywhere (e.g., at the edge, Fig. 8–11*D*). The cord is usually 1 to 2 cm in diameter and 30 to 90 cm in length (average 55 cm).

The umbilical cord usually contains two arteries and one vein. These vessels are surrounded by mucoid connective tissue, often called Wharton's jelly (Fig. 8–12*A*). Because the umbilical vein is longer than the arteries and the vessels are longer than the cord, twisting and bending of the vessels is common. The vessels frequently form loops, producing so-called *false knots,* which are of no significance.

True knots in the umbilical cord may be hazardous to the fetus (Fig. 8–13). Simple looping of the cord around the fetus occasionally occurs (Fig. 8–14). In

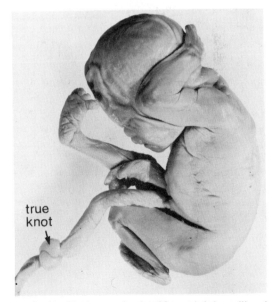

Figure 8–13. Photograph of a 20-week fetus with a true knot (arrow) in the umbilical cord. *Half actual size.* The diameter of the cord is greater in the portion closest to the fetus, indicating that there was an obstruction of blood flow in the umbilical arteries. The fetus died owing to a lack of oxygen. It was retained in the uterus for about four weeks. The patient then went into labor and delivered this dead fetus.

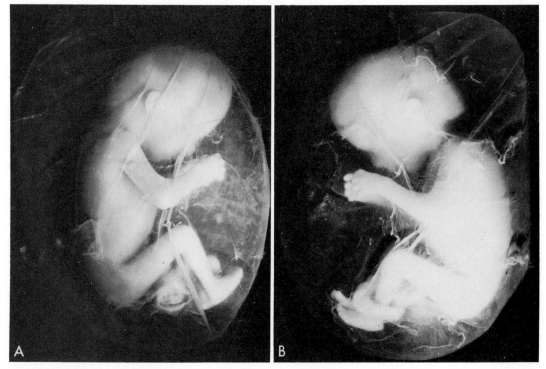

Figure 8–14. Photographs of a 12-week fetus within the amniotic sac. *Actual size.* Note in *B* that the umbilical cord is looped around the left foot of the fetus. Coiling of the cord around parts of the fetus affects development of them only when the coils are so tight that the circulation to them is affected. In this case the fetus appears normal, but the mother went into premature labor and spontaneously aborted the fetus.

about one fifth of all deliveries, the cord is looped once around the neck. If the cord becomes tightly looped around the neck or a limb, the circulation of blood to and from the embryo or fetus will be impeded. If the circulation is cut off, the embryo or fetus will die.

In up to 1 per cent of newborns, only one umbilical artery is present (Fig. 8–12*B*). This condition may be associated with abnormalities, particularly of the cardiovascular system.

THE AMNION AND AMNIOTIC FLUID

The amnion forms a fluid-filled, *membranous sac* that surrounds the embryo and later the fetus (Figs. 8–14 and 8–15). Formation of the amniotic cavity and early development of the amnion are described in Chapter 4.

Because the amnion is attached to the margins of the embryonic disc (Fig. 8–15*A*), its junction with the embryo becomes located on the ventral surface as a result of the folding of the embryo (see Chapter 6). As the amniotic sac enlarges, it gradually sheaths the

umbilical cord, forming its epithelial covering (Fig. 8–15*C* and *D*).

Origin of the Amniotic Fluid. Most fluid is derived from the maternal blood. Later, the fetus also makes a contribution by excreting urine into the amniotic fluid.

Amniotic fluid is normally swallowed by the fetus and absorbed by the gastrointestinal tract. In fetal conditions such as *renal agenesis* (absence of kidneys) or urethral obstruction, the volume of amniotic fluid may be abnormally small *(oligohydramnios)*. An excess of amniotic fluid *(polyhydramnios)* may occur when the fetus does not drink the usual amount of fluid. This condition is often associated with malformations of the central nervous system, e.g., *meroanencephaly* (anencephaly) and hydrocephalus (see Chapter 17). In other malformations, such as esophageal or duodenal atresia (see Chapter 13), amniotic fluid accumulates because it is unable to pass to the intestine for absorption.

Significance of the Amniotic Fluid. The embryo, suspended by the umbilical cord, floats freely in amniotic fluid. This buoyant medium (1) permits symmetrical growth and development of the embryo;

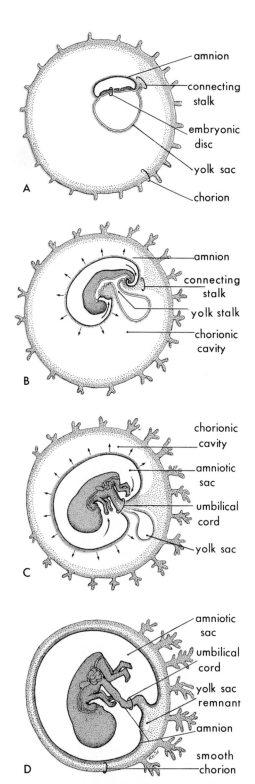

Figure 8–15. Drawings illustrating how the amnion forms the covering of the umbilical cord and how the yolk sac is partially incorporated into the embryo as the primitive gut. *A*, Three weeks. *B*, Four weeks. *C*, 10 weeks, *D*, 20 weeks.

(2) prevents adherence of the amnion to the embryo; (3) *cushions the embryo against jolts* by distributing impacts the mother may receive; (4) *helps to control the embryo's body temperature* by maintaining a relatively constant temperature; and (5) enables the fetus to move freely, thus aiding musculoskeletal development.

A very marked increase in the volume of amniotic fluid is called *polyhydramnios* (Gr. *polys*, much). This results in enlargement of the uterus and may result in premature labor. Most cases of polyhydramnios are caused by the inability of the fetus to swallow or absorb amniotic fluid normally.

A marked reduction in the volume of amniotic fluid is called *oligohydramnios* (Gr. *oligos*, few, or a little). This condition results from failure of the fetus to excrete urine into the amniotic fluid owing to abnormal kidney development or obstruction of the urethra.

THE YOLK SAC

Early development of the yolk sac is described in Chapters 4 and 5. By nine weeks, the yolk sac has shrunk to a pear-shaped remnant, about 5 mm in diameter. It is connected to the midgut by the narrow yolk stalk (Fig. 8–15C). Although the human yolk sac is nonfunctional as far as yolk storage is concerned, its development is essential for several reasons. (1) It appears to have a role in the transfer of nutrients to the embryo during the second and third weeks while the uteroplacental circulation is being established. (2) Blood develops on the walls of the yolk sac beginning in the third week and continues to form here until hemopoietic activity begins in the liver during the sixth week. (3) During the fourth week, the dorsal part of the yolk sac is incorporated into the embryo as the primitive gut (see Fig. 6–1); this gives rise to the epithelium of the trachea, bronchi, and lungs, and of the digestive tract. (4) Primordial germ cells appear in the wall of the yolk sac early in the third week and subsequently migrate to the developing sex glands or gonads, where they become the primitive germ cells (spermatogonia or oogonia—see Chapter 14).

Fate of the Yolk Sac (Fig. 8–15). The yolk sac shrinks as pregnancy advances and eventually becomes very small. The yolk stalk usually detaches from the gut by the end of the fifth week. In about 2 per cent of adults, the intra-abdominal part of the yolk stalk persists as a diverticulum of the ileum known as *Meckel's diverticulum* (see Chapter 13).

THE ALLANTOIS

The early development of the allantois is described in Chapter 5. Although the allantois does not function in human embryos, it is important for two reasons: (1) blood formation occurs in its walls during the first two months; and (2) its blood vessels become the umbilical vessels (Fig. 8–16A and B).

During the second month, the extraembryonic portion of the allantois degenerates. The intraembryonic portion of the allantois runs from the umbilicus to the urinary bladder with which it is continuous (Fig. 8–16B). As the bladder enlarges, the allantois involutes to form a thick tube called the *urachus*. After birth, the urachus becomes a fibrous cord called the *median umbilical ligament* (Fig. 8–16D).

MULTIPLE PREGNANCY

Multiple births are more common nowadays, owing to the stimulation of ovulation that occurs when human gonadotropins or other ovulation-inducing drugs are administered to women with *ovulatory failure* (failure of ovulation). See the discussion of *in vitro fertilization* on page 28.

Twins

Twins may originate from two zygotes (Fig. 8–17), in which case they are *dizygotic twins* (also called

nonidentical or fraternal twins). About one third of twins are derived from one zygote (Fig. 8–18). They are called *monozygotic twins* or identical twins.

Twins occur about once in 90 pregnancies; about two thirds of the total number are dizygotic twins. In addition, the rate of monozygotic twinning shows little variation with the mother's age, whereas dizygotic twinning increases with maternal age.

There is a tendency for dizygotic, but not monozygotic, twins to repeat in families. It has also been found that if the firstborn are twins, a repetition of twinning or some other form of multiple birth is about five times more likely to occur at the next pregnancy than it is in the general population.

The study of twins is important in human genetics because of their usefulness for comparing the effects of genes and environment on development. If an abnormal condition does not show a simple genetic pattern, comparison of its incidence in monozygotic and dizygotic twins can reveal that heredity is involved.

Dizygotic Twins (Fig. 8–17). Because they result from the fertilization of two ova by different sperms, *the twins may be of the same sex or of different sexes.* For the same reason, they are no more alike genetically than brothers or sisters born at different times. Dizygotic twins always have two amnions and two

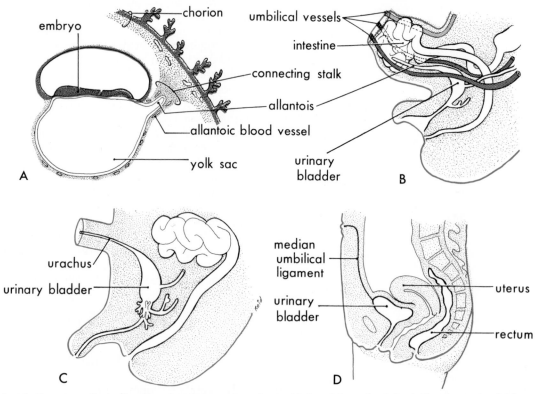

Figure 8–16. Drawings illustrating the development and usual fate of the allantois. *A,* Three weeks. *B,* Nine weeks. *C,* Three month male fetus. *D,* Woman.

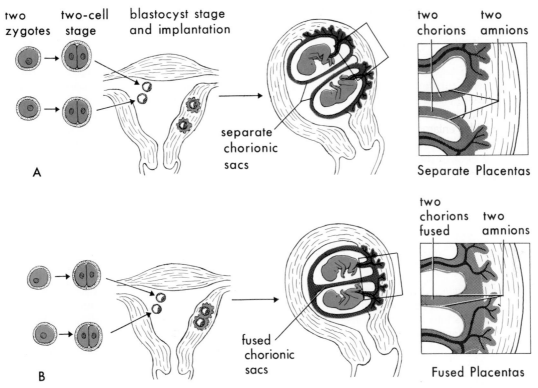

Figúre 8–17. Diagrams illustrating *how dizygotic twins develop* from two zygotes. The relations of the fetal membranes and placentas are shown for instances in which, *A*, the blastocysts implant separately, and *B*, the blastocysts implant close together. In both cases there are two amnions and two chorions, and the placentas may be separate or fused.

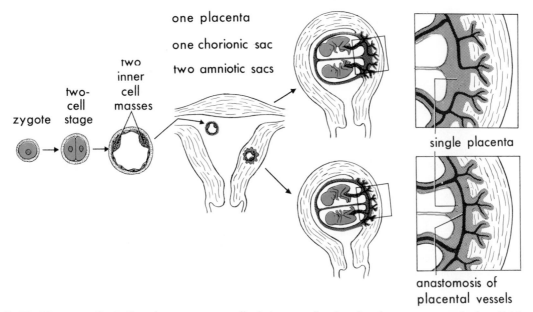

Figure 8–18. Diagrams illustrating *how monozygotic twins usually develop* from one zygote by division of the inner cell mass toward the end of the first week of development. Such twins always have separate amnions, a single chorion, and a common placenta.

chorions, but the chorions and placentas may be fused.

Monozygotic Twins (Figs. 8–18 and 8–19). Because they result from the fertilization of one ovum, monozygotic twins are (1) of the same sex, (2) genetically identical, and (3) very similar in physical appearance. Physical differences between identical twins are caused by environmental factors, e.g., anastomosis of placental vessels resulting in differences in blood supply from the placenta.

About 30 per cent of monozygotic twins *begin to develop early in the first week* and result from the separation of the blastomeres at two, four, or eight cell stages (see Fig. 3–3). Each blastomere or group of blastomeres gives rise to a blastocyst that implants separately in the endometrium and develops its own placenta. The placentas may remain separate or they may fuse in the same manner as dizygotic twins (see Fig. 8–17).

Monozygotic twinning usually begins around the end of the first week and results from early division of the inner cell mass into two embryonic primordia. Subsequently, two identical embryos, each in its own amniotic sac, develop within one chorionic sac. The twins have a common placenta, and often some placental vessels join (see Fig. 8–18).

In unusual cases, division of the embryonic cells occurs in the second week, after the amniotic sac has formed. As a result, both embryos develop within the same amniotic cavity. These monozygotic twins are in one amniotic sac and one chorionic sac (Fig. 8–19A). Such twins are rarely delivered alive because the umbilical cords are frequently entangled so that circulation ceases and one or both fetuses die.

Conjoined Twins (Figs. 8–19B and C and 8–20). If the embryonic disc does not divide completely, various types of conjoined twins ("siamese twins") may form. These are named according to the regions that are attached, e.g., "thoracopagus," which indicates that there is anterior union of the thoracic regions.

Most twins are born prematurely because the uterus becomes overdistended and the twins become crowded within the uterus. This crowding interferes with the growth of the twins during the late stages of pregnancy. In addition, the placenta ceases to provide sufficient nutrition. Hence, a twin is always smaller than a single infant at a comparable stage of gestation

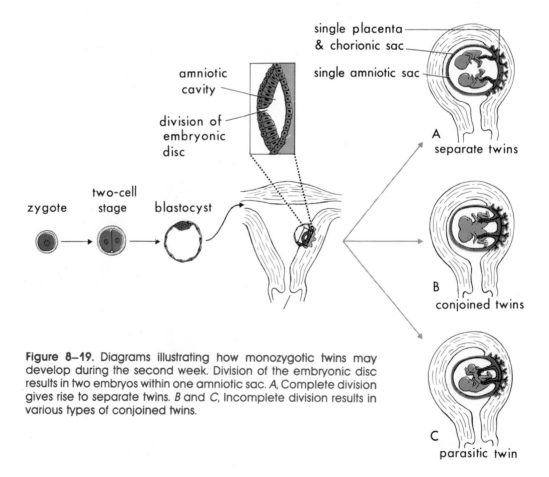

Figure 8–19. Diagrams illustrating how monozygotic twins may develop during the second week. Division of the embryonic disc results in two embryos within one amniotic sac. *A*, Complete division gives rise to separate twins. *B* and *C*, Incomplete division results in various types of conjoined twins.

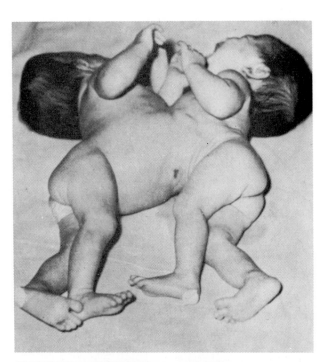

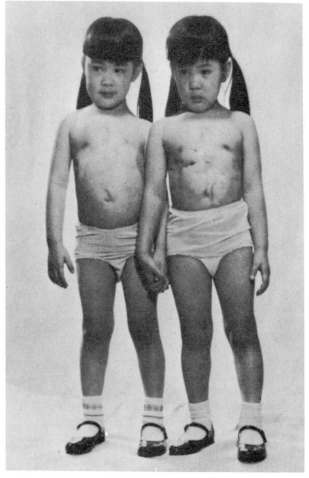

Figure 8–20. *A,* Photograph of newborn conjoined twins showing ventral union (thoracopagus). The twinning process began during the second week, but there was incomplete division of the embryonic disc (see Fig. 8–19). *B,* The twins about four years after separation. (From de Vries, P. A.: Case history—the San Francisco twins; in Bergsma, D. [Ed.]: *Conjoined Twins. Birth Defects. Original Article Series,* Vol. III, No. 1, April, 1967. © The National Foundation, New York.)

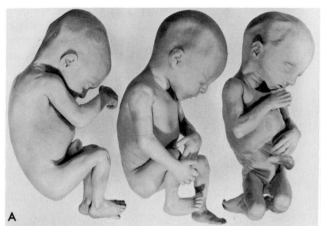
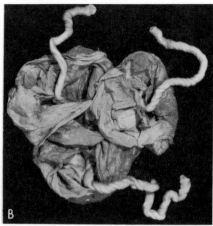

Figure 8–21. *A,* Photograph of 20-week triplets: monozygotic male twins (left) and a single female (right). *B,* Photograph of their fused placentas shows the twin placenta with two amnions (left) and the single placenta (upper right). These triplets developed from two zygotes. In many cases they develop from three zygotes.

(see Fig. 7–10). In addition, congenital malformations are more common in twins than in singletons.

Other Types of Multiple Birth

Triplets occur once in about 8100 pregnancies and may be derived from (1) one zygote and be identical, (2) two zygotes and consist of identical twins and a single infant (Fig. 8–21), or (3) three zygotes and be of the same sex or of different sexes. In the last case, the infants are no more similar than those from three separate pregnancies.

Similar possible combinations occur in *quadruplets, quintuplets, sextuplets, septuplets,* and so forth. Types of multiple births higher than triplets are normally uncommon, but they have occurred more often in recent years following the administration of gonadotropins to women with ovulatory failure.

SUMMARY

In addition to the embryo, the zygote gives rise to the fetal membranes and most of the placenta.

The placenta consists of two parts: (1) a fetal portion derived from the *villous chorion,* and (2) a maternal portion formed by the *decidua basalis.* The two parts are held together by *anchoring chorionic* villi and the cytotrophoblastic shell.

The fetal circulation is separated from the maternal circulation by a thin layer of fetal tissues known as the *placental membrane.* It is a permeable membrane that allows water, oxygen, nutrient substances, hormones, and noxious agents to pass from the mother to the embryo (fetus). Some products of excretion pass from the embryo (fetus) to the mother through the placental membrane.

The principal activities of the placenta are (1) metabolism, (2) transfer, and (3) endocrine secretion. These activities are essential for the maintenance of pregnancy and the growth and development of the embryo (fetus).

The fetal membranes and placenta(s) in multiple pregnancy vary considerably depending on the derivation of the embryos and when division of the embryonic cells occurs.

The common type of twins is dizygotic twins, with two amnions, two chorions, and two placentas which may or may not be fused. About a third of all twins are derived from one zygote; these *monozygotic twins* commonly have two amnions, one chorion, and one placenta. Other types of multiple birth (triplets and so forth) may be derived from one or more zygotes.

Although the yolk sac and allantois are vestigial structures, their formation is essential for normal embryonic development. Both are important early sites of blood formation, and part of the yolk sac is incorporated into the embryo as the primitive gut.

The amnion forms a sac for the amniotic fluid and provides a covering for the umbilical cord. The amniotic fluid provides a protective buffer for the embryo, room for fetal movements, and assistance in the regulation of fetal body temperature.

Commonly Asked Questions

1. What is meant by the term *"stillbirth"*? Do older women have more stillborn infants?
2. My sister's baby was born dead owing to a *"cord accident."* What does this mean?
3. What is the scientific basis of the pregnancy test kits that are sold in drug stores? Are they accurate?
4. What is the proper name for the *"bag of waters"*? What is meant by a *"dry birth"*? Does premature rupture of this "bag" induce the birth of the baby?
5. What does the term *"fetal distress"* mean? How is the condition recognized? What causes fetal distress?
6. I have heard that twins are born more commonly to older mothers. Is this true? I have also heard that twinning is hereditary. Is this true?
7. Can pregnant women with AIDS pass the virus to their babies?

Answers

1. A stillbirth is the birth of a fetus who, after 26 to 28 weeks of gestation, shows no evidence of life. The term *stillborn* denotes an infant that is *dead at birth*. Stillborn infants occur about three times more frequently among mothers over the age of 40 than in women in their 20s.
2. Sometimes the umbilical cord is abnormally long and becomes wrapped around the fetus' neck or a limb. This *"cord accident"* obstructs blood flow to and from the placenta. As a result, *the fetus does not receive sufficient oxygen and nutrients,* and soon dies. A true knot in the umbilical cord, formed when the fetus passes through a loop in it, also obstructs blood flow through the cord.
3. Most *pregnancy tests* are based on the presence of a hormone called *hCG* (human chorionic gonadotropin). These tests are capable of detecting the relatively large amounts of hCG that are in the woman's blood or urine. Such tests are positive a

short time (a week or so) after the first missed period. This hormone is produced by the syncytiotrophoblast of the chorion. These tests usually give an accurate diagnosis of pregnancy, but a doctor should be consulted as soon as possible because some tumors *(choriocarcinoma)* also produce this hormone.
4. The *"bag of waters"* is a layperson's term for the *amniotic sac* that is filled with amniotic fluid (largely composed of water). Sometimes this sac ruptures before birth, allowing the fluid to escape. *Premature rupture of the amnion is the most common event leading to premature labor (birth).* The premature rupture of the membranes may complicate the birth process (a dry birth) because normally the bulging amniotic sac helps to dilate the cervix of the uterus. Premature rupture of the membranes may also allow a vaginal infection to spread to the fetus.
5. The term *"fetal distress"* is synonymous with *fetal hypoxia* (a decrease below normal levels of oxygen in the fetal blood). Fetal distress exists when the fetal heart rate falls below 100 beats per minute. *Prolapse of the umbilical cord* (displacement of the cord into the cervix or vagina) causes fetal distress in about 1 to 200 deliveries, owing to impairment of blood supply to the fetus. In these cases the fetus compresses the umbilical cord as it passes through the cervix and vagina. Often the reason for the fetal distress is unknown.
6. Yes, this statement is true for dizygotic (fraternal) twins, but not for monozygotic (identical) twins. Dizygotic twinning is an autosomal-receptive trait that is carried by the daughters of mothers of twins. Hence, *dizygotic twinning is hereditary* or, as laypeople say, it "runs in the family." Monozygotic twinning, on the other hand, is a random occurrence that is not genetically controlled.
7. Yes. The human immunodeficiency virus *(HIV) can cross the placental membrane from the mother's blood and infect the fetus.* The HIV-infected fetus may develop AIDS 2 to 10 years after birth.

9

Congenital Malformations and Their Causes

Congenital malformations are anatomical or structural abnormalities present at birth. They may be macroscopic (visible with the unaided eye) or microscopic (visible with a microscope), on the surface or within the body.

About 20 per cent of deaths in the perinatal period (the period just before and just after birth) are attributed to congenital malformations. *Congenital malformations are the largest single cause of severe illness and death during infancy and childhood.*

The branch of embryology dealing with abnormal development and congenital malformations is called *teratology.* It is estimated that nearly 7 per cent of human developmental abnormalities result from the actions of drugs, viruses, and other environmental factors (Table 9–1). About 3 per cent of liveborn infants have one or more congenital malformations, and this figure is doubled by the end of the first year owing to the discovery of malformations that were present but indiscernible at birth.

Although it is customary to divide the causes of congenital malformations into (1) *genetic factors* (chromosomal abnormalities or mutant genes) and (2) *environmental factors,* it is not usually possible to separate clearly the factors which cause the abnormalities. Most common malformations result from an interaction of genetic and environmental factors, that is, *multifactorial inheritance* (Table 9–1).

Malformations may be single or multiple and of major or minor clinical significance. Single *minor malformations* are present in about 14 per cent of newborns. Such malformations are of no functional significance, but they should alert one to the possible

presence of associated major malformations. For example, a single umbilical artery (see Fig. 8–12) alerts the clinician to the possible presence of *cardiovascular malformations.* Major malformations are very common in early development, but most of these embryos are spontaneously aborted.

MALFORMATIONS CAUSED BY GENETIC FACTORS

Numerically, genetic factors are the major causes of congenital malformations (see Table 9–1). Genetic factors initiate mechanisms of malformation by biochemical or other means at the subcellular, cellular, or tissue level. The mechanism initiated by the genetic factor may be identical with or similar to the causal mechanism initiated by a *teratogen* (e.g., a drug or a virus).

Chromosomal abnormalities are common and are thought to be present in 6 per cent of all zygotes (Table 9–1). Many of these cells never become blas-

Table 9–1. Estimated Causes of Major Congenital Malformations

Chromosomal abnormalities	6.0%
Environmental factors	7.0%
Monogenic or single gene defects	8.0%
Multifactorial inheritance*	25.0%
Unknown etiology	54.0%

*Multiple genes at different loci on chromosomes that interact with environmental factors to produce congenital malformations.

tocysts and implant, and many more abort spontaneously during the first three weeks. Chromosome complements are subject to two kinds of changes—numerical and structural—and they may affect the sex chromosomes or the autosomes or both.

Persons with chromosomal abnormalities usually have characteristic *phenotypes* (e.g., the physical characteristics of the Down syndrome), and they often look more like other persons with the same chromosomal abnormality than like their own siblings (brothers or sisters). These characteristic appearances result from the genetic imbalance that disrupts normal development.

Numerical Chromosomal Abnormalities

Numerical abnormalities of chromosomes usually arise as the result of nondisjunction, an error in cell division in which there is failure of the paired chromosomes or sister chromatids to separate at anaphase. This error may occur during a mitotic division or during the first or second meiotic divisions (Fig. 9–1).

Normally the chromosomes exist in pairs (Fig. 9–2). Normal human females have 22 pairs of autosomes plus two X chromosomes, and normal males have 22 pairs of autosomes plus one X and one Y chromosome.

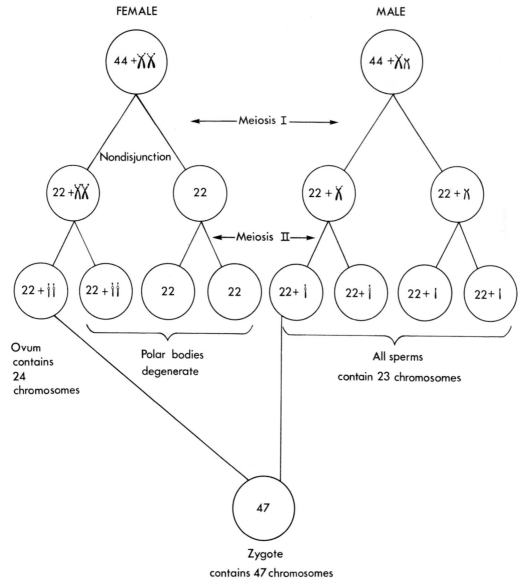

Figure 9–1. Diagram showing the first meiotic nondisjunction in a female resulting in an abnormal ovum with 24 chromosomes and how subsequent fertilization by a normal sperm produces a zygote with 47 chromosomes.

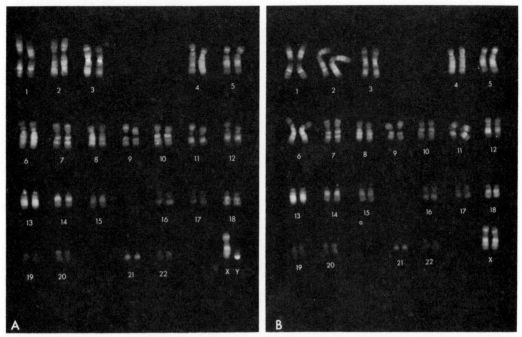

Figure 9–2. *A,* Normal male karyotype (chromosome set) showing chromosome banding. *B,* Similar bands in a normal female karyotype. When chromosomes are stained with quinacrine mustard or related compounds and examined by fluorescent microscopy, each pair of chromosomes stains in a distinctive pattern of bright and dim bands. They form the basis of the classification of chromosomes. (Courtesy of Dr. M. Ray, Department of Human Genetics, University of Manitoba, Winnipeg, Canada.)

Changes in chromosome number result in *aneuploidy,* which is any deviation from the diploid number of 46 chromosomes. The cells may be hypodiploid (usually 45) or hyperdiploid (usually 47).

Monosomy. Most embryos lacking a sex chromosome die, but some survive and develop characteristics of the *Turner syndrome* (Fig. 9–3). The incidence of the Turner syndrome is about 1 in 2500. The error (nondisjunction) in gametogenesis, when it can be traced, is usually during spermatogenesis (i.e., it is the paternal X chromosome that is missing). Maternal age is not advanced.

Embryos missing an autosome usually die; hence monosomy of an autosome is extremely rare in living persons.

Trisomy. If three chromosomes are present instead of the usual pair, the disorder is called trisomy. The usual cause of trisomy is *nondisjunction* or nonseparation of chromosomes, resulting in a germ cell with 24 instead of 23 chromosomes (see Fig. 9–1). If this cell is subsequently involved in fertilization, a zygote with 47 chromosomes forms.

Trisomy of the autosomes is primarily associated with three syndromes (Table 9–2). The most common condition is trisomy 21 or the Down syndrome (Fig. 9–4), in which three number 21 chromosomes are present. Trisomy 18 (Fig. 9–5) and trisomy 13 (Fig. 9–6) are less common. Infants with these abnormalities are severely malformed and mentally retarded. They usually die during early infancy.

Autosomal trisomies occur with increasing frequency as maternal age increases, particularly trisomy 21, which is present once in about 1550 births in mothers under 25, but one in about 25 mothers over the age of 45.

Trisomy of the sex chromosomes is a relatively common condition (Table 9–3); however, because there are no characteristic physical findings in infants or children, it is rarely detected until adolescence (Fig. 9–7).

Sex chromatin patterns are useful in detecting trisomy of the sex chromosomes because two masses of sex chromatin are present in XXX females (Fig. 9–8C), and cells of XXY males are chromatin-positive.

Tetrasomy and Pentasomy of the Sex Chromosomes. Some persons, usually mentally retarded, have four or five sex chromosomes. Usually the greater the number of X chromosomes present in males, the greater the severity of the mental retardation and physical impairment. The extra sex chromosomes do not accentuate male or female characteristics.

Text continued on page 114

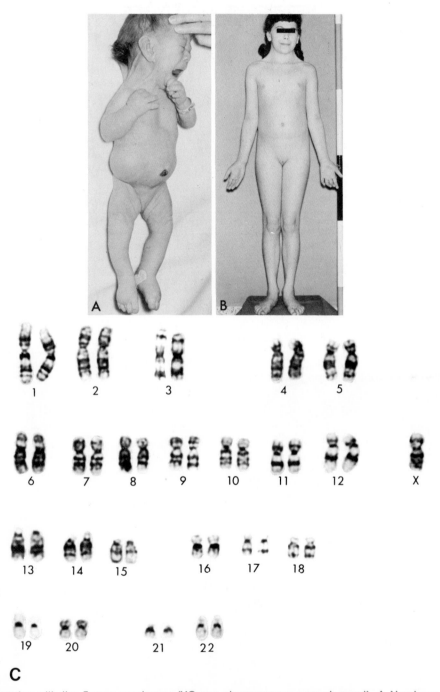

Figure 9–3. Females with the Turner syndrome (XO sex chromosome complement). *A*, Newborn infant. Note the webbed neck. *B*, 13-year-old girl showing the classic features of the syndrome: short stature, webbed neck, absence of sexual maturation, and broad, shield-like chest with widely spaced nipples. (From Moore, K. L.: *The Sex Chromatin*. Philadelphia, W. B. Saunders Company, 1966). *C*, Note the presence of only one X chromosome in the karyotype (chromosome set). (Courtesy of Dr. M. Ray, Department of Human Genetics, University of Manitoba, Winnipeg, Canada.)

Table 9–2. Trisomy of the Autosomes

Disorder	Incidence	Usual Characteristics
Trisomy 21 or Down syndrome*	1:700	Mental deficiency; hypotonia; flat nasal bridge; upward slant to palpebral fissures; protruding tongue; simian crease; congenital heart defects
Trisomy 18†	1:3000	Mental deficiency; growth retardation; prominent occiput; short sternum; ventricular septal defect; micrognathia; low-set malformed ears; flexed fingers
Trisomy 13†	1:5000	Mental deficiency; sloping forehead; malformed ears; microphthalmos; bilateral cleft lip and/or palate; polydactyly; posterior prominence of the heels

*The importance of this disorder in the overall problem of mental retardation is indicated by the fact that persons with the Down syndrome represent 10 to 15 per cent of institutionalized mental defectives. Down syndrome is by far the most common and best known of the chromosomal disorders. The old name, "mongolism," should not be used; it refers to the somewhat oriental appearance of the face caused by the apparent slanting of the eyes.

†Infants with this syndrome rarely survive beyond a few months.

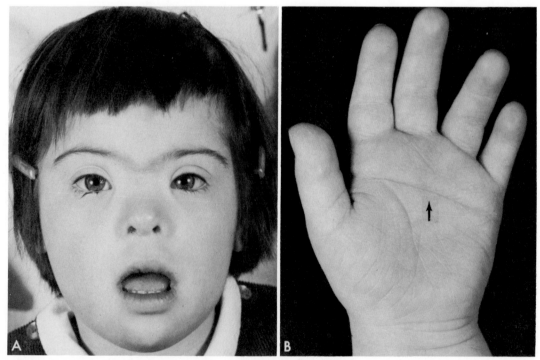

Figure 9–4. *A*, Photograph of a 3½-year-old girl, showing the typical facial appearance associated with the Down syndrome. Note the flat, broad face, oblique palpebral fissures, epicanthus, speckling of the iris, and furrowed lower lip. *B*, The typical short, broad hand of this child shows the characteristic single transverse palmar or simian crease (arrow). About half the palms of patients with Down syndrome have a single crease, and *about 1 per cent of normal persons have this unusual palm pattern*. (From Bartalos, M., and Baramki, T. A.: *Medical Cytogenetics.* Baltimore, Williams & Wilkins Company, 1967.)

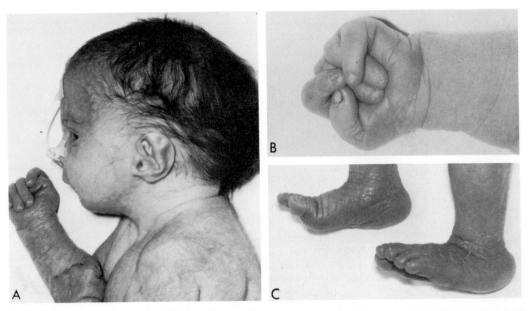

Figure 9-5. Photographs of an infant with the trisomy 18 syndrome. *A,* Prominent occiput and malformed ears. *B,* Typical flexed fingers. *C,* So-called rocker-bottom feet, showing posterior prominences of the heels. Most trisomy 18 fetuses abort spontaneously. The mean survival time of those who live after birth is two months. (Courtesy of Dr. Harry Medovy, Children's Centre, Winnipeg.)

Figure 9-6. Female infants with trisomy 13 syndrome. Note bilateral cleft lip, sloping forehead, and rocker-bottom feet. Trisomy 13 is a severe disorder and is fatal within the first month in about half of the liveborn infants. (From Smith, D. W.: *Am. J. Obstet. Gynecol. 90:*1055, 1964.)

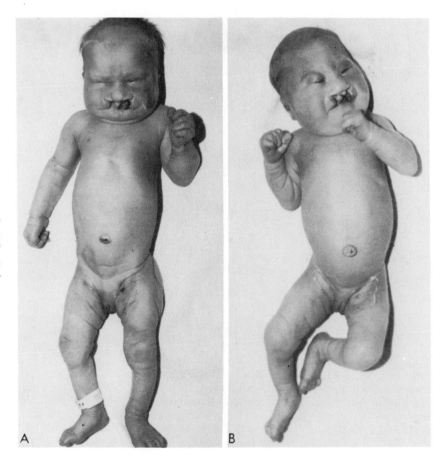

Table 9–3. Trisomy of the Sex Chromosomes

Chromosome Complement*	Sex	Incidence	Usual Characteristics
47,XXX	Female	1:1000	Normal in appearance; fertile; 15 to 25% are mentally retarded
47,XXY	Male	1:1000	Klinefelter syndrome: small testes and hyalinization of seminiferous tubules; aspermatogenesis; may be mentally retarded; often tall with long lower limbs
47,XYY	Male	1:1000	Normal in appearance, often tall; may have personality disorder

*The number designates the total number of chromosomes, including the sex chromosomes shown after the comma.

Mosaicism. A *mosaic* is a person derived from one zygote that has cells with *two or more different genotypes* (genetic constitutions). Either the autosomes or sex chromosomes may be involved. Usually the malformations are less serious than in persons with monosomy or trisomy, e.g., the features of the Turner syndrome are not as evident in mosaic females as in the usual 45,X females.

Mosaicism usually arises by nondisjunction during early cleavage divisions of the zygote. Mosaicism due to loss of a chromosome by so-called *anaphase lag*-ging is also known to occur. The chromosomes separate normally, but one chromosome is delayed in its migration and is eventually lost.

Polyploidy. Polyploid cells contain *multiples of the haploid number of chromosomes* (i.e., 69, 92, and so forth). Polyploidy is a significant cause of spontaneous abortion.

The most common type of polyploidy in human embryos is **triploidy** (69 chromosomes). This could result from the second polar body failing to separate from the oocyte during the second meiotic division (see Chapter 3). More likely, triploidy results from an ovum being fertilized by two sperms almost simultaneously. It has been estimated that 66 per cent of triploid embryos result from double fertilization (*dispermy*).

Triploidy occurs in about 2 per cent of embryos, but most of them abort spontaneously. Although fetuses with triploidy have been born alive, this occurrence is exceptional. They have all died within a few days owing to multiple malformations and low birth weight.

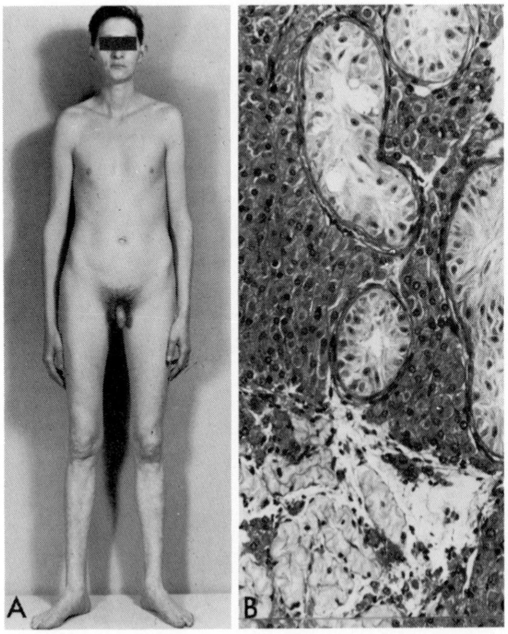

Figure 9–7. A, Adult male with the XXY Klinefelter syndrome. Note the relatively long lower limbs and normal trunk length. B, Section of a testicular biopsy showing some seminiferous tubules without germ cells and others that have degenerated. (From Ferguson-Smith, M. A.: *in* Moore, K. L. [Ed.]: *The Sex Chromatin.* Philadelphia, W. B. Saunders Company, 1966.)

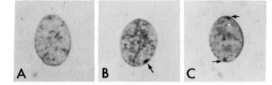

Figure 9–8. Oral epithelial nuclei stained with cresylecht violet (×2000). The sex chromatin (Barr body) represents a single X chromosome that is inactive in the metabolism of a cell. Normal females have sex chromatin; normal males do not. A, From normal male. No sex chromatin is visible (chromatin-negative). B, From normal female. The arrow indicates a typical mass of sex chromatin (chromatin-positive). C, From female with XXX trisomy. The arrows indicate two masses of sex chromatin. (A and B from Moore, K. L., and Barr, M. L.: *Lancet 2:57,* 1955.)

Structural Chromosomal Abnormalities

Most structural abnormalities of chromosomes result from chromosome breaks induced by environmental factors, e.g., radiation. The type of abnormality which results depends upon what happens to the broken pieces of chromosomes (Figs. 9–9 and 9–10). The only aberrations of chromosome structure that are likely to be transmitted from parent to child are the structural rearrangements of inversion and translocation.

Translocation. This is the transfer of a piece of one chromosome to a nonhomologous chromosome. If two nonhomologous chromosomes exchange pieces,

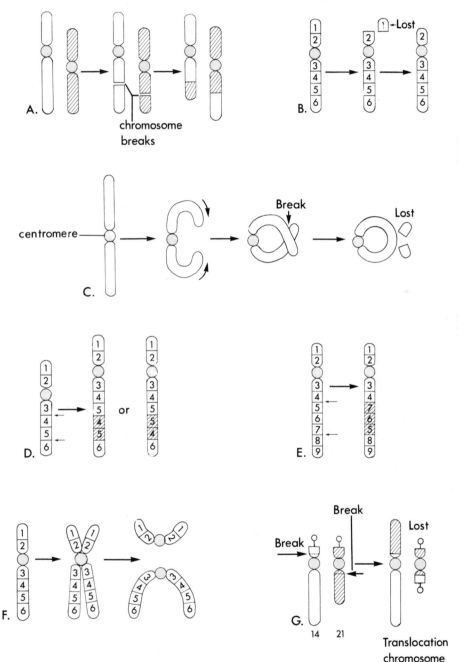

Figure 9–9. Diagrams illustrating structural abnormalities of chromosomes. *A,* Reciprocal translocation. *B,* Terminal deletion. *C,* Ring. *D,* Duplication. *E,* Paracentric inversion. *F,* Isochromosome. *G,* Robertsonian translocation. The only structural chromosome abnormalities that are likely to be transmitted from parent to child are rearrangements of the inversion or translocation type.

it is called a *reciprocal translocation* (Fig. 9–9A and G). Translocation does not necessarily lead to abnormal development. A person with a translocation—·for example, between a number 21 chromosome and a number 14 (Fig. 9–9G)—is phenotypically normal. Such persons are called *balanced translocation carriers*. They have a tendency, independent of age, to produce germ cells with an abnormal translocation chromosome. Three to 4 per cent of persons with the Down syndrome have translocation trisomies, i.e., the extra 21 chromosome is attached to another chromosome.

Deletion. When a chromosome breaks, a portion of the chromosome may be lost (Fig. 9–9B). A partial terminal deletion from the short arm end of a chromosome number 5 (Fig. 9–10B) causes the **cri du chat syndrome** (Fig. 9–10A). Affected infants have a weak catlike cry, microcephaly, severe mental retardation, and congenital heart disease. The only invariable feature is mental retardation.

A ring chromosome is a type of deletion chromosome from which both ends have been lost and the broken ends have rejoined to form a ring-shaped chromosome (Fig. 9–9C). These abnormal chromosomes have been described in persons with the Turner syndrome, trisomy 18, and other abnormalities.

Duplication. This abnormality may be represented as a duplicated portion of a chromosome: (1) within a chromosome (Fig. 9–9D), (2) attached to a chromosome, or (3) as a separate fragment. Duplications are more common than deletions and, because there is no loss of genetic material, they are less harmful. Duplication may involve part of a gene, whole genes, or a series of genes.

Inversion. This is a chromosomal aberration in which a segment of a chromosome is reversed. Paracentric inversion (Fig. 9–9E) is confined to a single arm of the chromosome, whereas pericentric inversion involves both arms and includes the centromere. Pericentric inversion has been described with the Down syndrome and other abnormalities.

Isochromosome. This abnormality results when the centromere divides transversely instead of longitudinally (Fig. 9–9F). It appears to be the most common structural abnormality of the X chromosome. Patients with this chromosomal abnormality are often short in stature and have other stigmata of the Turner syndrome. These characteristics are related to the loss of a short arm of one X chromosome.

Malformations Caused By Mutant Genes

About 8 per cent of congenital malformations are caused by gene defects (Table 9–1). A *mutation* usually involves a loss or *a change in the function of a gene*. Although a mutation could result in an improvement in development, most mutations are deleterious, and some are lethal.

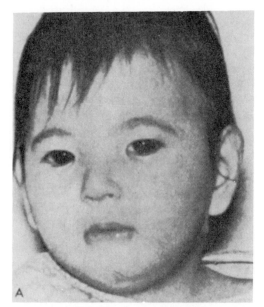
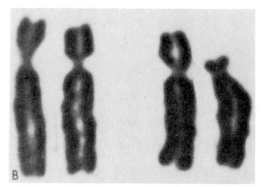

Figure 9–10. *A,* Male infant with cri du chat syndrome, showing the typical moon-faced appearance. *B,* The infant's chromosomes show a deletion of chromosome number 5 on the right. This syndrome received its name because of the resemblance of the cry of an affected child to the mewing of a cat. These children are severely mentally retarded. (Courtesy of Dr. J. de Grouchy, Paris.)

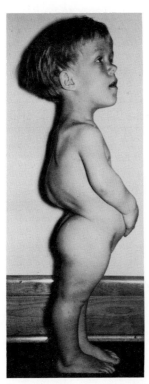

Figure 9–11. A child with achondroplasia, showing short limbs, large head, thoracic kyphosis (hump-back) and protrusion of the abdomen. (Courtesy of Dr. Harry Medovy, Children's Centre, Winnipeg.)

Because malformations caused by mutant genes are inherited according to mendelian laws, predictions can be made about the probability of their occurrence in the affected person's children and other relatives. Examples of *dominantly inherited* congenital malformations are achondroplasia (Fig. 9–11) and polydactyly or *extra digits* (see Chapter 16). Other malformations are attributed to *autosomal recessive inheritance*, e.g., microcephaly (see Chapter 17). Autosomal recessive genes manifest themselves only when homozygous; hence, many carriers of these genes go undetected.

The mutation rate can be increased by a number of environmental agents, e.g., large doses of radiation and many chemicals, especially carcinogenic (cancer-inducing) ones.

MALFORMATIONS CAUSED BY ENVIRONMENTAL FACTORS

The human embryo is well protected in the uterus, but certain agents, called *teratogens*, may induce congenital malformations when the tissues and organs are developing. The embryonic organs are most sensitive to teratogenic agents during periods of rapid differentiation.

Teratogenic agents cause about 7 percent of congenital malformations (Table 9–1). Because biochemical differentiation precedes morphological differentiation, the period during which structures are sensitive to interference often precedes the stage of their visible development by a few days (Fig. 9–12). Teratogens do not appear to be effective in causing malformations until cellular differentiation has begun. However, during the first two weeks they may cause the death of the embryo.

Six mechanisms can cause congenital malformations: (1) too little growth, (2) too little resorption, (3) too much resorption, (4) resorption in the wrong location, (5) normal growth in an abnormal position, and (6) overgrowth of a tissue or structure.

Critical Periods of Human Development

Environmental disturbances during the first two weeks after fertilization may interfere with implantation of the blastocyst or cause early death and/or abortion of the embryo (see Fig. 9–12).

Development of the embryo is most easily disturbed during the organogenetic period, particularly from days 15 to 60. During this period, teratogenic agents are most likely to produce congenital malformations. Each organ has a critical period during which its development may be deranged. For example, the critical period of upper limb development is from 24 to 42 days after fertilization.

The most critical period in the development of an embryo or in the growth of a particular tissue or organ is during the *time of most rapid cell division.* The critical period varies in accordance with the timing and duration of the period of increasing cell numbers for the tissue or organ concerned.

The critical period for brain growth and development is from 3 to 16 weeks (Fig. 9–12). Major morphological malformations (e.g., *neural tube defects*; see Chapter 17) develop during the third and fourth weeks. The brain is growing and differentiating rapidly at birth and continues to do so throughout the first two years after birth.

Tooth development also continues long after birth (see Chapter 19); hence, development of the permanent teeth may be affected by *tetracyclines* from 18 weeks (prenatal) to 16 years.

The skeletal system has a prolonged critical period of development, extending into adolescence and early adulthood. Hence, growth of skeletal tissues provides a very good gauge of general growth.

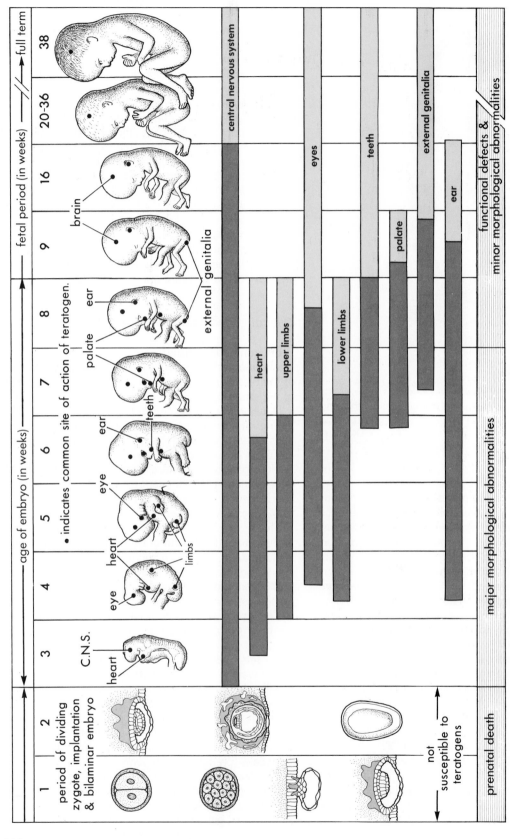

Figure 9–12. Schematic illustration of the critical periods in human development. Red denotes highly sensitive periods; yellow indicates stages that are less sensitive to teratogens. Note that each organ or structure has a critical period during which its development may be deranged, and that physiological defects, functional disturbances, and minor morphological changes are likely to result from disturbances during the fetal period. Severe mental retardation may result from exposure of the developing human to high levels of radiation during the 8- to 16-week period. Note that the embryo is not susceptible to teratogens (malformation-producing substances) during the first two weeks. During these early stages of development, a teratogen either kills the embryo or damages a few cells, allowing the embryo to recover without developing defects.

Teratogens and Human Malformations

A teratogen is any agent that can induce a congenital malformation or increase the incidence of a congenital malformation. The general objective of teratogenicity testing of drugs, food additives, and pesticides is to attempt to identify agents that may be teratogenic during human development.

Drugs vary considerably in their teratogenicity. Some drugs cause severe malformations (e.g., thalidomide); other commonly used drugs may produce mental and growth retardation (e.g., alcohol). It has been estimated that pregnant women take an average of four drugs, excluding nutritional supplements, and that 40 per cent of these women take the drugs during the critical period of embryonic human development.

Less than 2 per cent of congenital malformations are caused by drugs and chemicals. Few drugs have been positively implicated as teratogenic agents during human development (Table 9–4). Their use should be avoided by pregnant women and by those likely to conceive.

Alcohol (Fig. 9–13). Alcoholism is the most common drug abuse problem and affects 1 to 2 per cent of women of childbearing age. Infants born to chronic alcoholic mothers exhibit prenatal and postnatal growth deficiency, mental retardation, and congenital malformations. Short palpebral fissures, maxillary hypoplasia, abnormal palmar creases, joint anomalies, and congenital heart disease are present in most infants. This set of symptoms is known as the fetal alcohol syndrome. Even moderate maternal alcohol consumption (e.g., 2 to 3 ounces per day) may produce fetal alcohol effects (e.g., slight mental retardation), especially if the drinking is associated with malnutrition.

"Binge drinking" (heavy consumption of alcohol for one to three days) during pregnancy is very likely to harm the embryo.

Androgenic Agents (Fig. 9–14). The administration of synthetic progestins to prevent abortion has produced masculinization of female fetuses (see Table 9–4).

Any hormone that has masculinizing activities may affect development of the external genitalia of female fetuses.

Antibiotics. Tetracyclines pass the placental membrane and are deposited in the embryo's bones and teeth at sites of active calcification. Tetracycline therapy during the second and third trimesters of pregnancy may cause minor tooth defects and yellow to brown discoloration of the deciduous or primary teeth.

Penicillin appears to be harmless to the human embryo.

Anticoagulants. All anticoagulants, except heparin, cross the placental membrane (see Fig. 8–7) and may cause hemorrhage in the fetus. Warfarin is a teratogen. There are several reports of infants born with hypoplasia of the nasal bones and other abnormalities whose mothers took this anticoagulant during the critical period of their embryo's development. Second- and third-trimester exposure may result in mental retardation, optic atrophy, and microcephaly.

As heparin does not cross the placental membrane, it is not a teratogen and does not affect the embryo or fetus.

Anticonvulsants. There is now strong suggestive evidence that trimethadione (Tridione) and paramethadione (Paradione) may cause fetal facial dysmorphia, cardiac defects, cleft palate, and intrauterine growth retardation (IUGR) when given to pregnant women. Seven cases of hypoplasia of the terminal phalanges in infants of epileptics have been reported. All mothers had taken phenytoin and a barbiturate.

Phenytoin (diphenylhydantoin) is definitely a teratogen. A fetal hydantoin syndrome is now recognized, consisting of the following abnormalities: IUGR, microcephaly, mental retardation, a ridged metopic suture, inner epicanthal folds, eyelid ptosis, a broad depressed nasal bridge, nail and/or distal phalangeal hypoplasia, and hernias.

Phenobarbital appears to be a safe antiepileptic drug for use during pregnancy.

Antitumor Agents. Most tumor-inhibiting chemicals are highly teratogenic.

Aminopterin is a potent teratogen which can induce major congenital malformations (Fig. 9–15), especially of the central nervous system. Methotrexate, a derivative of aminopterin, is also teratogenic.

Environmental Chemicals. In recent years there has been increasing concern over the possible teratogenicity of environmental chemicals, including industrial pollutants and food additives. Most of these chemicals have not been positively implicated as teratogens in humans.

Infants of mothers whose main diet during pregnancy consisted of fish containing abnormally high levels of organic mercury acquire fetal Minamata disease and exhibit neurological and behavioral disturbances resembling cerebral palsy. In some cases, severe brain damage, mental retardation, and blindness have been present in the infants of mothers who received methylmercury in their food. Similar observations have been made in infants of mothers who

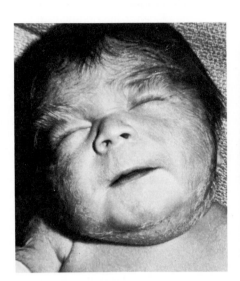 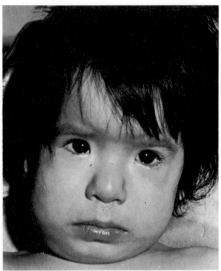

Figure 9–13. Photographs showing the facial appearance of an infant with the *fetal alcohol syndrome*. The characteristic triad of abnormalities includes growth deficiency, mental retardation, and abnormal facial features. *A,* At birth. *B,* At one year. (*A* is from Jones, K. L., and Smith, D. W.: *Lancet 2:999,* 1973; *B,* is from Jones, K. L., et al.: *Lancet 1:1267,* 1973.)

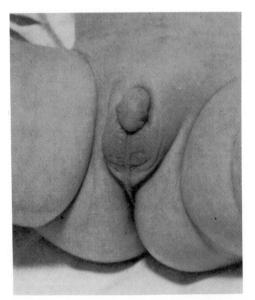 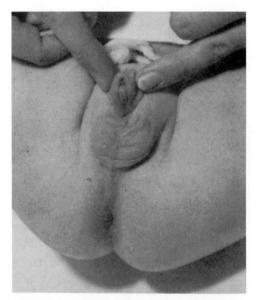

Figure 9–14. The external genitalia of a newborn female infant showing fusion of the labia majora to form a scrotum-like structure and enlargement of the clitoris. These abnormalities were caused by an androgenic agent given to the infant's mother during the first trimester. (From Jones, H. W., and Scott, W. W.: *Hermaphroditism, Genital Anomalies and Related Endocrine Disorders.* Baltimore, Williams & Wilkins Company, 1958.)

Table 9–4. Teratogens Known to Cause Human Malformations

Teratogens	Common Congenital Malformations
Androgenic Agents	
Ethisterone	Varying degrees of masculinization of female fetuses: ambiguous
Norethisterone	external genitalia owing to labial fusion and clitoral hypertrophy
Testosterone	(see Fig. 9–14)
Drugs and Chemicals	
Alcohol	*Fetal alcohol syndrome:* intrauterine growth retardation (IUGR); mental retardation; microcephaly; ocular anomalies; joint abnormalities; short palpebral fissures
Aminopterin	Wide range of skeletal defects; IUGR; malformations of the central nervous system, notably meroanencephaly or anencephaly (partial absence of the brain) (see Fig. 9–15)
Busulfan	Stunted growth; skeletal abnormalities; corneal opacities; cleft palate; hypoplasia of various organs
Phenytoin (diphenylhydantoin)	*Fetal hydantoin syndrome:* IUGR; microcephaly; mental retardation; ridged metopic suture; inner epicanthal folds; eyelid ptosis; broad depressed nasal bridge; phalangeal hypoplasia
Lithium carbonate	Various malformations, usually involving the heart and great vessels
Methotrexate	Multiple malformations, especially skeletal, involving the face, skull, limbs, and vertebral column
Large doses of retinoic acid (vitamin A)	Facial abnormalities and neural tube defects
Tetracycline	Stained teeth and enamel hypoplasia
Thalidomide	Amelia, meromelia, and other limb deformities; external ear, cardiac, and gastrointestinal malformations (see Fig. 9–16)
Warfarin	Nasal hypoplasia; chondroplasia punctata; mental retardation; optic atrophy; microcephaly
Infectious Agents	
Cytomegalovirus	Microcephaly; hydrocephaly; microphthalmia; microgyria; mental retardation; cerebral calcifications
Herpes simplex virus	Microcephaly; microphthalmia; retinal dysplasia
Rubella virus	Cataracts; glaucoma; chorioretinitis; deafness; microphthalmia; congenital heart defects
Toxoplasma gondii	Microcephaly; microphthalmia; hydrocephaly; chorioretinitis; cerebral calcifications
Treponema pallidum	Hydrocephalus; congenital deafness; mental retardation
High Levels of Ionizing Radiation	Microcephaly; mental retardation; skeletal malformations

ate pork that became contaminated when the pigs ate corn grown from seed that had been sprayed with a mercury-containing fungicide. *Methylmercury is a teratogen* that causes cerebral atrophy, spasticity, seizures, and *mental retardation.*

Thyroid Drugs. *Potassium iodide* and *radioactive iodine* may cause congenital goiter. Propylthiouracil interferes with thyroxine formation in the fetus and may cause goiter.

Thalidomide. A mass of evidence has shown that this drug is a potent teratogen. As a result, it has been withdrawn from the market. It has been estimated that 7000 infants were malformed by thalidomide (Fig. 9–16). The malformations ranged from amelia (absence of limbs) through intermediate stages of development (rudimentary limbs) to micromelia (short limbs). Thalidomide also causes malformations of other structures.

Lysergic Acid Diethylamide (LSD). This socially used drug may be teratogenic. Of 161 infants born to women who ingested LSD before conception and/or during the pregnancy, five infants had limb deficiency anomalies. These observations *suggest* that LSD may be teratogenic and that ingestion of it should be avoided during pregnancy.

Marijuana. There is no evidence that this drug is teratogenic in humans, but there is no assurance that heavy usage of it does not affect the mental development of the embryo.

Phencyclidine (PCP, "Angel Dust"). An infant with several malformations and behavioral abnormalities was born to a mother who used PCP throughout her pregnancy. This suggests, but does not prove, a causal association.

Retinoic Acid (Vitamin A). This is a well-established teratogen in animals. Its teratogenicity in hu-

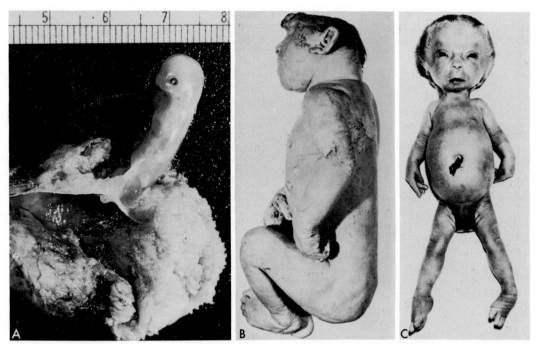

Figure 9–15. Aminopterin-induced congenital malformations. *A,* Grossly malformed embryo and its membranes. (Courtesy of Dr. J. B. Thiersch, Seattle, Washington.) *B,* Newborn infant with meroanencephaly or partial absence of the brain. (From Thiersch, J. B.: *in* Wolstenholme, G. E. W., and O'Connor, C. M. [Eds.]: *Ciba Foundation Symposium on Congenital Malformations.* London, J. & A. Churchill, Ltd. 1960, pp. 152–154.) *C,* Newborn infant showing marked intrauterine growth retardation, a large head, a small mandible, deformed ears, clubhands, and clubfeet. (From Warkany, J., Beaudry, P. H., and Hornstein, S.: *Am. J. Dis. Child.* 97:274, 1960.)

mans was established in 1983. *Isotretinoin (ITR), used for the oral treatment of acne, is teratogenic at very low doses in humans.* The critical period for exposure to retinoic acid appears to be from the third week to the fifth week of development. The most common malformations observed are craniofacial dysmorphism (microtia, micrognathia), cleft palate and/or thymic aplasia defects, and neural tube defects. *Vitamin A is a valuable and necessary nutrient during pregnancy,* but long-term exposure to large doses is unwise.

Salicylates. There is some evidence that *aspirin,* the most commonly ingested drug during pregnancy, is potentially harmful to the embryo or fetus when administered to the mother in *large doses.*

Drug Testing in Animals. Although the testing of drugs in pregnant animals is important, the results are of limited value for predicting drug effects on human embryos. Animal experiments can only suggest similar effects in humans.

Infectious Agents

Three viruses are known to be teratogenic in humans: rubella virus, cytomegalovirus, and herpes simplex virus.

Rubella Virus (German Measles). About 15 to 20 per cent of infants born to women who have had German measles during the first trimester of pregnancy are congenitally malformed. The usual triad of malformations is *cataract* (Fig. 9–17A), *cardiac malformations,* and *deafness,* but other malformations occur occasionally, e.g., glaucoma (Fig. 9–17B).

The earlier in pregnancy the maternal rubella infection occurs, the greater is the danger of the embryo being malformed. Most infants have congenital malformations if the disease occurs during the first five weeks after fertilization. This is understandable because this period includes the most susceptible organogenetic periods of the eye, ear, heart and brain (see Fig. 9–12). Malformations may result from infections during the second and third trimesters, but usually functional defects of the central nervous system (mental retardation) and internal ear (hearing loss) result.

Cytomegalovirus. Infection with cytomegalovirus (CMV) is probably the most common viral infection of the human fetus. Because the disease seems to be fatal when it affects the embryo or young fetus, it is believed that most pregnancies end in abortion when the infection occurs during the first trimester. Infection with this virus during the second and third trimesters

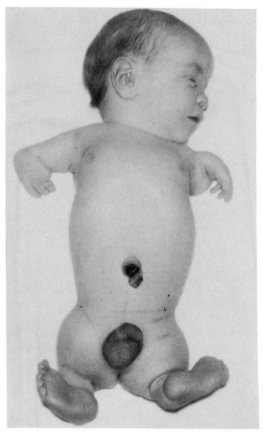

Figure 9–16. Newborn male infant showing typically malformed limbs (meromelia) caused by thalidomide. (From Moore, K. L.: *Manitoba Med. Rev. 43*:306, 1963.)

causes abnormalities of the brain (microcephaly) and of the eyes (microphthalmia).

Herpes Simplex Virus. Infection of the fetus with this virus usually occurs late in pregnancy, probably most often during delivery. The congenital abnormalities that have been observed in fetuses infected before birth are microcephaly, microphthalmia, retinal dysplasia, and mental retardation.

Two other microorganisms are known to be teratogens in humans, *Toxoplasma gondii* and *Treponema pallidum*.

Toxoplasma Gondii. This intracellular parasite can be contracted from eating raw or poorly cooked meat (usually pork or mutton), by contact with infected animals (usually cats), or from the soil. This organism may cross the placental membrane and infect the fetus, causing destructive changes in the brain and eye, resulting in microcephaly, microphthalmia, and hydrocephaly (see Chapters 17 and 18).

Syphilis. *Treponema pallidum,* the small spiral-shaped microorganism that causes syphilis, rapidly penetrates the placental membrane after the twentieth week of gestation, when the cytotrophoblast disappears (see Chapter 8).

Untreated *primary maternal infections* (acquired during pregnancy) nearly always cause serious fetal infection, but adequate treatment of the mother before the sixteenth week kills the organism, thereby preventing it from crossing the placental membrane and infecting the fetus.

Secondary maternal infections (acquired before pregnancy) seldom result in fetal disease and malformations. If the mother is untreated, stillbirths result in one fourth of cases. The tissues most often extensively involved in the dead fetuses are bone, bone marrow, lungs, liver, and spleen, but any organ system may be involved.

Radiation

Ionizing radiations are potent teratogens. Exposure to radiation may injure embryonic cells, resulting in cell death, chromosome injury, and retardation of growth. The severity of embryonic damage is related to the absorbed dose, the dose rate, and the stage of embryonic or fetal development during which the exposure occurs.

Large amounts of ionizing radiation produce congenital malformations and mental retardation. Large doses of radiation (over 25,000 millirads) are *harmful to the developing central nervous system.*

There is no proof that human congenital malformations have been caused by diagnostic levels of radiation. Scattered radiation from an x-ray examination of a part of the body that is not near the uterus (e.g., chest, sinuses, teeth) produces only a dose of a few millirads, which is not teratogenic to the embryo.

It is prudent to be cautious during diagnostic examinations of the pelvic region in pregnant women (x-ray examinations and medical diagnostic tests using radioisotopes) because they result in exposure of the embryo to 0.3 to 2 rads.

Mechanical Factors

The significance of mechanical influences in the uterus on congenital postural deformities is still an open question. The amniotic fluid absorbs mechanical pressures, thereby protecting the embryo from most external trauma. It is generally accepted that congenital abnormalities caused by external injury to the mother are extremely uncommon, but possible.

Congenital dislocation of the hip and clubfoot may

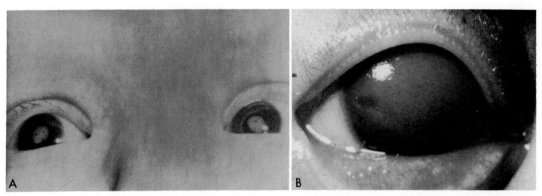

Figure 9–17. Congenital malformations of the eye caused by the rubella virus. *A,* Cataracts. (From Cooper, L. Z., et al.: *Am. J. Dis. Child. 110:416,* 1965. Courtesy of Dr. Richard Baragry, Department of Ophthalmology, Cornell-New York Hospital.) *B,* Glaucoma. (From Cooper, L. Z., et al.: *Am. J. Dis. Child. 110:416,* 1965. Courtesy of Dr. Daniel I. Weiss, Department of Ophthalmology, New York University School of Medicine.)

be caused by mechanical forces, particularly in a malformed uterus. Such deformations may be caused by any factor that restricts the mobility of the fetus, thereby causing prolonged compression in an abnormal posture.

A significantly reduced quantity of amniotic fluid *(oligohydramnios)* may result in mechanically induced abnormalities of the fetal limbs, e.g., hyperextension of the knee. Intrauterine amputations or other malformations caused by local constriction during fetal growth may result from amniotic bands or fibrous rings, presumably formed as a result of rupture of the fetal membranes (amnion and chorion) during early pregnancy.

SUMMARY

A congenital malformation is an anatomical or structural abnormality present at birth. Much progress has been made in recent years in the search for causes of congenital malformations, but satisfactory explanations are still lacking for most of them. Developmental abnormalities may be macroscopic or microscopic, on the surface or within the body.

Some congenital malformations are caused by *genetic factors* (chromosomal abnormalities and mutant genes) and a few are caused by *environmental factors* (infectious agents and teratogenic drugs), but most common malformations result from a complex interaction of genetic and environmental factors *(multifactorial inheritance).*

During the first two weeks of development, teratogenic agents may kill the embryo, but they are not known to cause congenital malformations.

During the *organogenetic period,* particularly from days 15 to 60, teratogenic agents may cause major congenital malformations. During the *fetal period,* teratogens may produce minor morphological and functional abnormalities, particularly of the brain and the eyes.

Mental retardation may result from infectious agents and from high levels of radiation.

Commonly Asked Questions

1. If a pregnant woman takes *aspirin* (acetylsalicylic acid or ASA) in normal doses, will it cause congenital malformations?
2. If *a woman is a drug addict,* will her child show signs of drug addiction?
3. Are all drugs tested for teratogenicity (the ability to produce congenital malformations) before they are marketed? If the answer is "yes," why are human teratogens still sold?
4. Is *cigarette smoking during pregnancy* harmful to the embryo or fetus? If the answer is "yes," would refraining from inhalation of the smoke be safer?
5. *Are there any drugs that are safe to take during pregnancy?* If so, what are they?

Answers

1. Almost certainly not. There is no evidence that the occasional use of aspirin *in the usual recommended dosages* is harmful during pregnancy. However, large doses at subtoxic levels (e.g., for rheumatoid arthritis) have not been proved to be harmless to the embryo and fetus.

2. Yes. A woman who is addicted to a habit-forming drug (e.g., morphine and heroin) and uses the drug during pregnancy is almost certain to give birth to a child who shows signs of drug addiction. However, the fetus's chances of survival until birth are not good; the mortality and premature birth rates are high among fetuses of drug-addicted mothers.

3. *All drugs prescribed in Canada and the United States are tested for teratogenicity before they can be marketed.* However, the thalidomide tragedy clearly demonstrated the need for improved methods for detecting potential human teratogens. Thalidomide was not teratogenic in pregnant mice and rats, but it was extraordinarily potent in humans during the fourth to sixth weeks of pregnancy. Because it would be unethical to test the effects of drugs on embryos who are to be aborted, there is no way of preventing some human teratogens from being marketed. Human teratological evaluation depends on retrospective epidemiological studies and the reports of astute physicians. This is the way thalidomide teratogenicity was detected. Most new drugs contain a disclaimer in the accompanying package insert such as, "This drug has not been proven safe for pregnant women." Some drugs may be used if "in the opinion of the physician the potential benefits outweigh the possible hazards." All teratogenic drugs that are likely to be taken by a pregnant woman are available only through prescription by a physician.

4. *Cigarette smoking during pregnancy is clearly harmful to the embryo and fetus.* Therefore, abstinence from smoking during the embryo's critical period of development (third to eighth weeks) will not prevent its most adverse effect, *intrauterine growth retardation.* Women who stop smoking during the first half of pregnancy have infants with birth weights closer to those of nonsmokers. Decreased placental blood flow, thought to be a nicotine-mediated effect, is believed to cause decreased intrauterine blood flow. *There is no conclusive evidence that maternal smoking causes congenital malformations in infants.* The growth of the fetus of a woman who smokes but does not inhale is still endangered because nicotine, carbon monoxide, and other harmful substances are absorbed into the bloodstream through the mucous membranes of the mouth and throat, as well as through the lungs. Hence, refraining from inhalation of the smoke is safer, but smoking in any manner is not advisable.

5. There is ample evidence to indicate that most drugs do not cause congenital malformations in human embryos. However, *a pregnant women should not take any drugs that are not essential for her health.* This should be determined by her physician. A pregnant woman with a severe lower respiratory infection, for example, would be unwise to refuse drugs recommended by her doctor (e.g., antibiotics) to cure her illness. Otherwise, her health and that of her embryo or fetus could be endangered. Most drugs, including sulfonamides, meclizine, penicillin, antihistamines, and bendectin, are considered safe. Similarly, local anesthetic agents, dead vaccines, and salicylates (e.g., aspirin) in low doses are not known to cause congenital malformations.

10

Body Cavities, Primitive Mesenteries, and the Diaphragm

Early development of the **intraembryonic coelom** or embryonic body cavity is described in Chapter 5. By the fourth week it appears as a horseshoe-shaped cavity in the cardiogenic and lateral mesoderm (Fig. 10–1A). The curve or bend of the "horseshoe" represents the future *pericardial cavity,* and its limbs or lateral extensions indicate the future *pleural and peritoneal cavities.*

The intraembryonic coelom provides room for organ development and movement. For a while, the intraembryonic coelom communicates with the extraembryonic coelom at the lateral edges of the embryonic disc (Fig. 10–1A and B). This communication is largely occluded during folding of the embryonic disc into a cylindrical embryo, but persists for awhile around the stalk of the yolk sac (Fig. 10–2E). This communication is important because, as described in Chapter 13, most of the midgut herniates through this communication into the umbilical cord (see Figs. 7–3 and 13–6), where it develops into most of the small intestine and part of the large intestine.

During horizontal folding of the embryo, the lateral limbs or extensions of the intraembryonic coelom come together and fuse on the ventral aspect of the embryo (Fig. 10–2C and F). In the region of the future peritoneal cavity, the ventral mesentery degenerates, forming a large peritoneal cavity extending from inferior to the heart to the pelvic region.

Three body cavities are now recognizable: (1) a large *pericardial cavity* around the heart (Fig. 10–2B and E); (2) two relatively small *pericardioperitoneal canals* (or pleural canals) connecting the pericardial and peritoneal cavities (Fig. 10–3); and (3) a large

peritoneal cavity containing the abdominal and pelvic viscera (see Figs. 10–2F and 13–6).

With formation of the head fold, the heart and pericardial cavity move or "swing" ventrally beneath the foregut (see Fig. 10–2B and E). The pericardial cavity then opens dorsally into the pericardioperitoneal canals, which pass dorsal to the septum transversum on each side of the foregut (Fig. 10–3).

The *septum transversum* is a transverse sheet of mesoderm that separates the pericardial cavity from the peritoneal cavity, forming a partial diaphragm or partition between them.

DIVISION OF THE COELOM

Partitions form at both ends of the pericardioperitoneal canals and separate the pericardial cavity from the pleural cavities, and the pleural cavities from the peritoneal cavity.

The *pleuropericardial membranes* (Fig. 10–4) separate the pericardial cavity from the pleural cavities. Initially, this pair of membranes appears as ridges or bulges containing the *common cardinal veins* which pass to the heart (Fig. 10–4A). These veins drain the primitive venous system into the sinus venosus of the primitive heart (see Chapter 15).

At first the pleuropericardial membranes are free dorsally and project into the cranial ends of the pericardioperitoneal canals; however, after expansion of the pleural cavities, the pleuropericardial membranes fuse with one another and with the mesoderm ventral to the esophagus (Fig. 10–4C).

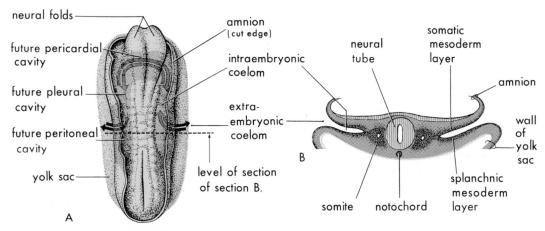

Figure 10–1. *A,* Embryo of about 22 days showing the outline of the horseshoe-shaped intraembryonic coelom. The amnion has been removed and the coelom is shown as if the embryo were translucent. The continuity of the intraembryonic coelom and the communication of its right and left extremities with the extraembryonic coelom is indicated by arrows. *B,* Transverse section through the embryo at the level shown in *A.*

The *pleuroperitoneal membranes* separate the pleural cavities from the peritoneal cavity (Fig. 10–5). This pair of membranes is mainly produced as the developing lungs and pleural cavities expand by invading the body wall. They are attached dorsolaterally to the body wall, and their crescentic free edges initially project into the caudal ends of the pericardioperitoneal canals (Fig. 10–5B). Later they fuse with other diaphragmatic components to form the diaphragm (Fig. 10–5C to E).

DEVELOPMENT OF THE DIAPHRAGM

The diaphragm is a dome-shaped musculotendinous partition separating the thoracic and abdominopelvic cavities. It *develops from four structures* (Fig. 10–5).

The Septum Transversum (Figs. 10–2E, 10–3, and 10–5). This *transverse septum,* composed of mesodermal tissue, initially forms a thick incomplete partition or diaphragm between the pericardial and peritoneal cavities. Later it fuses dorsally with the mesoderm ventral to the esophagus and with the pleuroperitoneal membranes. Eventually, it forms the *central tendon* of the adult diaphragm (Fig. 10–5E).

The Pleuroperitoneal Membranes (Fig. 10–5). These membranes fuse with the dorsal mesentery of the esophagus and the dorsal portion of the septum transversum, thereby completing the partition between the thoracic and abdominopelvic cavities. Although the pleuroperitoneal membranes form large portions of the primitive diaphragm, they represent relatively small intermediate portions of the fully developed diaphragm (Fig. 10–5E).

Dorsal Mesentery of the Esophagus (Figs. 10–4 and 10–5). This mesentery constitutes the median portion of the diaphragm. The *crura of the diaphragm* form from developing muscle fibers that grow into the dorsal mesentery of the esophagus (mesoesophagus).

The Body Wall (Fig. 10–5). As the lungs grow, the pleural cavities enlarge and burrow into the lateral body walls (see Fig. 10–4). During this "excavation" process, body-wall tissue is split into two layers: (1) an external layer that will form part of the definite body wall, and (2) an internal layer that contributes to peripheral portions of the diaphragm, external to the portions derived from the pleuroperitoneal membranes.

Positional Changes and Innervation of the Diaphragm

During the fourth week, the septum transversum lies opposite the third, fourth, and fifth *cervical somites* (Fig. 10–6A). During the fifth week, myoblasts (primitive muscle cells) from the *myotomes* of these cervical somites migrate into the developing diaphragm and bring their nerves with them. Thus, *the nerve supply of the diaphragm is from the third, fourth, and fifth cervical nerves,* which are contained in the **phrenic nerves.** These nerves pass to the septum transversum via the pleuropericardial membranes. This explains why the phrenic nerves subsequently come to lie on the fibrous pericardium (see Fig. 10–4C and D).

Rapid growth of the dorsal part of the embryo's

Text continued on page 132

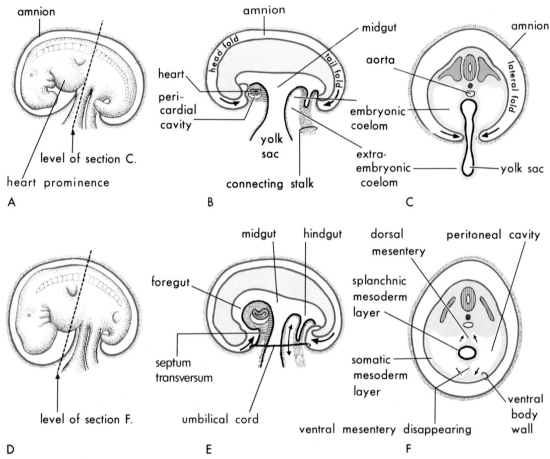

Figure 10–2. Drawings illustrating folding of the embryo and its effect on the intraembryonic coelom and other structures. *A,* Lateral view of an embryo of about 26 days. *B,* Schematic sagittal section of this embryo showing the head and tail folds. *C,* Transverse section at the level shown in *A* indicating how the lateral folds give the embryo a cylindrical form. *D,* Lateral view of a 28-day embryo. *E,* Schematic sagittal section of this embryo showing the reduced communication between the intraembryonic and extraembryonic coeloms (double-headed arrow). *F,* Transverse section as indicated in *D,* illustrating formation of the ventral body wall and disappearance of the ventral mesentery. The arrows indicate the junction of the somatic and splanchnic mesoderm layers. The somatic mesoderm layer will become the parietal peritoneum, which lines the abdominal wall, and the splanchnic mesoderm layer will become the visceral peritoneum covering the organs (e.g., the stomach).

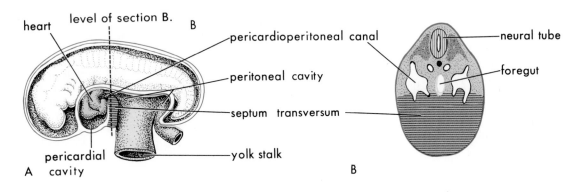

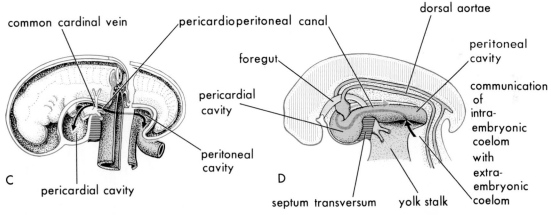

Figure 10–3. Schematic drawings of a four-week embryo (about 24 days). *A,* The lateral wall of the pericardial cavity has been removed to show the heart. *B,* Transverse section illustrating the relationship of the pericardioperitoneal canals to the septum transversum (primordium of part of the diaphragm) and the foregut. *C,* Lateral view with the heart removed. The embryo has been sectioned transversely to show the continuity of the intraembryonic and extraembryonic coeloms. *D,* Sketch showing the pericardioperitoneal canals arising from the dorsal wall of the pericardial cavity and passing on each side of the foregut to join the peritoneal cavity. The arrows show the communication of the extraembryonic coelom with the intraembryonic coelom and the continuity of the intraembryonic coelom at this stage.

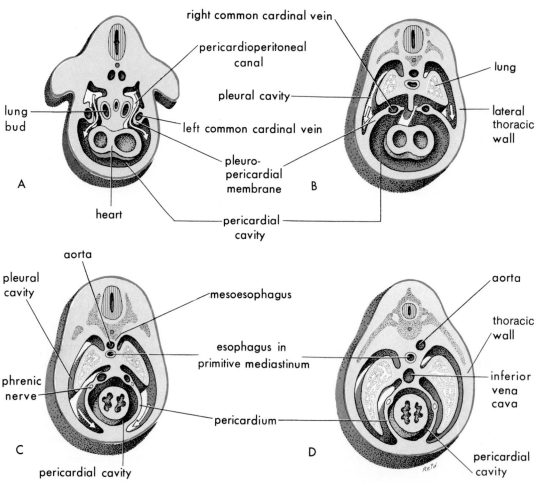

Figure 10–4. Schematic drawings of transverse sections through an embryo cranial to the septum transversum, illustrating successive stages in the separation of the pleural cavities from the pericardial cavity. Growth and development of the lungs, expansion of the pleural cavities, and formation of the fibrous pericardium are also shown. *A*, Five weeks. The arrows indicate the communications between the pericardioperitoneal canals and the pericardial cavity. *B*, Six weeks. The arrows indicate development of the pleural cavities as extensions of the pericardioperitoneal canals and as expansion of the pleural cavities into the body wall. *C*, Seven weeks. Expansion of the pleural cavities ventrally around the heart is shown. The pleuropericardial membranes are now fused in the midline with each other and with the mesoderm ventral to the esophagus. *D*, Eight weeks. Continued expansion of the lungs and pleural cavities and formation of the fibrous pericardium and chest wall are illustrated.

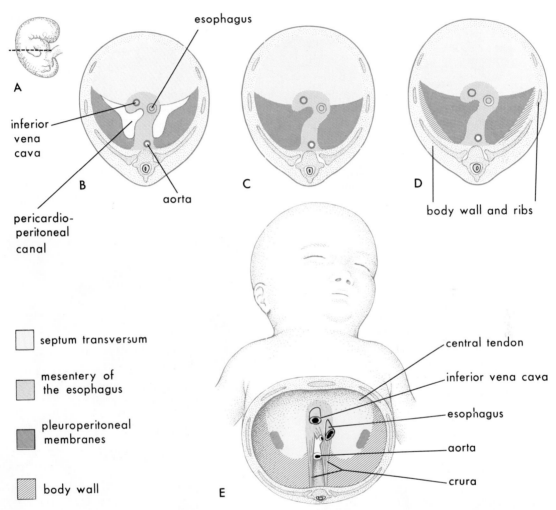

Figure 10–5. Drawings illustrating development of the diaphragm as viewed from below. *A,* Sketch of a lateral view of an embryo during the fifth week *(actual size)* indicating the level of the sections. *B,* Transverse section showing the unfused pleuroperitoneal membranes. *C,* Similar section at the end of the sixth week after fusion of the pleuroperitoneal membranes with the other two diaphragmatic components. *D,* Transverse section through a 12-week embryo after ingrowth of the fourth diaphragmatic component from the body wall. *E,* View of the diaphragm of a newborn infant, indicating the probable embryological origin of its components.

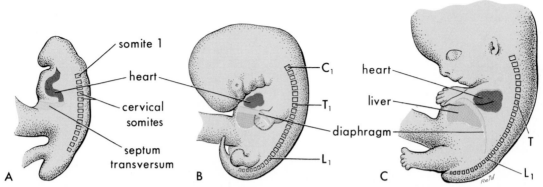

Figure 10–6. Diagrams illustrating positional changes of the developing diaphragm. *A,* About 24 days. The septum transversum (primordium of part of the diaphragm) is at the level of the third, fourth, and fifth cervical segments. *B,* About 41 days. *C,* About 52 days.

body compared with the ventral part results in an apparent migration or descent of the diaphragm. By the sixth week, the developing diaphragm is at the level of the thoracic somites (Fig. 10–6B). The phrenic nerves now take a descending course, and, as the diaphragm "moves" relatively farther caudally in the body, these nerves are correspondingly lengthened. By the beginning of the eighth week, the dorsal part of the diaphragm lies at the level of the first lumbar vertebra (Fig. 10–6C).

As the parts of the diaphragm fuse (Fig. 10–5), mesenchyme of the septum transversum extends into the other parts and forms myoblasts that differentiate into the muscle of the diaphragm. Hence, *the motor nerve supply to the diaphragm is via the phrenic nerves (ventral rami of C3, 4, and 5).*

The phrenic nerve is also sensory to the central region of the diaphragm, but its peripheral region,

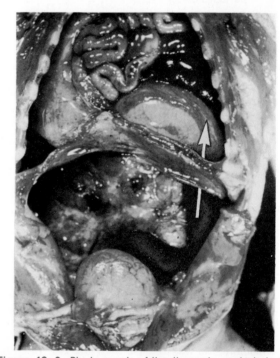

Figure 10–8. Photograph of the thoracic and abdominopelvic cavities of an infant with a large left posterolateral diaphragmatic defect similar to that shown in Figure 10–7. The thoracic and abdominal cavities were opened at autopsy to show the intestines and other viscera in the thoracic cavity. The liver has been removed to show that only distal parts of the large intestine have remained in the abdominal cavity. The arrow passes through the diaphragmatic defect. (Courtesy of Dr. Jan Hoogstraten, Children's Centre, Winnipeg, Canada.)

Figure 10–7. Photograph of a transverse section through the thoracic region of a stillborn infant, viewed from the thorax. Note the large left posterolateral defect of the diaphragm. *Half actual size.*

which develops from the body wall (see Fig. 10–5E), receives sensory nerves from the lower six or seven intercostal nerves.

Congenital Diaphragmatic Hernia

A *posterolateral defect of the diaphragm* is a relatively common developmental abnormality (Fig. 10–7). It occurs about once in 2000 births and results from failure of the pleuroperitoneal membrane on the affected side to fuse with other diaphragmatic components. The defect, *usually on the left side,* consists of a large opening in the posterolateral region of the diaphragm, usually in the region of the kidney. There is free communication between the abdominal and pleural cavities. As a result, the intestines and other abdominal organs pass into the thorax (Fig. 10–8). Because of the presence of the abdominal viscera in the chest, the heart is pushed anteriorly and the lungs are compressed.

SUMMARY

The *intraembryonic coelom* or embryonic body cavity begins to develop near the end of the third week. By the beginning of the fourth week, it appears as a continuous horseshoe-shaped cavity in the cardiogenic and lateral mesoderm.

During folding of the embryonic disc in the fourth week, the lateral limbs or extensions of the coelom are brought together on the ventral aspect of the embryo. When the caudal part of the ventral mesentery disappears, the right and left parts of the intraembryonic coelom merge to form the peritoneal cavity.

As the peritoneal portions of the intraembryonic coelom come together, the splanchnic mesoderm encloses the primitive gut and suspends it from the dorsal body wall by a double-layered membrane known as the *dorsal mesentery.*

Until the seventh week, the *pericardial cavity* communicates with the peritoneal cavity through paired *pericardioperitoneal canals.* During the fifth and sixth weeks, partitions or membranes form at the cranial and caudal ends of these canals. The cranial *pleuropericardial membranes* separate the pericardial cavity from the pleural cavities, and the caudal *pleuroperitoneal membranes* separate the pleural cavities from the peritoneal cavity.

The diaphragm develops from four main structures: (1) the septum transversum, (2) the pleuroperitoneal membranes, (3) the dorsal mesentery of the esophagus, and (4) the body wall.

Posterolateral defect of the diaphragm is the common type of congenital diaphragmatic malformation. It is associated with herniation of abdominal viscera into the thoracic cavity.

Congenital diaphragmatic hernia occurs five times more often on the left side than on the right. It results from failure of the pleuroperitoneal membrane on the affected side to fuse with the other diaphragmatic components, thereby separating the pleural and peritoneal cavities.

Commonly Asked Questions

1. I heard about a baby who was born with its liver in its chest. Is this possible?
2. Can a baby with most of its abdominal viscera in its chest survive?
3. Do the lungs develop normally in babies who are born with diaphragmatic hernias?
4. A friend of mine had a routine chest x-ray about a year ago, and was told that a small part of his small intestine was in his chest. He is the type that "has never been sick a day in his life." Is it possible for this to occur without the person being aware of this abnormality?

Answers

1. Yes. When a baby is born with *a congenital diaphragmatic hernia,* its liver may be in its chest. This is uncommon, however. Usually the abnormally placed viscera are hollow ones (e.g., the stomach and the small or large intestine). The viscera enter the chest through a defect in the diaphragm, usually on the left side (see Fig. 10–8).

2. Yes, but the treatment must be effected immediately. A feeding tube is inserted into the stomach and, with continuous suction, the air and gastric contents are aspirated. The displaced viscera are then replaced into the abdominal cavity and the defect in the diaphragm is surgically repaired. Infants with large diaphragmatic hernias, operated on within 24 hours after birth, have survival rates of 40 to 70 per cent.

3. It depends upon the degree of herniation of the abdominal viscera. With a moderate degree of herniation, the lungs may be mature but small. With a severe degree of herniation, lung development is reduced, but the lungs often develop normally following surgery.

4. Yes, it is possible. Some diaphragmatic hernias remain completely asymptomatic into adulthood and are discovered only in the course of a routine radiographic examination of the chest.

The Branchial Apparatus and the Head and Neck

The branchial apparatus consists of: (1) *branchial arches,* (2) *pharyngeal pouches,* (3) *branchial grooves,* and (4) *branchial membranes* (Fig. 11–1). The derivatives of the branchial apparatus contribute greatly to the formation of the head and neck.

The cranial region of an early human embryo somewhat resembles a fish embryo of a comparable stage. This explains why the adjective *branchial* is used to describe this apparatus. The Greek term *branchia* means "gill." By the end of the embryonic period, these primitive branchial structures have either been rearranged and adapted to new functions or they have disappeared.

Most congenital malformations of the head and neck originate during transformation of the branchial apparatus into its adult derivatives.

In fish and larval amphibians, the branchial apparatus forms a system of gills for exchanging oxygen and carbon dioxide between the blood and the water. The branchial arches support the gills. A branchial apparatus develops in human embryos, but no gills form.

THE BRANCHIAL ARCHES

Branchial arches begin to develop early in the fourth week and appear as ridges on the future head and neck region (Figs. 11–1 and 11–2). The arches are separated from each other by *branchial grooves* (Fig. 11–1D), and are numbered in a craniocaudal sequence.

The mouth initially appears as a slight depression of the surface ectoderm, called the *stomodeum* or

primitive mouth (Fig. 11–1D to G). At first this cavity is separated from the foregut or primitive pharynx by a bilaminar membrane, the *oropharyngeal membrane* (buccopharyngeal membrane). This membrane ruptures at about 24 days, bringing the digestive tract into communication with the amniotic cavity (Fig. 11–1F and 11–1J).

Initially, each branchial arch is composed of mesenchyme derived from the intraembryonic mesoderm, and is covered externally by ectoderm and internally by endoderm (Fig. 11–2). Cells from the *neural crest* (see Fig. 5–6) migrate into the arches and surround the central core of mesenchymal cells. It is the migration of these *neural crest cells* into the branchial arches that causes them to enlarge. These cells form the skeletal structures in the arches which later form bones in the head and neck (see Fig. 11–4).

Fate of the Branchial Arches

The first branchial arch or *mandibular arch* is involved with development of the face (Fig. 11–3). It develops two elevations called the *mandibular prominence* and the *maxillary prominence.* The mandibular prominence forms the lower jaw or *mandible* (Fig. 11–3G), and the maxillary prominence forms the upper jaw or *maxilla,* the zygomatic bone, and the squamous part of the temporal bone (see Fig. 16–6).

During the fifth week, the second branchial arch (hyoid arch) overgrows the third and fourth arches, forming a deep ectodermal depression known as the *cervical sinus* (Fig. 11–3A to D). During the sixth and seventh weeks, the second to fourth branchial grooves

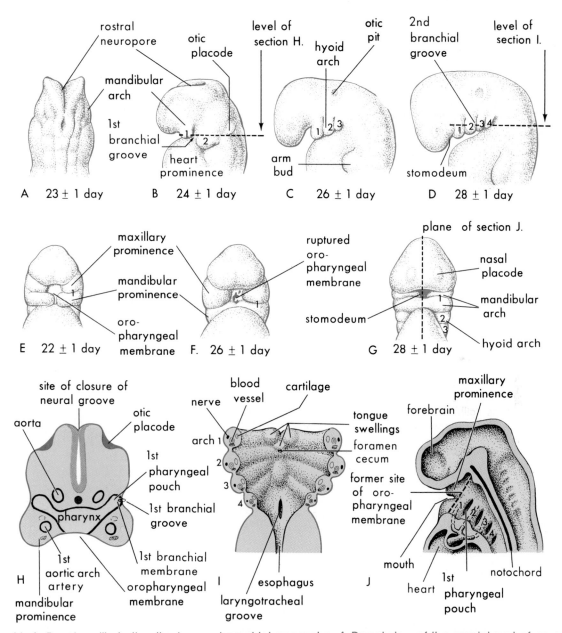

Figure 11-1. Drawings illustrating the human branchial apparatus. *A,* Dorsal view of the cranial part of an early embryo. *B* to *D,* Lateral views, showing later development of the branchial arches. *E* to *G,* Ventral views illustrating the relationship of the first or mandibular arch to the stomodeum or primitive mouth. *H,* Transverse section through the cranial region of an embryo. *I,* Horizontal section through the cranial region of an embryo, illustrating the branchial arch components and the floor of the primitive pharynx. *J,* Sagittal section of the cranial region of an embryo, illustrating the openings of the pharyngeal pouches in the lateral wall of the primitive pharynx.

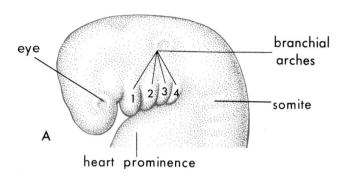

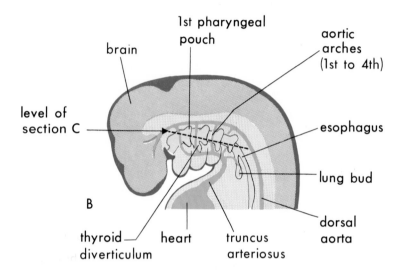

Figure 11–2. *A,* Drawing of the head and neck region of a 28-day embryo, illustrating the human branchial apparatus. *B,* Schematic drawing showing the pharyngeal pouches and aortic arches (arteries in the branchial arches), exposed by removal of the ectoderm and mesoderm. *C,* Horizontal section through the embryo, illustrating the germ layer of origin of the branchial arch components.

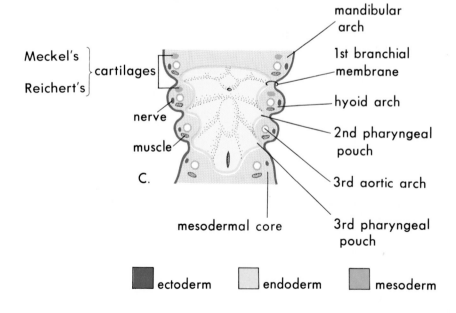

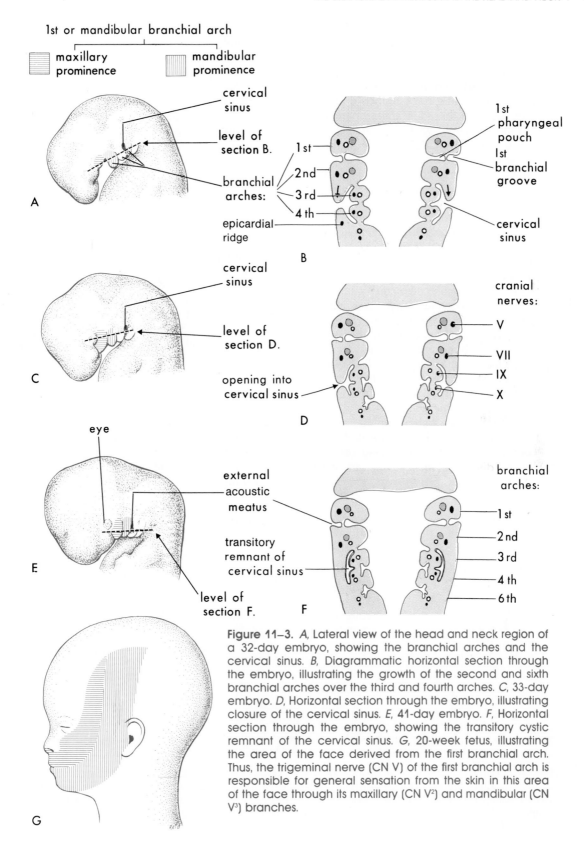

1st or mandibular branchial arch

maxillary prominence   mandibular prominence

A
cervical sinus
level of section B.
branchial arches:
1st
2nd
3rd
4th
epicardial ridge

B
1st pharyngeal pouch
1st branchial groove
cervical sinus

C
cervical sinus
level of section D.
opening into cervical sinus

D
cranial nerves:
V
VII
IX
X

E
eye
external acoustic meatus
transitory remnant of cervical sinus
level of section F.

F
branchial arches:
1st
2nd
3rd
4th
6th

G

Figure 11–3. A, Lateral view of the head and neck region of a 32-day embryo, showing the branchial arches and the cervical sinus. B, Diagrammatic horizontal section through the embryo, illustrating the growth of the second and sixth branchial arches over the third and fourth arches. C, 33-day embryo. D, Horizontal section through the embryo, illustrating closure of the cervical sinus. E, 41-day embryo. F, Horizontal section through the embryo, showing the transitory cystic remnant of the cervical sinus. G, 20-week fetus, illustrating the area of the face derived from the first branchial arch. Thus, the trigeminal nerve (CN V) of the first branchial arch is responsible for general sensation from the skin in this area of the face through its maxillary (CN V²) and mandibular (CN V³) branches.

and the cervical sinus are obliterated, giving the neck a smooth contour (Fig. 11–3F and G). The branchial arches caudal to the second one make little contribution to the skin of the neck (Fig. 11–3G).

Derivatives of the Branchial Arch Arteries. The transformation of the arteries in the branchial arches, called *aortic arches,* into the adult arterial pattern is described with the circulatory system in Chapter 15.

Derivatives of the Branchial Arch Cartilages (Fig. 11–4). The dorsal end of the *first arch cartilage* (Meckel's cartilage) becomes ossified to form two middle ear bones, the *malleus* and *incus.* The intermediate portion of the cartilage regresses, and its perichondrium forms the *anterior ligament of the malleus* and the *sphenomandibular ligament.* The ventral portion of the first arch cartilage largely disappears as the mandible develops around it by intramembranous ossification.

The dorsal end of the *second arch cartilage* (Reichert's cartilage) also ossifies and forms the *stapes* of the middle ear and the *styloid process* of the temporal bone. The portion of cartilage between the styloid process and the hyoid bone regresses, and its perichondrium forms the *stylohyoid ligament.* The ventral end of the second arch cartilage ossifies to form part of the *hyoid bone* (lesser cornu) and the superior part of the body of the hyoid bone (Fig. 11–4).

The *third arch cartilages* also contribute to the formation of the *hyoid bone.* They are located in the ventral portions of the arches where they ossify to form the greater cornua and the inferior part of the body of the hyoid bone.

The *fourth and sixth arch cartilages* also persist in the ventral regions of the arches. They fuse to form the *laryngeal cartilages.* The rudimentary fifth branchial arch, if present, has no recognizable adult derivative.

Derivatives of the Branchial Arch Muscles (Fig. 11–5). The muscle components of the branchial arches form various striated muscles in the head and neck (e.g. *the muscles of facial expression*).

THE PHARYNGEAL POUCHES

The primitive pharynx, derived from the foregut, is wide cranially and narrow caudally. The endoderm of the pharynx lines the internal surfaces of the branchial arches and passes into balloon-like out-growths called *pharyngeal pouches* (see Figs. 11–1H to J and 11–2B and C). The pouches develop in a craniocaudal sequence between the branchial arches, e.g., the first pharyngeal pouch lies between the first and second branchial arches. There are four well-defined pairs of pharyngeal pouches. The fifth pharyngeal pouch is rudimentary.

Derivatives of the Pharyngeal Pouches

The First Pharyngeal Pouch (Fig. 11–6). This pouch expands into an elongate *tubotympanic recess,* which forms the *tympanic cavity* and *mastoid antrum.* Its connection with the pharynx gradually elongates to form the *auditory tube* (pharyngotympanic tube).

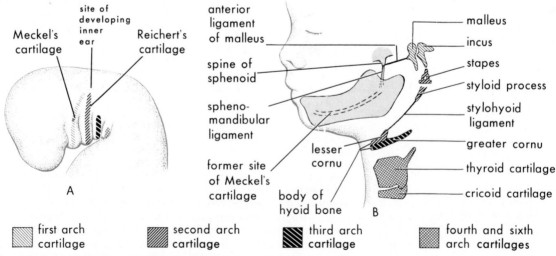

Figure 11–4. *A,* Schematic lateral view of the head and neck region of a four-week embryo, illustrating the location of the branchial arch cartilages. *B,* Similar view of a 24-week fetus, illustrating the adult derivatives of the branchial arch cartilages. Note that the mandible is formed by membranous ossification of the mesenchymal tissue surrounding Meckel's cartilage. This cartilage acts as a template, or guide, but does not contribute much to the formation of the mandible.

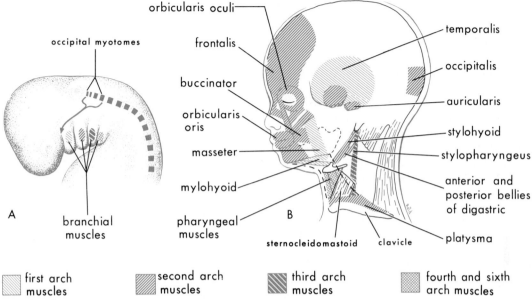

first arch muscles

second arch muscles

third arch muscles

fourth and sixth arch muscles

Figure 11–5. *A,* Sketch of lateral view of the head and neck region of a four-week embryo, showing the branchial muscles. The arrow shows the pathway taken by myoblasts from the occipital myotomes to form the tongue musculature. *B,* Sketch of the head and neck of a 20-week fetus dissected to show the muscles derived from the branchial arches. Parts of the platysma and sternocleidomastoid muscles have been removed to show the deeper muscles. Note that myoblasts from the second branchial arch migrate from the neck region to the head and give rise to the muscles of facial expression. Thus, these muscles are supplied by the facial nerve, the nerve of the second branchial arch.

The Second Pharyngeal Pouch (Fig. 11–6). The endoderm of this pouch proliferates and forms buds that grow into the underlying mesenchyme. The central parts of these buds break down, forming the *tonsillar crypts.* The pouch endoderm forms the surface epithelium and the *lining of the crypts of the palatine tonsil.* The mesenchyme surrounding the crypts differentiates into lymphoid tissue and soon becomes organized into *lymphatic nodules.* Although it is largely obliterated as the palatine tonsil develops, part of the cavity of this pouch remains as the *intratonsillar cleft or tonsillar fossa* (Fig. 11–6C).

The Third Pharyngeal Pouch (Fig. 11–6). This pouch expands into a solid dorsal bulbar portion and a hollow ventral elongate portion. Each dorsal bulbar portion differentiates into an *inferior parathyroid gland.* The elongate ventral portions form two masses that eventually meet and fuse to form the *thymus.*

The thymus and parathyroid glands migrate caudally. Later the parathyroid glands separate from the thymus gland and come to lie on the dorsal surface of the thyroid gland, which has descended from the foramen cecum of the tongue (see Fig. 11–10).

The Fourth Pharyngeal Pouch (Fig. 11–6). This pouch also expands into a dorsal bulbar portion and a ventral elongate portion. Each dorsal portion devel-

ops into a *superior parathyroid gland.* The ventral elongate portion of each fourth pouch develops into an *ultimobranchial body* which becomes incorporated into the thyroid gland and gives rise to its *parafollicular* or *C cells.* These cells produce *calcitonin,* a hormone involved in the regulation of the normal calcium level in body fluids.

The Fifth Pharyngeal Pouch. This is a rudimentary structure which, if present, is partially incorporated into the fourth pouch.

THE BRANCHIAL GROOVES

The early neck region of the human embryo exhibits four branchial grooves on each side during the fourth and fifth weeks (see Figs. 11–1 and 11–3). These grooves *separate the branchial arches externally.* Only one pair of branchial grooves contributes to adult structures. The ectoderm of the first branchial groove persists as the epithelium of the *external acoustic meatus* (Fig. 11–6C). The other branchial grooves come to lie in a depression called the *cervical sinus.* These are normally obliterated with it as the neck develops.

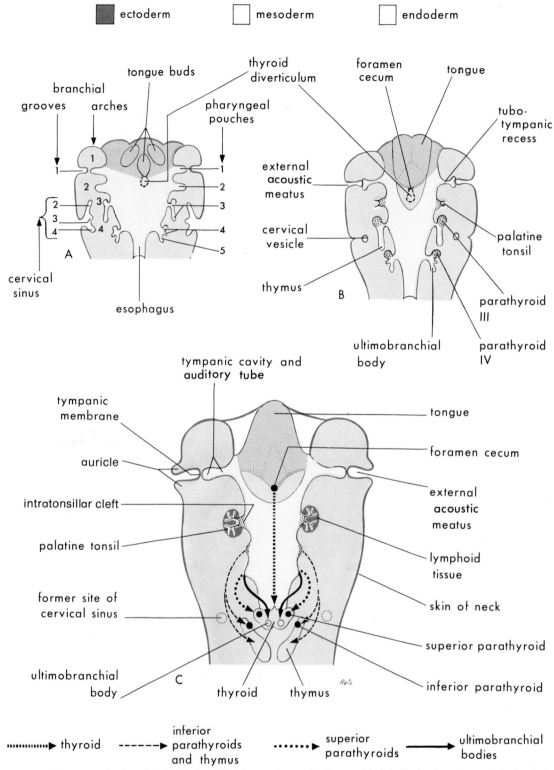

Figure 11–6. Schematic horizontal sections at the level shown in Figure 11–3*A*, illustrating the adult derivatives of the pharyngeal pouches. *A*, Five weeks. *B*, Six weeks. *C*, Seven weeks.

THE BRANCHIAL MEMBRANES

Four branchial membranes appear in the bottoms of the branchial grooves on each side of the future neck region of the human embryo during the fourth week (see Figs. 11–1H and 11–2C).

The branchial membranes form where the epithelia of a branchial groove and a pharyngeal pouch approach each other. They are temporary structures in the human embryo. The endoderm of the pharyngeal pouches and the ectoderm of the branchial grooves are soon separated by mesoderm. Only one pair of branchial membranes contributes to the formation of adult structures. The first branchial membrane, along with the intervening layer of mesoderm, gives rise to the *tympanic membrane*, or eardrum (Fig. 11–6C).

BRANCHIAL MALFORMATIONS

Congenital malformations of the head and neck originate mainly during transformation of the branchial apparatus into adult structures (Fig. 11–7). Most of these abnormalities represent *remnants of the branchial apparatus* that normally disappear as these structures develop. *Most branchial malformations are uncommon.*

Congenital Auricular Sinuses and Cysts (Fig. 11–7F). Small blind pits, or cysts, in the skin are commonly found in a triangular area anterior to the ear, but they may occur in other sites around the auricle or in the lobule. Most of these auricular sinuses and cysts are remnants of the first branchial groove.

Branchial Sinus, or Lateral Cervical Sinus (Figs. 11–7D and 11–8). Branchial sinuses are uncommon, and almost all that open externally on the side of the neck result from failure of the second branchial groove and the cervical sinus to obliterate. A blind sinus then remains, which typically opens on the line of the anterior border of the sternocleidomastoid muscle in the inferior third of the neck. Often there is an intermittent discharge of mucus from the opening.

External branchial sinuses are commonly detected during infancy owing to the discharge of mucus from their orifices on the neck. Branchial sinuses are bilateral in about 10 per cent of cases and are commonly associated with auricular sinuses.

Internal branchial sinuses opening into the pharynx are uncommon (Fig. 11–7D). Because they usually open into the intratonsillar cleft (tonsillar fossa), or near the palatopharyngeal arch, almost all these sinuses result from persistence of part of the second pharyngeal pouch.

Branchial Fistula (Fig. 11–7E). An abnormal tract (canal) opening on the side of the neck and in the pharynx is called a *branchial fistula*. It results from persistence of parts of the second branchial groove and second pharyngeal pouch. The fistula ascends from its opening on the neck, through the subcutaneous tissue, the platysma muscle, and the deep fascia to reach the carotid sheath. It then passes between the internal and external carotid arteries and opens in the intratonsillar cleft (tonsillar fossa).

Branchial Cysts or Lateral Cervical Cysts (Fig. 11–7F). The third and fourth branchial arches are normally buried in the *cervical sinus*. Remnants of the cervical sinus and/or the second branchial groove may persist and form spherical or elongate cysts. Although they may be associated with branchial sinuses and drain through them, these cysts often lie free in the neck just inferior to the angle of the mandible. They may, however, develop anywhere along the anterior border of the sternocleidomastoid muscle.

Branchial cysts often do not become apparent until late childhood or early adulthood, when they produce a slowly enlarging, painless swelling in the neck. The cysts enlarge owing to the accumulation of fluid and cellular debris derived from desquamation of their epithelial linings.

Branchial Vestiges (Fig. 11–7F). Normally the branchial arch cartilages disappear, except for parts that form ligaments or bones (see Fig. 11–4B). In very unusual cases, cartilaginous or bony remnants of branchial arch cartilages appear under the skin on the side of the neck. These are usually found anterior to the inferior third of the sternocleidomastoid muscle.

The First Arch Syndrome (Fig. 11–9). Maldevelopment of the components of the first branchial arch results in various congenital malformations of the eyes, ears, mandible, and palate that together constitute the first arch syndrome. This set of symptoms *results from insufficient migration of cranial neural crest cells into the first branchial arch* during the fourth week. There are two main manifestations of the first arch syndrome as follows: the *Treacher Collins syndrome* and the *Pierre Robin syndrome.*

THE THYROID GLAND

The thyroid gland appears during the fourth week as a median endodermal thickening in the floor of the primitive pharynx (Figs. 11–6 and 11–10). It is the first endocrine gland to form in the embryo.

The thickening indicating the thyroid gland soon forms a downgrowth known as the *thyroid diverticulum*. The developing thyroid descends in the neck, retaining its connection to the tongue by a narrow *thyroglossal duct*. This duct's opening in the tongue is called the *foramen cecum* (Fig. 11–10C).

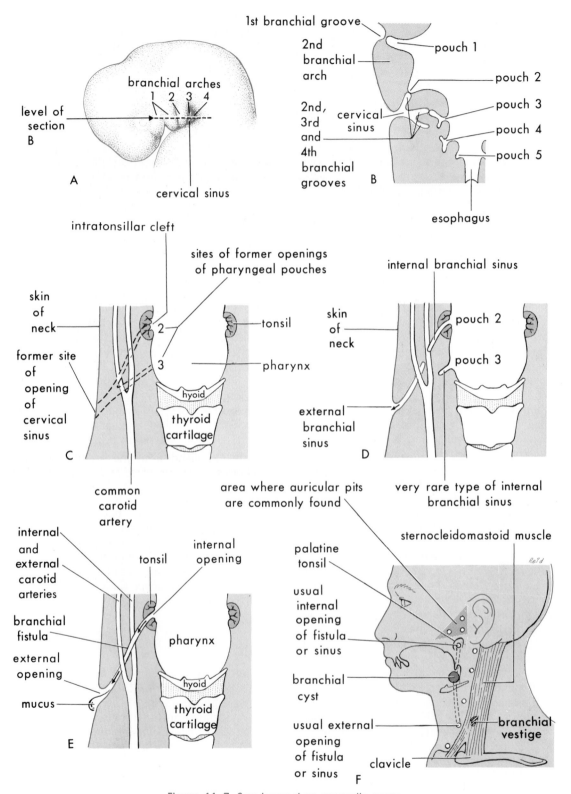

Figure 11-7 *See legend on opposite page*

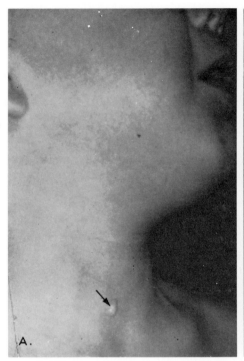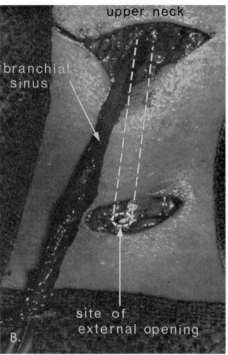

Figure 11-8. *A,* Photograph of a child's neck showing mucus dripping from an external branchial sinus (arrow). *B,* Photograph of a branchial sinus taken during excision. The external opening in the skin of the neck and the original course of the sinus in the subcutaneous tissue are indicated by broken lines. (From Swenson, O.: *Pediatric Surgery,* 1958. Courtesy of Appleton-Century-Crofts, Publishing Division of Prentice-Hall, Inc., Englewood Cliffs, New Jersey.)

By seven weeks the thyroid gland has usually reached its final site in the neck, and the thyroglossal duct has normally disappeared. The original opening of the thyroglossal duct persists as a vestigial pit, the *foramen cecum of the tongue* (Figs. 11–10D and 11–12C).

Congenital Malformations of the Thyroid Gland

Thyroglossal Duct Cysts and Sinuses (Fig. 11–11). Cysts may form anywhere along the course followed by the thyroglossal duct during descent of the thyroid gland from the tongue. Normally the thyroglossal duct atrophies and disappears, but remnants of it may persist and give rise to cysts in the tongue or in the midline of the neck, usually just inferior to the hyoid bone. The swelling produced by a thyroglossal cyst usually develops as a painless, progressively enlarging, and movable mass. In some cases, an opening through the skin exists as a result of perforation following infection of the cyst. This forms a *thyroglossal duct sinus* that usually opens in the midline of the neck anterior to the laryngeal cartilages (Fig. 11–11A).

Ectopic Thyroid Gland and Accessory Thyroid Tissue. Uncommonly, the thyroid fails to descend,

Figure 11-7. *A,* Drawing of the head and neck region of a five-week embryo. *B,* Horizontal section through the embryo, illustrating the relationship of the cervical sinus to the branchial arches and pharyngeal pouches. *C,* Diagrammatic sketch of the adult neck region, indicating the former sites of openings of the cervical sinus and the pharyngeal pouches. The broken lines indicate possible courses of branchial fistulas. *D,* Similar sketch showing the embryological basis of various types of branchial sinus. *E,* Drawing of a branchial fistula resulting from persistence of parts of the second branchial groove and the second pharyngeal pouch. *F,* Sketch showing possible sites of branchial cysts and openings of branchial sinuses and fistulas. A branchial vestige is also illustrated.

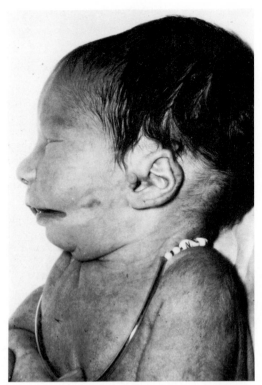

Figure 11–9. Photograph of an infant with the first arch syndrome, a pattern of malformations resulting from insufficient migration of neural crest cells into the first branchial arch. Note the following: deformed auricle of the external ear, preauricular appendage, defect in cheek between the ear and the mouth, hypoplasia of the mandible, and large mouth. (Courtesy of Dr. T. V. N. Persaud, Professor and Head of Anatomy, University of Manitoba, Winnipeg, Canada.)

resulting in a *lingual thyroid.* Incomplete descent may result in the thyroid gland appearing high in the neck at or just inferior to the hyoid bone.

Accessory thyroid tissue results from remnants of the thyroglossal duct. This glandular tissue may be functional, but it is often of insufficient size to maintain normal function if the thyroid gland is removed.

Accessory thyroid tissue may be found anywhere from the tongue to the usual site of the thyroid gland in the neck.

THE TONGUE

The first indication of tongue development appears around the end of the fourth week as a median elevation, the *median tongue bud* (tuberculum impar) in the floor of the primitive pharynx, just rostral to the foramen cecum (Fig. 11–12A).

Two oval *distal tongue buds* (lateral lingual swellings) soon develop on each side of the median tongue bud. The distal tongue buds rapidly increase in size, merge with each other, and overgrow the median tongue bud. The fused distal tongue buds form the *anterior two thirds, or oral part, of the tongue* (Fig. 11–12C). The plane of fusion of the distal tongue buds is indicated by the *median sulcus of the tongue.* The median tongue forms no identifiable adult derivative.

The *posterior third, or pharyngeal part, of the tongue* is initially indicated by two elevations that develop caudal to the foramen cecum (Fig. 11–12A). One elevation, called the *copula* (L. a bond), is formed by fusion of the ventromedial parts of the second branchial arches. The other elevation, called the *hypobranchial eminence,* develops caudal to the copula from mesoderm in the ventromedial parts of the third and fourth branchial arches.

As the tongue develops, the copula is gradually overgrown by the hypobranchial eminence (Fig. 11–12B and C). As a result, the posterior third of the tongue develops from the rostral part of the hypobranchial eminence. The line of fusion of the anterior and posterior parts of the tongue is roughly indicated by the V-shaped groove called the *terminal sulcus* (Fig. 11–12C).

Branchial arch mesenchyme forms the connective tissue and the lymphatic and blood vessels of the tongue. Most of the tongue musculature is derived from myoblasts that migrate from the *myotomes of the occipital somites* (see Fig. 11–5A). These myoblasts (primitive muscle cells) migrate into the tongue, where they differentiate into muscle fibers. The hypoglossal nerve *(cranial nerve XII)* accompanies the myoblasts during their migration and innervates the *tongue muscles* when they develop.

Congenital Malformations of the Tongue

Malformations of the tongue are uncommon, except for the fissures associated with the *Down syndrome* (see Chapter 9).

Congenital Cysts and Fistulas (see Fig. 11–11). *Cysts in the tongue,* often just superior to the hyoid bone, are usually derived from *remnants of the thyroglossal duct.* They may enlarge and produce symptoms of pharyngeal discomfort and/or *dysphagia* (difficulty in swallowing).

Fistulas in the tongue are also derived from persistence of the thyroglossal duct, and they open through the *foramen cecum* into the mouth.

Ankyloglossia (Tongue-Tie). The frenulum normally connects the inferior surface of the anterior part

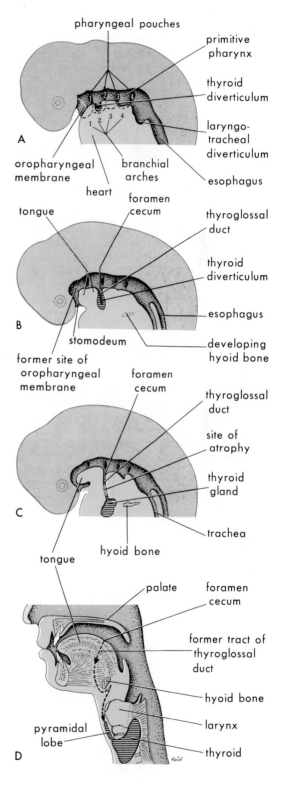

Figure 11–10. *A, B,* and *C,* Schematic sagittal sections of the head and neck region of embryos at four, five, and six weeks, respectively, illustrating successive stages of development of the thyroid gland. *D,* Similar section of an adult head, showing the path taken by the thyroid gland during its descent and the former tract of the thyroglossal duct.

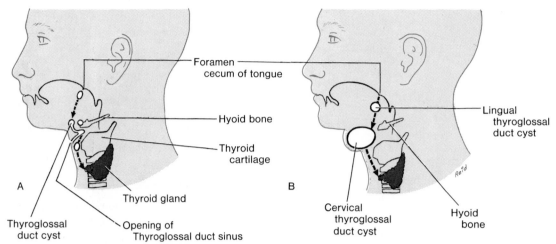

Figure 11-11. *A,* Diagrammatic sketch of the head, showing the possible locations of thyroglossal duct cysts. A thyroglossal duct sinus is also illustrated. The broken line indicates the course taken by the thyroglossal duct during descent of the thyroid gland from the foramen cecum to its final position in the anterior part of the neck. *B,* A similar sketch illustrating lingual and cervical thyroglossal duct cysts. Most cysts are located close to or in the median plane, near the hyoid bone.

of the tongue to the floor of the mouth. In tongue-tie, the frenulum extends to the tip of the tongue and interferes with its free protrusion. Usually, the frenulum stretches with time, but surgical correction of the malformation may be necessary.

Macroglossia. An excessively large tongue is not common and results from generalized hypertrophy of the tongue. These cases usually result from lymphangioma or muscular hypertrophy.

Microglossia. An abnormally small tongue is rare and is usually associated with micrognathia (underdeveloped mandible with recession of the chin).

Cleft Tongue. Incomplete fusion of the distal tongue buds posteriorly may result in a median groove, or *cleft of the tongue;* usually, the cleft does not extend to the tip. Complete failure of fusion of the distal tongue buds results in a cleft in the oral part of the tongue. This malformation is referred to as *bifid tongue.*

DEVELOPMENT OF THE FACE

The five facial primordia appear around the stomodeum or primitive mouth early in the fourth week (Figs. 11–1E and 11–13A).

The large *frontonasal prominence* (swelling) constitutes the cranial boundary of the stomodeum. The paired *maxillary prominences* (swellings) of the first branchial arch form the lateral boundaries of the stomodeum, and the paired *mandibular prominences*

of this same arch constitute the caudal boundary of the stomodeum.

Bilateral oval-shaped thickenings of the surface ectoderm, called *nasal placodes,* develop on each side of the caudal part of frontonasal elevation (Fig. 11–13B). Horseshoe-shaped *medial and lateral nasal prominences* develop at the margins of the nasal placodes (Fig. 11–13C and D). As a result, the nasal placodes lie in depressions called *nasal pits* (Fig. 11–13C). The maxillary prominences grow rapidly and soon approach each other and the medial nasal prominences (Fig. 11–13D and E).

The face develops mainly between the fifth and eighth weeks. By the end of the embryonic period (eight weeks), the face has an unquestionably human appearance (see Fig. 6–14). Facial proportions develop during the fetal period.

During the sixth and seventh weeks, the medial nasal prominences merge with each other and the maxillary prominences (Fig. 11–13F and G). As the medial nasal prominences merge with each other, they form an *intermaxillary segment* of the maxilla (Fig. 11–13H). This segment gives rise to (1) the middle portion of the upper lip called the *philtrum;* (2) the premaxillary part of the maxilla and its associated gingiva (gum); and (3) the *primary palate.*

The lateral parts of the upper lip, most of the maxilla, and the *secondary palate* form from the maxillary prominences (Figs. 11–13H and I and 11–14). These prominences merge laterally with the mandibular prominences.

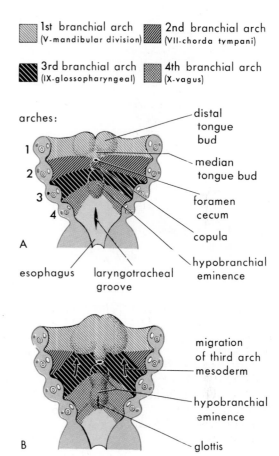

1st branchial arch (V-mandibular division)

2nd branchial arch (VII-chorda tympani)

3rd branchial arch (IX-glossopharyngeal)

4th branchial arch (X-vagus)

arches:

1
2
3
4

A

distal tongue bud

median tongue bud

foramen cecum

copula

hypobranchial eminence

esophagus

laryngotracheal groove

migration of third arch mesoderm

hypobranchial eminence

glottis

B

Figure 11–12. *A* and *B*, Schematic horizontal sections through the pharynx at the level shown in Figure 11–3*A*, showing successive stages in the development of the tongue during the fourth and fifth weeks. *C*, Adult tongue showing the branchial arch derivation of the nerve supply of the mucosa.

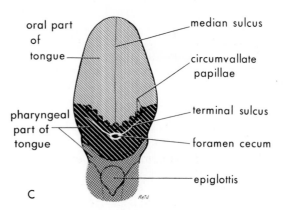

oral part of tongue

median sulcus

circumvallate papillae

terminal sulcus

foramen cecum

pharyngeal part of tongue

epiglottis

C

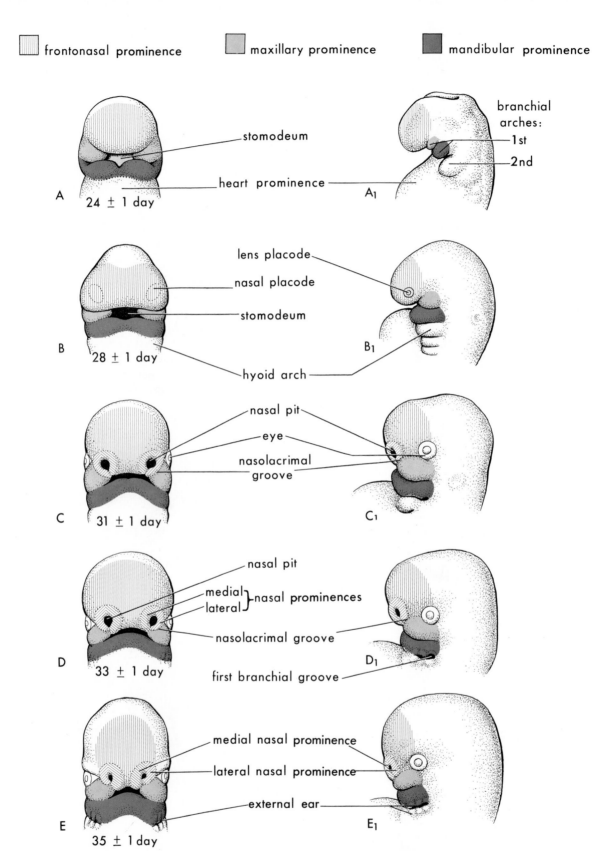

Figure 11-13. Diagrams illustrating progressive stages in the development of the human face.

Illustration continued on following page

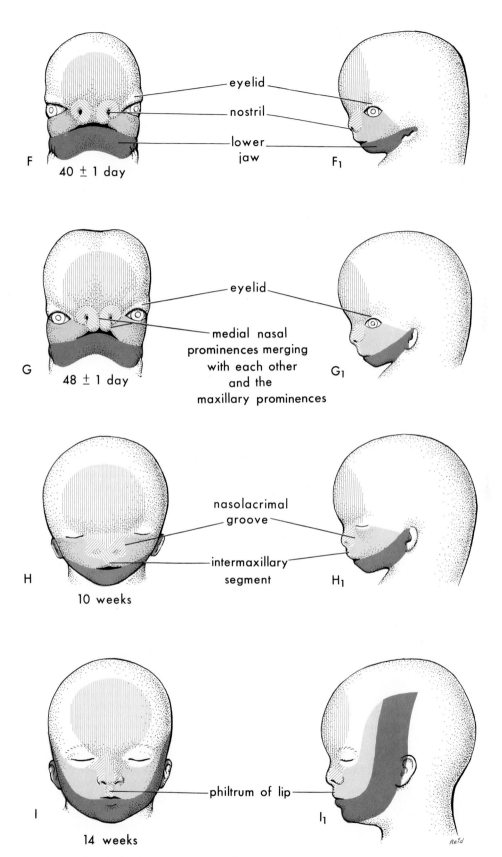

F   eyelid

   nostril

   lower jaw

F $_1$

40 ± 1 day

G   eyelid

   medial nasal prominences merging with each other and the maxillary prominences

G $_1$

48 ± 1 day

H   nasolacrimal groove

   intermaxillary segment

H $_1$

10 weeks

I   philtrum of lip

I $_1$

14 weeks

Figure 11–13 *Continued*

The *frontonasal prominence* (Fig. 11–13) forms the forehead and the dorsum and apex of the nose. The sides of the nose are derived from the lateral nasal prominences (Fig. 11–13H and I).

The mandibular prominences merge with each other in the fourth week and the groove between them disappears before the end of the fifth week (Fig. 11–13D). The mandibular prominences give rise to the mandible (lower jaw), lower lip, and the inferior part of the face. Final development of the face occurs slowly and results mainly from changes in the proportion and relative position of the facial components.

The smallness of the face at birth results from (1) the rudimentary upper and lower jaws, (2) the unerupted teeth, and (3) the small size of the nasal cavities and maxillary sinuses.

DEVELOPMENT OF THE NASAL CAVITIES

As the face develops, the *nasal placodes* are surrounded by the *nasal prominences*. They then form the floors of depressions called *nasal pits* (Fig. 11–13C). Growth of the surrounding mesenchyme results in deepening of the nasal pits and formation of *nasal sacs*. The nasal sacs are the primordia of the nasal cavities (Fig. 11–14).

The growth of the *paranasal sinuses* is important in altering the size and shape of the face during infancy and childhood, and in adding resonance to the voice during adolescence. Most of these sinuses develop after birth.

DEVELOPMENT OF THE PALATE

The palate develops from the *primary palate* and the *secondary palate*. Although palatogenesis begins toward the end of the fifth week, fusion of the palate's parts is not complete until the twelfth week.

The Primary Palate (Fig. 11–14). The primary palate, or *median palatine process,* develops at the end of the fifth week from the innermost part of the *intermaxillary segment* of the maxilla. It forms a wedge-shaped mass of mesoderm between the maxillary prominences of the developing maxilla.

The Secondary Palate (Fig. 11–14). The secondary palate develops from two internal projections from the maxillary prominences, called the *lateral palatine processes* (Fig. 11–14B). These shelflike structures initially project inferomedially on each side of the tongue (Fig. 11–14C). As the jaws develop, the tongue moves inferiorly and the lateral palatine processes gradually grow toward each other and fuse (Fig. 11–14E and G). They also fuse with the primary palate and the *nasal septum* (Fig. 11–14D to H).

The fusion of the palatal processes begins anteriorly during the ninth week and ends posteriorly in the region of the *uvula* by the twelfth week. The uvula (L. little grape) is the last part of the palate to form. The *palatine raphe* indicates the line of fusion of the lateral palatine processes (Fig. 11–14H).

Bone gradually develops in the primary palate, forming the *premaxillary part of the maxilla,* which carries the incisor teeth. Concurrently, bone extends from the maxillae and palatine bones into the lateral palatine processes to form the *hard palate* (Fig. 11–14). The posterior portions of the lateral palatine processes do not become ossified. They extend beyond the nasal septum and fuse to form the *soft palate* and *uvula* (Fig. 11–14D, F, and H).

Cleft Lip and Cleft Palate

Cleft lip and cleft palate are common malformations of the face and palate. Although often associated, cleft lip and cleft palate are embryologically and etiologically distinct malformations. They originate at different times during development and involve different developmental processes.

Cleft Lip (Figs. 11–15 to 11–19). This malformation of the upper lip, without or with cleft palate, occurs about once in 1000 births. The defect may be unilateral or bilateral and is *more common in males.* The clefts vary from a small notch in the lip to complete division of the lip and alveolar part of the maxilla. This defect is also inappropriately called *harelip.*

Unilateral cleft lip results from failure of the maxillary prominences on the affected side to merge with the merged medial nasal prominences (Fig. 11–16).

Bilateral cleft lip results from failure of the maxillary prominences to meet and merge with the medial nasal prominences. In complete bilateral cleft of the upper lip and alveolar part of the maxilla, the intermaxillary segment hangs free (Fig. 11–15C and D). The defects may be similar or dissimilar, with varying degrees of defect on each side.

A *median cleft of the upper lip,* resulting from incomplete merger of the medial nasal prominences, is unusual (Fig. 11–19).

Cleft Palate (Figs. 11–17 and 11–18). Cleft palate, with or without cleft lip, occurs about once in 2500 births. The clefts may be unilateral or bilateral and are *more common in females.* A cleft may involve only the uvula, or it may extend through the soft and hard regions of the palate. In severe cases associated with cleft lip, the cleft in the anterior and posterior regions of the palate extends through the alveolar part of the maxilla and the lip on both sides.

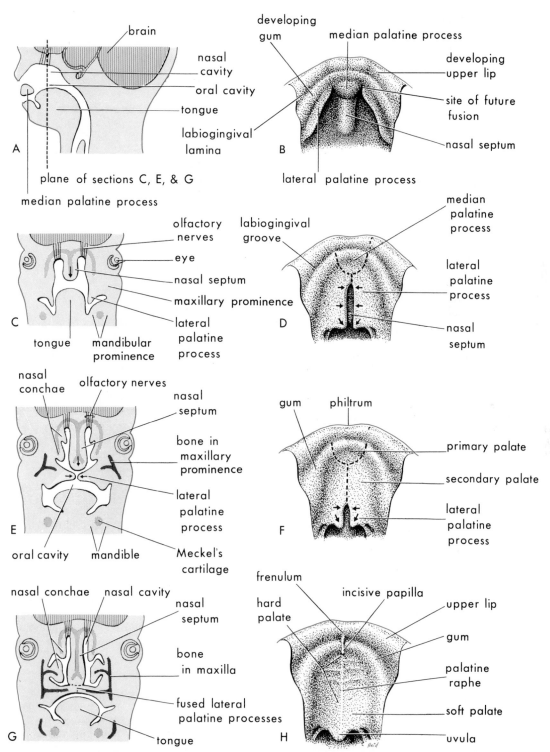

Figure 11-14. *A*, Sketch of a sagittal section of the embryonic head at the end of the sixth week showing the primary palate. *B*, *D*, *F*, and *H*, Drawings of the roof of the mouth from the sixth to twelfth weeks illustrating development of the palate. The broken lines in *D* and *F* indicate sites of fusion of the palatine processes; the arrows indicate medial and posterior growth of the lateral palatine processes. *C*, *E*, and *G*, Drawings of frontal sections of the head illustrating fusion of the lateral palatine processes with each other and the nasal septum, and separation of the nasal and oral cavities.

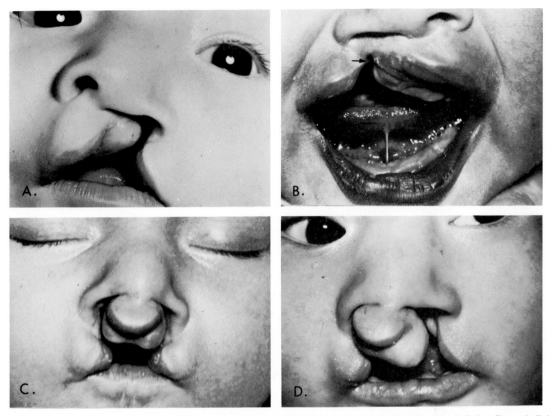

Figure 11–15. Photographs illustrating the various types of cleft lip. *A* and *B*, Unilateral cleft lip. The cleft in *B* is incomplete; the arrow indicates a band of tissue (Simonart band) connecting the parts of the lip. *C* and *D*, Bilateral cleft lip. Note that the intermaxillary segment of the maxilla protrudes between the clefts in the lip. Deformed, supernumerary, or absent teeth are often associated abnormalities. (Courtesy of Dr. D. A. Kernahan, The Children's Memorial Hospital, Chicago.)

The embryological basis of cleft palate is failure of the mesenchymal masses of the lateral palatine processes to meet and fuse with each other, with the nasal septum, and/or with the median palatine process or primary palate.

Most cases of cleft lip and cleft palate are determined by multiple factors, genetic and nongenetic, each causing only a minor developmental disturbance. This is called *multifactorial inheritance.* These factors seem to operate by influencing the number of neural crest cells that migrate into the embryonic facial primordia. If the number is insufficient, clefting of the lip and/or palate occurs.

Studies of twins indicate that genetic factors are of more importance in cleft lip, with or without cleft palate, than in cleft palate alone. A sibling of a child with a cleft palate has an elevated risk of having a cleft palate, but no increased risk of having a cleft lip.

Text continued on page 157

Figure 11–16. Drawings illustrating the embryological basis of complete unilateral cleft lip. *A,* Five-week embryo. *B,* Horizontal section through the head, illustrating the grooves between the maxillary prominences and the merging medial nasal prominences. *C,* Six-week embryo, showing a persistent labial groove on the left side. *D,* Horizontal section through the head, showing the groove gradually filling in on the right side because of proliferation of mesenchyme (arrows). *E,* Seven-week embryo. *F,* Horizontal section through the head, showing that the epithelium on the right has almost been pushed out of the groove between the maxillary prominence and medial nasal prominence. *G,* 10-week fetus with a complete unilateral cleft lip. *H,* Horizontal section through the head after stretching of the epithelium and breakdown of the tissues in the floor of the persistent labial groove on the left side, forming a complete unilateral cleft lip. (From Moore, K. L.: *The Developing Human: Clinically Oriented Embryology,* 4th ed. Philadelphia, W. B. Saunders Company, 1988.)

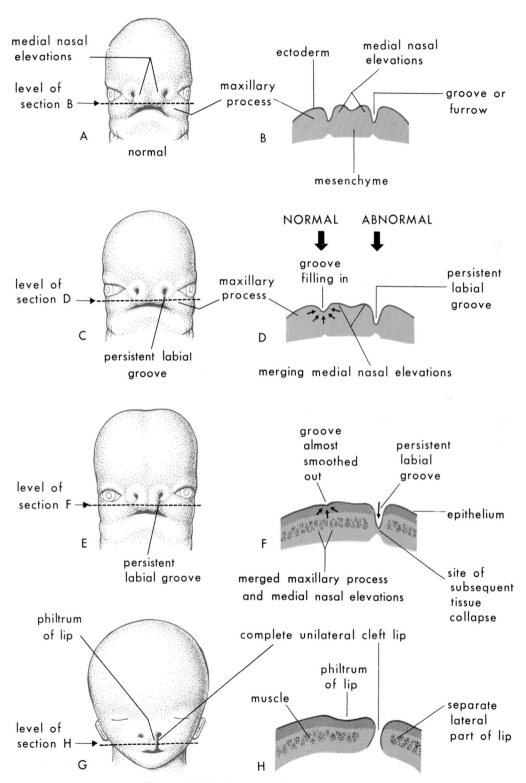

Figure 11-16 *See legend on opposite page*

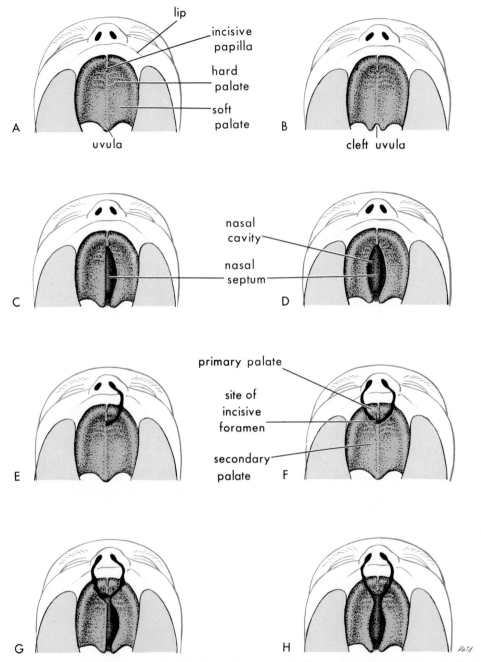

Figure 11–17. Drawings of various types of cleft lip and palate. *A*, Normal lip and palate. *B*, Cleft uvula. *C*, Unilateral cleft of the posterior or secondary palate. *D*, Bilateral cleft of the posterior palate. *E*, Complete unilateral cleft of the lip and alveolar process of the maxilla with a unilateral cleft of the anterior or primary palate. *F*, Complete bilateral cleft of the lip and alveolar process with bilateral cleft of the anterior palate. *G*, Complete bilateral cleft of the lip and alveolar process with bilateral cleft of the anterior palate and unilateral cleft of the posterior palate. *H*, Complete bilateral cleft of the lip and alveolar process with complete bilateral cleft of the anterior and posterior parts of the palate.

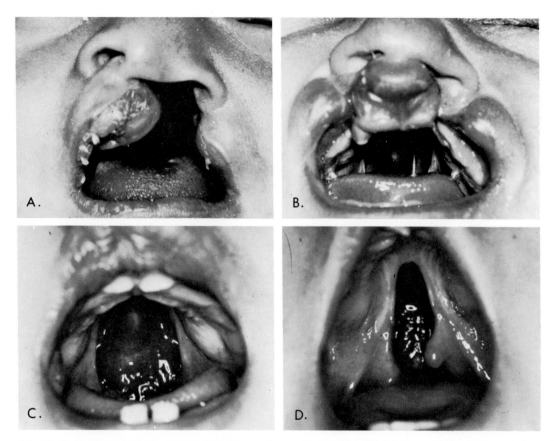

Figure 11–18. Photographs illustrating congenital malformations of the lip and/or palate. *A,* Complete unilateral cleft of the lip and alveolar process of the maxilla. *B,* Complete bilateral cleft of the lip and alveolar processes of the maxillae with bilateral cleft of the anterior palate. Note the protruding intermaxillary segment between the clefts in the lip. *C* and *D,* Bilateral cleft of the posterior or secondary palate.

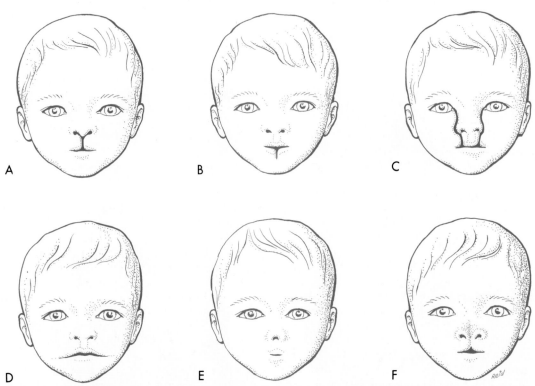

Figure 11–19. Drawings of uncommon malformations of the face. *A*, Median cleft of the upper lip. *B*, Median cleft of the lower lip and jaw. *C*, Bilateral oblique facial clefts with complete bilateral cleft lip. *D*, Macrostomia or lateral facial cleft. *E*, Single nostril and microstomia; these malformations are not usually associated. *F*, Bifid nose and incomplete median cleft of the upper lip.

Unusual Facial Clefts

Various types of facial cleft occur, but they are all uncommon. Severe facial clefts are usually associated with gross malformations of the head.

In *median cleft of the lower lip and mandible* (Fig. 11–19B), there is a deep cleft resulting from failure of the mandibular prominences of the first branchial arch to merge completely with each other.

Oblique facial clefts are often bilateral and extend from the upper lip to the medial margin of the eye (Fig. 11–19C). They result from failure of the maxillary prominences to merge with the lateral and medial nasal prominences.

Lateral or *transverse facial clefts* run from the mouth toward the external ear. Bilateral clefts result in a very large mouth, a condition called *macrostomia* (Fig. 11–19D).

Other Uncommon Facial Malformations

Congenital microstomia (small mouth) results from excessive merging of the maxillary and mandibular prominences of the first arch (Fig. 11–19E).

A *single nostril* results when only one nasal placode forms (Fig. 11–19E).

Bifid nose results from failure of the medial nasal prominences to merge completely (Fig. 11–19F). In mild forms of bifid nose, a small groove is present in the tip of the nose.

SUMMARY

During the fourth and fifth weeks, the primitive pharynx is bounded laterally by barlike *branchial arches*. Each arch consists of a core of mesenchymal tissue, which is covered externally by *surface ectoderm* and internally by *endoderm*. Each branchial arch also contains an artery called an *aortic arch*, a cartilage bar, a nerve, and a muscle component.

Externally, between the arches, are *branchial grooves*. Internally, between the arches, are extensions of the pharynx called *pharyngeal pouches*. Where the ectoderm of each branchial groove contacts the endoderm of each pharyngeal pouch, *branchial membranes* are formed. The pharyngeal pouches and the branchial arches, grooves, and membranes make up the *branchial apparatus*.

Development of the tongue, face, lips, jaws, palate, pharynx, and neck largely involves transformation of the branchial apparatus into adult structures. The branchial grooves disappear except for the first pair, which persists as the *external acoustic meatus*.

The branchial membranes also disappear, except for the first, which becomes the *tympanic membrane*.

The first pharyngeal pouch gives rise to the *tympanic cavity*, *mastoid antrum*, and *auditory tube*. The second pharyngeal pouch is associated with development of the *palatine tonsil*. The *thymus gland* is derived from the third pair of pharyngeal pouches, and the *parathyroid glands* are formed from the third and fourth pairs of pharyngeal pouches. The thyroid gland develops from a downgrowth from the floor of the pharynx in the region where the tongue develops.

Most congenital malformations of the head and neck originate during transformation of the branchial apparatus into adult structures.

Branchial cysts, sinuses, or *fistulas* may develop from parts of the second branchial groove, the *cervical sinus*, or the second pharyngeal pouch which fail to obliterate.

An *ectopic thyroid gland* results when the thyroid gland fails to descend, or only partially descends, from its site of origin in the tongue.

The thyroglossal duct may persist or remnants of it may give rise to *thyroglossal duct cysts*; these cysts, if infected, may perforate and form *thyroglossal duct sinuses* which open anteriorly in the midline of the neck.

Cleft lip is the most common congenital malformation of the face. Although frequently associated with cleft palate, cleft lip and cleft palate are etiologically distinct malformations which involve different developmental processes that occur at different times.

Cleft lip results from failure of mesenchymal masses of the medial nasal prominences and maxillary prominences to merge, whereas *cleft palate* results from failure of the mesenchymal masses of the palatine processes to fuse.

Most cases of cleft lip, with or without cleft palate, are caused by a combination of genetic and environmental factors (i.e., *multifactorial inheritance*). These factors appear to act by interfering with the migration of *neural crest cells* into the maxillary prominences of the first branchial arch. If the number of cells is insufficient, clefting of the lip and/or palate may occur.

Commonly Asked Questions

1. My mother said that my uncle had a *"harelip."* What is meant by this term?
2. I was told that embryos have cleft lips, and that this common facial malformation represents a persistence of this embryonic condition. Are these statements accurate?
3. Neither my husband nor I have a cleft lip or cleft palate, and no one in our families is known to have or to have had these malformations. What are our chances of having a child with a cleft lip with or without cleft palate?
4. I have a son with cleft lip and cleft palate. My brother has a similar malformation of his lip and palate. Although I do not plan to have any more children, my husband says that I am "entirely to blame" for our son's malformations. Was the defect likely inherited only from my side of the family?
5. My sister's son has minor malformations of his external ears, but he does not have hearing abnormalities or facial malformations. Would the ear abnormalities be considered *branchial malformations?*

Answers

1. *"Harelip"* is the old term for cleft lip that many lay persons still use. It was given this name because the hare (a mammal like a large rabbit) has a divided upper lip. It is not an accurate comparison, however, because the cleft in the hare's lip is a median one. Median cleft of the upper lip is very uncommon in humans.
2. No, both statements are inaccurate. All embryos have grooves in their upper lips where the maxillary prominences meet the merged medial nasal prominences (Fig. 11–16A and B), but normal embryos do not have cleft lips. When lip development is abnormal, the tissue in the floor of the lip groove breaks down and a cleft lip forms (Fig. 11–16E to H). This malformation usually results from a combination of genetic and environmental factors.
3. The risk in your case is the same as for the general population, that is, 1 per 1000.
4. Although environmental factors may be involved, it is reasonable to assume that your son's cleft lip and cleft palate were hereditary and recessive in their expression. This would mean that your husband also carried a concealed gene for cleft lip and that his family was equally responsible for your son's malformations.
5. Minor malformations of the auricle of the external ear are common, and usually they are of no serious medical or cosmetic consequence. About 14 per cent of newborn infants have minor morphological abnormalities, and less than 1 per cent of them have other defects. The child's abnormal ears could be considered branchial malformations because the external ears develop from six small swellings of the first two pairs of branchial arches (see Fig. 18–8); however, such minor abnormalities of shape would not normally be classified in this way.

12

The Respiratory System

The respiratory system begins to form during the fourth week. A median *laryngotracheal groove* develops in the caudal end of the ventral wall of the primitive pharyngeal floor (Fig. 12–1). Soon this groove deepens to form a *laryngotracheal diverticulum* or outpouching ventral to the primitive pharynx (Fig. 12–2A). As this diverticulum grows caudally, it gradually separates from the pharynx; however, it maintains open communication with the pharynx through the *primitive laryngeal aditus* (Fig. 12–2C), the future inlet of the larynx.

Tracheoesophageal folds grow toward each other and fuse to form the *tracheoesophageal septum* (Fig. 12–2E). This septum divides the cranial part of the foregut into the *laryngotracheal tube* and the *esophagus* (Fig. 12–2F). The laryngotracheal tube is the primordium of the epithelium of the internal lining of the larynx, trachea, bronchi, and lungs.

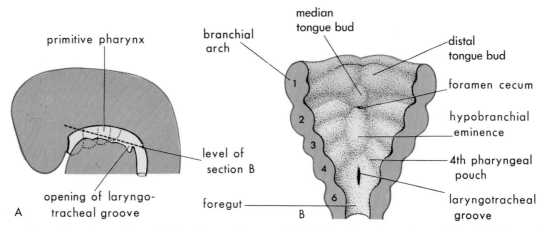

Figure 12–1. *A,* Diagrammatic sagittal section of the cranial half of a human embryo of about 26 days showing the laryngotracheal groove in the caudal end of the floor of the primitive pharynx (develops from the cranial part of the foregut). *B,* Horizontal section at the level shown in *A,* illustrating the floor of the primitive pharynx and the location of the laryngotracheal groove.

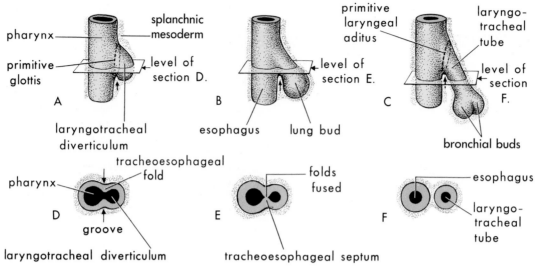

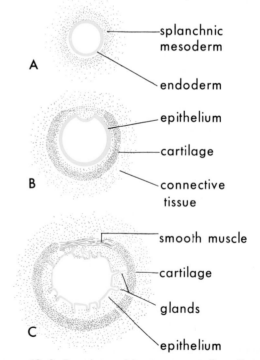

Figure 12–2. Successive stages of development of the tracheoesophageal septum during the fourth week. *A, B,* and *C,* Lateral views of the caudal part of the primitive pharynx illustrating partitioning of the foregut into the esophagus and laryngotracheal tube. *D, E,* and *F,* Transverse sections illustrating development of the tracheoesophageal septum and division of the cranial part of the foregut into the laryngotracheal tube and esophagus.

DEVELOPMENT OF THE LARYNX

The endodermal lining of the cranial end of the laryngotracheal tube and the surrounding mesenchyme from the fourth and sixth pairs of branchial arches develop into the larynx. The *laryngeal cartilages* develop from the fourth and sixth pairs of branchial arch cartilages (see Fig. 11–4). The epiglottis develops from the caudal half of the *hypobranchial eminence* (see Fig. 11–12). Folds of mucous membrane of the larynx become the *vocal folds* (vocal cords). The *laryngeal muscles* develop from muscle elements in the fourth and sixth pairs of branchial arches.

DEVELOPMENT OF THE TRACHEA

The endodermal lining of the laryngotracheal tube distal to the larynx gives rise to the epithelium and glands of the trachea (Fig. 12–3). The cartilage, connective tissue, and muscle of the trachea are derived from the surrounding splanchnic mesenchyme.

Tracheoesophageal Fistula (Fig. 12–4). A communication, or fistula, connecting the trachea and esophagus occurs about once in every 2500 births; most affected infants are male.

Tracheoesophageal fistula is usually associated with *esophageal atresia;* in all cases, there is an abnormal communication between the trachea and the esophagus (Fig. 12–4).

Tracheoesophageal fistula results from incomplete division of the foregut into respiratory and digestive portions during the fourth week. Incomplete fusion of the tracheoesophageal folds results in a defective

Figure 12–3. Drawings of transverse sections through the laryngotracheal tube illustrating progressive stages of development of the trachea. *A,* 4 weeks. *B,* 10 weeks. *C,* 11 weeks.

tracheoesophageal septum, leaving a communication between the trachea and the esophagus.

There are four main varieties of tracheoesophageal fistula. The most common abnormality is for the cranial portion of the esophagus to end blindly (esophageal atresia) and for the caudal portion to join the trachea near its bifurcation (Fig. 12–4A). Other varieties of this malformation are illustrated in Figure 12–4B to D.

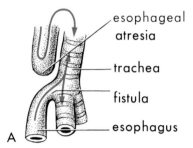

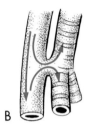

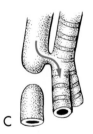

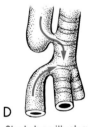

Figure 12–4. Sketches illustrating the four main varieties of tracheoesophageal fistula. Possible direction of flow of contents is indicated by arrows. Esophageal atresia, as illustrated in A, occurs in about 90 per cent of cases. The abdomen rapidly becomes distended as the intestines fill with air. In C, air cannot enter the lower esophagus and the stomach.

Infants with esophageal atresia and tracheoesophageal fistula cough and choke on swallowing owing to excessive amounts of saliva accumulating in the mouth and upper respiratory tract. When the infant swallows milk, it rapidly fills the esophageal pouch and is regurgitated. Some of this milk passes into the trachea, resulting in gagging, coughing, and *respiratory distress.* Gastric contents may also reflux through the fistula into the trachea and lungs from the stomach. This may result in pneumonia or pneumonitis (inflammation of the lungs).

Normal fetuses swallow amniotic fluid, which is absorbed through the intestines into their blood. It then passes via the placenta into the maternal blood via the placenta (see Chapter 8) and is excreted by her kidneys.

An excess of amniotic fluid *(polyhydramnios)* may be associated with esophageal atresia and tracheoesophageal fistula, because amniotic fluid may not pass to the stomach and intestines for absorption and subsequent placental transfer to the mother's blood for disposal.

DEVELOPMENT OF THE BRONCHI AND LUNGS

The bulb-shaped *lung bud* at the caudal end of the laryngotracheal tube (Fig. 12–5A) soon divides into two knoblike *bronchial buds* (Fig. 12–5B). These endodermal buds differentiate into the bronchi and lungs and grow laterally into the *pericardioperitoneal canals, i.e.,* the primitive pleural cavities (Fig. 12–6A).

The bronchial buds enlarge to form the primordia of the *primary bronchi.* Soon the primary bronchi subdivide into *secondary bronchi* (Fig. 12–5C to F). On the right, the superior secondary bronchus will supply the superior lobe of the lung, whereas the inferior secondary bronchus soon subdivides into two bronchi, one to the middle lobe of the right lung and the other to the inferior lobe. On the left, the two secondary bronchi supply the superior and inferior lobes of the lung (Fig. 12–5G).

Each secondary bronchus subsequently undergoes progressive branching; each branch bifurcates repeatedly into branches. Tertiary or segmental bronchi, 10 in the right lung and eight or nine in the left, begin to form by the seventh week. As this occurs, the surrounding mesenchymal tissue divides.

Each tertiary or *segmental bronchus* with its surrounding mass of mesenchyme will form a *bronchopulmonary segment.*

By 24 weeks, about 17 orders of branches have formed and the respiratory bronchioles are present (Fig. 12–7A). Additional orders of airways develop after birth.

As the bronchi develop, cartilaginous plates develop

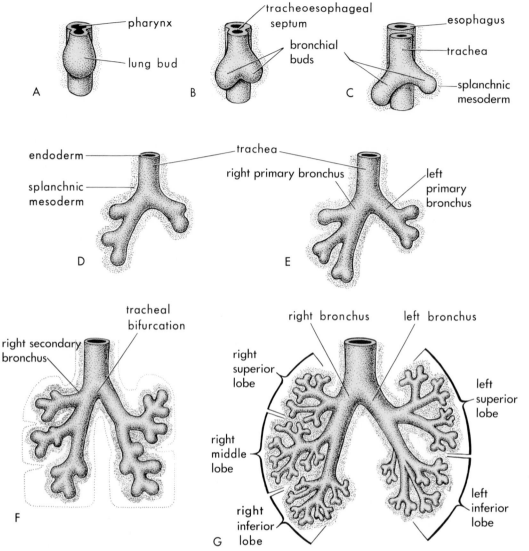

Figure 12–5. Drawings of ventral views illustrating successive stages in the development of the bronchi and lungs. *A* to *D*, four weeks. *E*, five weeks. *F*, six weeks. *G*, eight weeks.

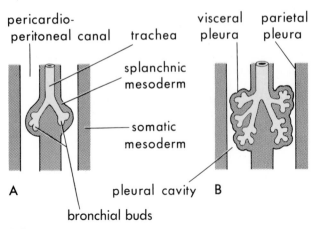

Figure 12–6. Diagrams illustrating growth of the developing lungs into the splanchnic mesoderm of the medial walls of the pericardioperitoneal canals (primitive pleural cavities). The development of the layers of the pleura is also shown. *A*, five weeks. *B*, six weeks.

from the surrounding mesenchyme. This splanchnic mesenchyme also gives rise to the bronchial smooth musculature and connective tissue, and to the pulmonary connective tissue and capillaries.

As the lungs develop, they acquire a layer of *visceral pleura* from the splanchnic mesenchyme (Fig. 12–6*B*). With expansion, the lungs and pleural cavities grow caudally into the mesenchyme of the body wall and soon come to lie close to the heart (see Fig. 10–4). The thoracic body wall becomes lined by a layer of *parietal pleura*, derived from the somatic mesoderm (see Fig. 12–6*B*). Lung development may be divided into four stages.

The Pseudoglandular Period (5 to 17 Weeks). Microscopically, the developing lung somewhat resembles an exocrine gland. The air-conducting system develops during this period, but respiration is not possible. Hence, *embryos or fetuses born during this period cannot survive.*

The Canalicular Period (16 to 25 Weeks). This period overlaps the pseudoglandular period because cranial segments of the lung develop faster than caudal ones. During the canalicular period the lumina of the bronchi and terminal bronchioles enlarge, and the lung tissue becomes highly vascular.

Each terminal bronchiole gives rise to two or more *respiratory bronchioles* (Fig. 12–7*A*). Each of these then divides into three to six tubular passages called *alveolar ducts*. Toward the end of this period, the lining cells of these ducts become attenuated, permitting the blood capillaries to project as capillary loops into the future air spaces.

Respiration is possible toward the end of the canalicular period because some thin-walled saccules, called *terminal sacs* (primitive alveoli), have developed at the ends of the respiratory branchioles, and these regions are well vascularized (Fig. 12–7*A*). Although a fetus born toward the end of this period may survive if given intensive care, death often occurs because the respiratory and other systems are still immature.

The Terminal Sac Period (24 Weeks to Birth). The alveolar ducts give rise to clusters of thin-walled terminal air sacs or primitive *pulmonary alveoli* (Fig. 12–7*B* and *C*). The capillary network proliferates rapidly in the mesenchyme around the developing alveoli, and *some capillaries bulge into these thin-walled air sacs.* There is concurrent active development of lymphatic capillaries.

By 28 weeks, sufficient terminal air sacs are usually present to permit survival of a prematurely born infant. The development of an adequate pulmonary vasculature is critical to the survival of premature infants.

During this period the type II alveolar epithelial cells or pneumocytes produce **surfactant,** a substance that covers the internal surface of the alveoli before birth.

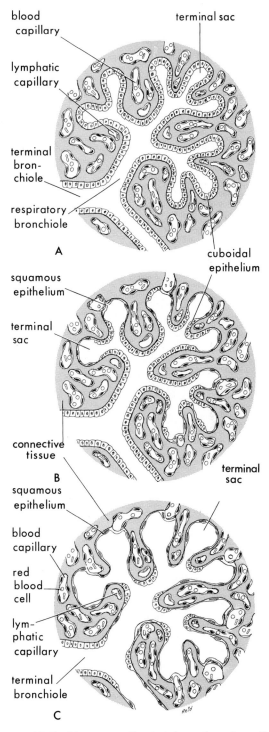

Figure 12–7. Diagrammatic sketches of sections illustrating progressive stages of lung development. *A,* 24 weeks (late canalicular period). *B,* 26 weeks (early terminal sac period). *C,* Newborn infant (early alveolar period).

It is capable of lowering the surface tension at the air-alveolar interface, thereby maintaining patency of the alveoli and facilitating expansion of the lungs at birth.

The Alveolar Period (Late Fetal Period to About Eight Years). The lining of the terminal air sacs becomes extremely thin, thus forming *characteristic pulmonary alveoli* (Fig. 12–7C). One eighth to one sixth of the adult number of alveoli are present at birth; their number increases until about the eighth year.

The lungs at birth are about half inflated with liquid derived from the lungs, the amniotic cavity, and the tracheal glands. Consequently, aeration of the lungs at birth involves rapid replacement of intra-alveolar fluid by air.

Respiratory Distress Syndrome. Infants born prematurely are most susceptible to the *respiratory distress syndrome (RDS)*. Shortly after birth, the infant develops rapid and labored breathing.

A deficiency of pulmonary surfactant appears to be a major cause of *hyaline membrane disease,* a common cause of death in the perinatal period. The lungs are underinflated and the alveoli contain a fluid of high protein content that resembles a hyaline (glassy) membrane.

Congenital malformations of the lungs are uncommon. Abnormal fissures or lobes are occasionally observed, but they are usually unimportant clinically.

SUMMARY

The lower respiratory system begins to develop around the middle of the fourth week from a median *laryngotracheal groove* in the floor of the primitive pharynx. This groove deepens to produce a *laryngotracheal diverticulum* which is soon separated from the foregut by a *tracheoesophageal septum.* This results in the formation of the esophagus and the *laryngotracheal tube.*

The endodermal lining of the laryngotracheal tube gives rise to the epithelium of the lower respiratory organs and the tracheobronchial glands. The splanchnic mesenchyme surrounding this tube forms the connective tissue, cartilage, muscle, and blood and lymphatic vessels of these organs.

Branchial arch mesenchyme contributes to the formation of the epiglottis and the connective tissue of the larynx. The laryngeal muscles and the cartilage skeleton of the larynx are derived from mesenchyme in the caudal branchial arches.

The laryngotracheal tube divides at its termination into two *bronchial buds* (lung buds). Each bud soon enlarges to form a *primary bronchus* and then each of these gives rise to two new bronchial buds, which develop into *secondary bronchi.* The right inferior secondary bronchus soon divides into two bronchi. The secondary bronchi supply the lobes of the developing lungs. Branching continues until about 17 orders of branches have formed. Additional airways are formed after birth, until about 24 orders of branches are formed.

Each secondary bronchus undergoes progressive branching. The tertiary or *segmental bronchi* begin to form by the seventh week.

Lung development may be divided into four stages: (1) the *pseudoglandular period,* 5 to 17 weeks, when the bronchi and terminal bronchioles form; (2) the *canalicular period,* 16 to 25 weeks, when the lumina of the bronchi and terminal bronchioles enlarge, the respiratory bronchioles and alveolar ducts develop, and the lung tissue becomes highly vascular; (3) the *terminal sac period,* 24 weeks to birth, when the alveolar ducts give rise to terminal air sacs (primitive alveoli); and (4) the final stage of lung development, the *alveolar period,* from the late fetal period to about eight years of age, when the characteristic pulmonary alveoli develop.

The respiratory system develops so that it is capable of immediate function at birth. To be capable of respiration, the lungs must acquire an *alveolocapillary membrane* that is sufficiently thin, and an adequate amount of *surfactant* must be present. Surfactant is formed by secretory epithelial cells or type II pneumocytes.

Major congenital malformations of the lower respiratory system are uncommon, except for *tracheoesophageal fistula,* which is usually associated with *esophageal atresia.* These malformations result from faulty partitioning of the foregut into the esophagus and trachea during the fourth and fifth weeks.

Commonly Asked Questions

1. I recently read in the newspaper about *fetal breathing*. Is it true that the fetus breathes before birth?
2. What stimulates the baby to start breathing when it is born?
3. My sister's baby died about 72 hours after birth from *hyaline membrane disease*. What is this condition? Is its cause genetic or environmental?
4. Can an infant born 22 weeks after fertilization survive?
5. I heard a doctor on the television talking about babies born with their intestines in their chests. How does this happen, and can they survive?

Answers

1. No, the fetus cannot breathe before birth, because the airways and terminal air sacs are distended with liquid. The fetal lungs do not function as organs of gas exchange, but *breathing movements are practiced by the fetus*. Rapid, irregular respiratory movements occur during the terminal stages of pregnancy. The lungs must develop in such a way that they can assume their breathing role as soon as the baby is born. There is a rapid replacement of the intra-alveolar fluid by air.
2. The stimuli that initiate breathing at birth are multiple. Slapping the buttocks used to be a common physical stimulus, but this is usually unnecessary. Under normal circumstances, the infant's breathing begins so promptly after birth as to suggest that it is a reflex response to the sensory stimuli of exposure to air and touching. *The changes in blood gases after interruption of the placental circulation are important*, e.g., the fall in oxygen tension and pH, and the rise in P_{CO_2}.
3. *Hyaline membrane disease*, also referred to as *respiratory distress syndrome* (RDS), occurs after the onset of breathing in infants with lung immaturity and a *deficiency of pulmonary surfactant*. The incidence of RDS is about 1 per cent of all live births and is the leading cause of death in newborn infants. It occurs mainly in infants who are born prematurely, and its incidence tends to decrease as term approaches.
4. A 22-week-old fetus is viable and, if born prematurely and given special care in a neonatal intensive care unit, may survive. However, chances of survival are poor for infants who weigh less than 600 gm, because the lungs are immature and incapable of adequate alveolar-capillary gas exchange. Furthermore, the fetus's brain is not differentiated sufficiently to allow for regular respiration.
5. When development of the diaphragm is abnormal, a large defect develops that allows the abdominal viscera to pass into the thoracic cavity. This is called a *congenital diaphragmatic hernia* (see Fig. 10–8). Usually the abnormally placed viscera are the hollow ones, such as the stomach and intestines. If the volume of intrathoracic abdominal viscera is great, respiratory distress appears soon after birth. Replacement of the viscera into the abdomen and surgical correction of the congenital defect permits survival of the infant. The percentage of cure depends largely on the promptness with which the diagnosis is made and corrective surgery is performed.

13

The Digestive System

The primitive gut forms during the fourth week, as the dorsal part of the yolk sac is incorporated into the embryo during folding (Chapter 6). The endoderm of the primitive gut gives rise to most of the epithelium and glands of the digestive tract. The epithelium at the cranial and caudal extremities of the tract is derived from ectoderm of the *stomodeum* (primitive mouth) and the *proctodeum* (anal pit), respectively (Fig. 13–1). The muscular and fibrous elements of the digestive tract are derived from the splanchnic mesenchyme surrounding the endodermal primitive gut.

For descriptive purposes, the primitive gut is divided into three parts: *foregut, midgut,* and *hindgut* (Fig. 13–1).

THE FOREGUT

The derivatives of the foregut are the pharynx (discussed in Chapter 11), lower respiratory system (discussed in Chapter 12), esophagus, stomach, part of the duodenum, the liver and biliary apparatus, and the pancreas.

The Esophagus. The partitioning of the trachea from the esophagus by the *tracheoesophageal septum* is described in Chapter 12 and is illustrated in Figure 12–2. Initially the esophagus is very short (Fig. 13–1), but it soon reaches its final relative length as the embryo grows. The smooth muscle of the esophagus develops from the surrounding splanchnic mesenchyme.

The epithelium of the esophagus and the esophageal glands is derived from endoderm. The epithelium of the esophagus proliferates and almost obliterates the lumen, but recanalization of the esophagus normally occurs by the end of the embryonic period.

Esophageal Atresia (see Fig. 12–4A). Esophageal atresia is usually associated with *tracheoesophageal fistula.* It may occur as a separate malformation, but this is uncommon.

Atresia probably results from deviation of the *tracheoesophageal septum* (see Fig. 12–2) in a posterior direction, but atresia could also result from failure of esophageal recanalization to occur during the embryonic period.

When there is esophageal atresia, amniotic fluid cannot pass to the intestines for absorption and transfer via the placenta to the maternal blood for disposal. This results in *polyhydramnios,* the accumulation of an excessive amount of amniotic fluid.

Newborn infants with esophageal atresia usually appear healthy, and their first one or two swallows are normal. Suddenly fluid returns through the nose and mouth, and then *respiratory distress* occurs. Confirmation of the presence of esophageal atresia can be made by demonstrating that a radiopaque catheter cannot pass into the stomach.

Esophageal Stenosis. Congenital stenosis or narrowing of the esophagus is usually present in the distal third as either a web or a long segment of esophagus with only a threadlike lumen. Esophageal stenosis results from incomplete recanalization of the esophagus during the eighth week of development.

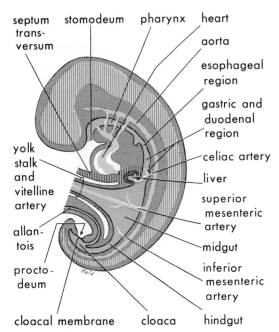

septum trans-versum · stomodeum · pharynx · heart · aorta · esophageal region · gastric and duodenal region · celiac artery · liver · superior mesenteric artery · midgut · inferior mesenteric artery · yolk stalk and vitelline artery · allan-tois · procto-deum · cloacal membrane · cloaca · hindgut

Figure 13–1. Drawing of a median section of a four-week embryo showing the primitive gut or early digestive system and its blood supply. At this stage the primitive gut is a long tube that extends the length of the embryo. It was formed by incorporation of the dorsal part of the yolk sac (see Fig. 6–1.) Its blood vessels are derived from those that originally supplied the yolk sac.

The Stomach. The stomach first appears as a fusiform dilatation of the caudal part of the foregut (Figs. 13–1 and 13–2A). This primordium soon enlarges and broadens ventrodorsally (Fig. 13–2B). The dorsal border grows faster than the ventral border, producing the *greater curvature* (Fig. 13–2C). As the stomach acquires its adult shape, it rotates in a clockwise direction around its longitudinal axis.

The stomach is suspended from the dorsal wall of the abdominal cavity by the dorsal mesentery or *dorsal mesogastrium* (Fig. 13–2A). The dorsal mesogastrium is carried to the left during rotation of the stomach and formation of a cavity known as the *omental bursa* or *lesser sac* of peritoneum (Fig. 13–2A to C). The lesser sac communicates with the main peritoneal cavity or *greater peritoneal sac* through a small opening, called the *epiploic foramen* (Fig. 13–2D).

A ventral mesentery or *ventral mesogastrium* (Fig. 13–2B) persists only in the region of the inferior end of the esophagus, the stomach, and the superior part of the duodenum. It attaches the stomach and duodenum to the developing liver and the ventral abdominal wall (Fig. 13–2D).

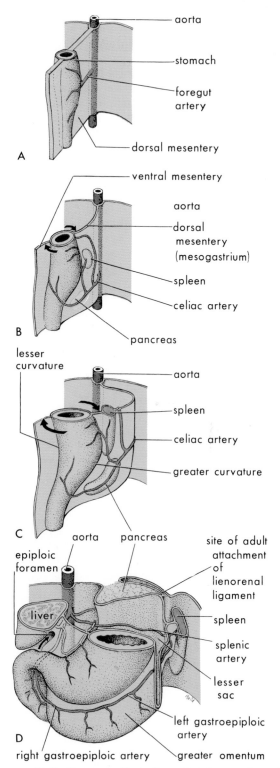

A · aorta · stomach · foregut artery · dorsal mesentery

B · ventral mesentery · aorta · dorsal mesentery (mesogastrium) · spleen · celiac artery · pancreas

C · lesser curvature · aorta · spleen · celiac artery · greater curvature

D · epiploic foramen · aorta · pancreas · liver · site of adult attachment of lienorenal ligament · spleen · splenic artery · lesser sac · left gastroepiploic artery · right gastroepiploic artery · greater omentum

Figure 13–2. Drawings illustrating development and rotation of the stomach and formation of the greater omentum. *A,* About 30 days. *B,* About 35 days. *C,* About 40 days. *D,* About 48 days.

Congenital Pyloric Stenosis. Malformations of the stomach are uncommon, except for hypertrophic pyloric stenosis. It affects 1 in every 150 male infants and 1 in every 750 female infants.

Babies with this abnormality have a *marked thickening of the pylorus,* the distal sphincteric region of the stomach. The circular and, to a lesser degree, the longitudinal muscle in the pyloric region are hypertrophied. This results in *severe narrowing (stenosis)* of the pyloric canal and obstruction to the passage of food.

Although the cause of congenital pyloric stenosis is unknown, the high incidence of the condition in both infants of monozygotic twins suggests the involvement of genetic factors.

The Duodenum. The duodenum develops from the caudal part of the foregut and the cranial part of the midgut. These parts grow rapidly and form a C-shaped loop that projects ventrally (Fig. 13–3B to D). The junction of the two embryonic parts of the duodenum in the adult is just distal to the entrance of the bile duct (common bile duct).

During the fifth and sixth weeks, the lumen of the duodenum becomes reduced and may be temporarily

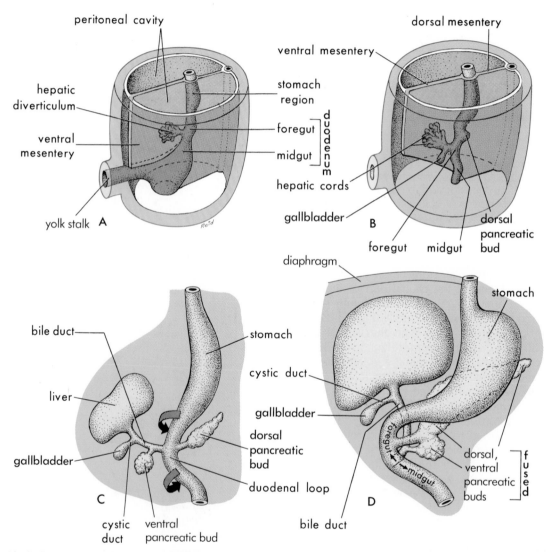

Figure 13–3. Drawings illustrating progressive stages in the development of the duodenum, liver, pancreas and extrahepatic biliary apparatus. *A,* Four weeks. *B* and *C,* Five weeks. *D,* Six weeks. The pancreas develops from dorsal and ventral buds that fuse to form the pancreas. Note that, as the result of the positional changes of the duodenum, the entrance of the bile duct into the duodenum gradually shifts from its initial position to a posterior one. This explains why the bile duct in the adult passes posterior to the duodenum and the head of the pancreas.

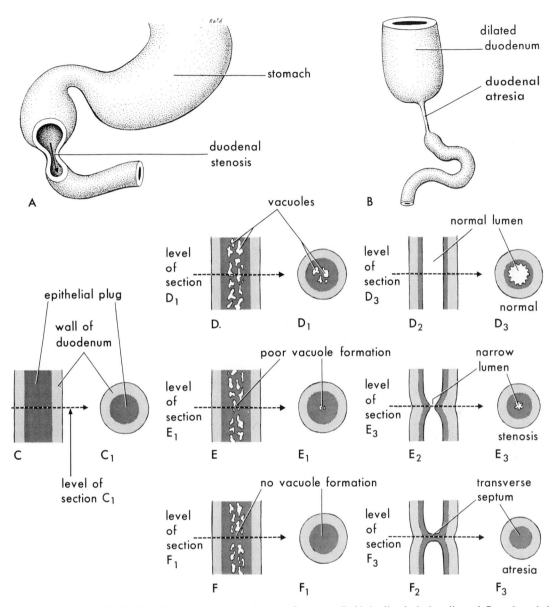

Figure 13–4. Diagrams illustrating the two common types of congenital intestinal obstruction. *A*, Duodenal stenosis. *B*, Duodenal atresia. *C* to *F*, Diagrammatic longitudinal and transverse sections of the duodenum showing: (1) normal recanalization (*D* to *D₃*), (2) stenosis (*E* to *E₃*), and (3) atresia (*F* to *F₃*).

obliterated by epithelial cells, but it normally recanalizes by the end of the embryonic period.

Duodenal Stenosis (Fig. 13–4A and E_3). Narrowing of the duodenal lumen usually results from incomplete recanalization of the duodenum. Most stenoses involve the horizontal (third) and/or ascending (fourth) parts of the duodenum. The vomitus usually contains bile.

Duodenal Atresia (Fig. 13–4B). Blockage of the lumen of the duodenum is not common, except in premature infants and in those with the Down syndrome (see Fig. 9–4). During the solid stage of duodenal development, the lumen is completely filled with epithelial cells. If reformation of the lumen fails to occur by a process of vacuolization (Fig. 13–4D), a short segment of the duodenum is occluded.

The Liver and Biliary Apparatus. The liver, gallbladder, and biliary duct system arise as a bud from the most caudal part of the foregut (see Fig. 13–3A). The *hepatic diverticulum* grows between the layers of

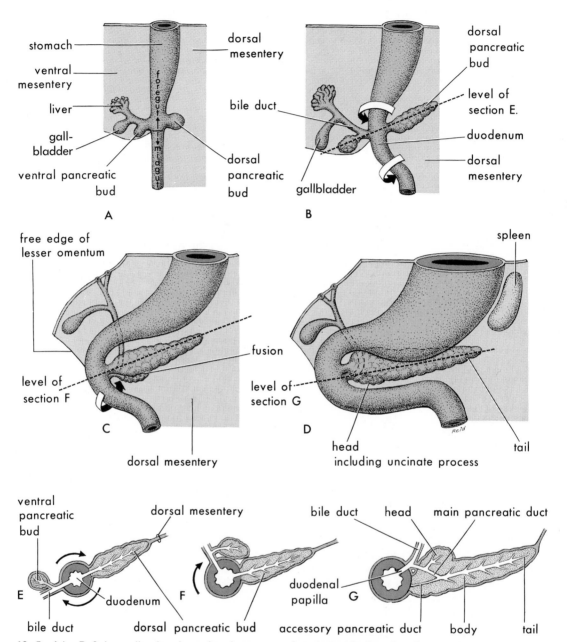

Figure 13–5. *A* to *D,* Schematic drawings showing successive stages in the development of the pancreas from the fifth to the seventh weeks. *E* to *G,* Diagrammatic transverse sections through the duodenum and developing pancreas. Growth and rotation (arrows) of the duodenum bring the ventral pancreatic bud toward the dorsal bud where they subsequently fuse. Note that the bile duct initially attaches to the ventral aspect of the duodenum, and is carried around to the dorsal aspect as the duodenum rotates.

the ventral mesentery, where it rapidly enlarges and divides into two parts (Fig. 13–3B).

The large cranial part is the primordium of the liver. The endodermal cells of the hepatic diverticulum give rise to the parenchymal or *hepatic cells,* which soon become arranged in a series of branching and anastomosing plates. The fibrous and *hemopoietic tissue* and *Kupffer cells* of the liver are derived from the splanchnic mesenchyme of the septum transversum (see Fig. 13–1).

The liver grows rapidly and soon fills most of the abdominal cavity (see Fig. 6–10B). Hemopoiesis (formation and development of blood cells) begins during the sixth week. This activity is mainly responsible for the relatively large size of the liver (see Fig. 13–3D). By nine weeks, the liver represents about 10 per cent of the total weight of the fetus.

The small caudal portion of the hepatic diverticulum expands to form the *gallbladder* (see Fig. 13–3C). The stalk connecting the hepatic and cystic ducts to the duodenum becomes the *bile duct* (common bile duct).

The Pancreas. The pancreas develops from *dorsal and ventral pancreatic buds* of endodermal cells that arise from the caudal part of the foregut (Fig. 13–5A). When the duodenum grows and rotates to the right (clockwise), the ventral bud is carried dorsally and fuses with the dorsal bud (Fig. 13–5D and G).

The Spleen. Development of the spleen is described here because this organ is derived from a mass of mesenchymal cells located between the layers of the dorsal mesogastrium. The spleen, a large, vascular, lymphatic organ, acquires its characteristic shape early in the fetal period (see Figs. 13–2 and 13–5D).

THE MIDGUT

The derivatives of the midgut are the small intestines, including most of the duodenum; cecum; vermiform appendix; ascending colon; and right half to two thirds of the transverse colon.

Rotation and Fixation of the Midgut Loop. At first the midgut communicates widely with the yolk sac (see Fig. 13–1), but this connection soon becomes reduced to the narrow *yolk stalk* (see Figs. 6–10A and 13–6A).

Herniation of the Midgut Loop. As the midgut elongates, it forms a ventral U-shaped *midgut loop* which projects into the umbilical cord (Fig. 13–6A). This "herniation" is a normal migration of the midgut into the extraembryonic coelom which occurs because there is not enough room in the abdomen. The space shortage is caused mainly by the relatively massive liver and kidneys.

Within the umbilical cord, the *midgut loop rotates counterclockwise,* as viewed from the ventral aspect of the embryo (Fig. 13–6B), around the axis of the *superior mesenteric artery.* This brings the cranial limb of the midgut loop to the right and the caudal limb to the left (Fig. 13–6B and B_1).

Return of the Midgut. During the tenth week, the intestines return to the abdomen, the so-called reduction of the midgut hernia. As the intestines return, they undergo further rotation (Fig. 13–6C_1 and D_1).

The decrease in the relative size of the liver and kidneys and enlargement of the abdominal cavity are likely important factors related to the return of the intestines to the abdomen. When the colon returns to the abdominal cavity, its cecal end rotates to the right side and enters the lower right quadrant of the abdomen (Fig. 13–6D and E).

Fixation of the Intestines. Lengthening of the proximal part of the colon gives rise to the hepatic flexure and the ascending colon (Fig. 13–6D and E). As the ascending colon assumes its final position, its mesentery is pressed against the posterior abdominal wall. The mesentery of the ascending colon gradually disappears. The other derivatives of the midgut loop retain their mesenteries.

The Cecum and Appendix. The primordium of the cecum and vermiform appendix is the *cecal diverticulum,* which appears during the fifth week. This conical pouch appears on the caudal limb of the midgut loop (Fig. 13–6B). The distal end or apex of this blind sac does not grow rapidly, and the appendix therefore forms (Fig. 13–6E). By birth it is a long blind tube, relatively longer than in the adult.

Omphalocele (Fig. 13–7). This condition occurs once in about 6000 births and results from failure of the intestines to return to the abdomen during the tenth week. The hernia may consist of a single loop of bowel, or it may contain most of the intestines. The covering of the hernial sac is the amniotic epithelium of the umbilical cord.

Umbilical Hernia. When the intestines return normally to the abdominal cavity and then herniate either prenatally or postnatally through an inadequately closed umbilicus, an umbilical hernia forms.

An umbilical hernia differs from an omphalocele in that *the protruding mass (omentum, or loop of bowel) is covered by subcutaneous tissue and skin.* The hernia usually does not reach its maximum size until the end of the first month after birth. It ranges in size from that of a marble to a grapefruit.

Nonrotation of the Midgut (Fig. 13–8A). This relatively common condition, often called "left-sided colon," is generally asymptomatic, but volvulus (twisting) of the intestines may occur. In nonrotation, the midgut loop does not rotate as it enters the abdomen; as a result, the caudal limb of the loop returns to the

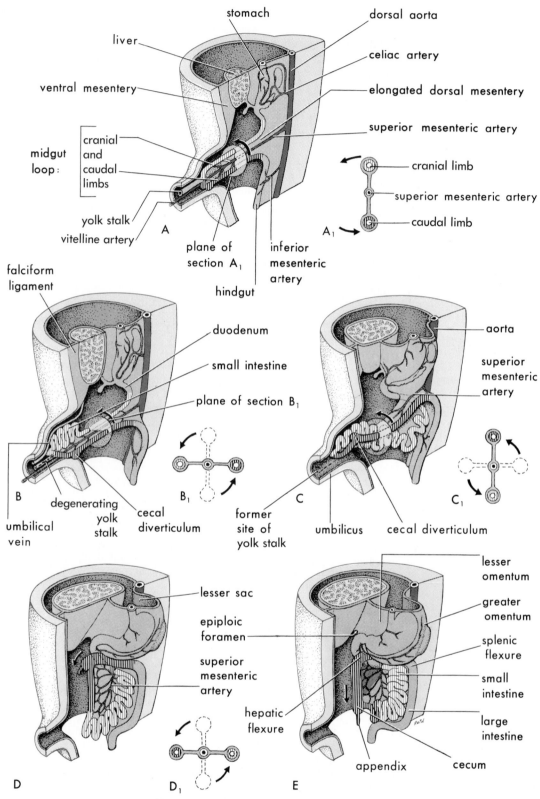

Figure 13–6 *See legend on opposite page*

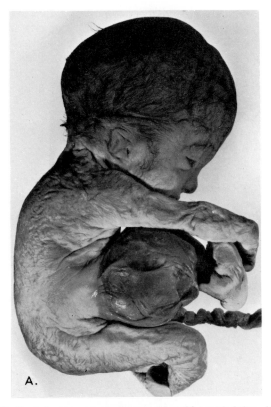

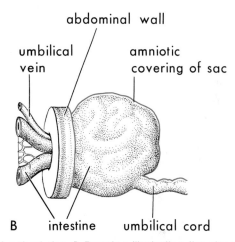

abdominal wall

umbilical
vein

amniotic
covering of sac

B   intestine   umbilical cord

Figure 13–7. *A,* Large omphalocele in a 28-week fetus. *Half actual size. B,* Drawing illustrating the structure and contents of the hernial sac. This condition results when the intestines do not return to the abdominal cavity from the umbilical cord during the tenth week.

abdomen first and the small intestine lies on the right side of the abdomen and the entire large intestine on the left.

When volvulus occurs, the superior mesenteric artery may be obstructed by the twisting. This results in *infarction* and gangrene of the bowel supplied by it.

Mixed Rotation and Volvulus (Fig. 13–8*B*). In this condition, the cecum lies inferior to the pylorus and is fixed to the posterior abdominal wall by peritoneal bands that pass over the duodenum. These bands and the frequent presence of volvulus of the intestines usually cause *duodenal obstruction.* This type of mal-

rotation results from failure of the midgut loop to complete the final 90 degrees of rotation. Consequently, the terminal part of the ileum returns to the abdomen first.

Subhepatic Cecum and Appendix (Fig. 13–8*D*). Failure of the proximal part of the ascending colon to elongate during the third stage of rotation results in the cecum remaining near the liver as the abdomen enlarges. More common in males, this condition occurs in about 6 per cent of fetuses and results in the cecum and appendix being located in the subcostal region, near the inferior surface of the liver. Some

Figure 13–6. Drawings showing rotation of the midgut, as seen from the left. *A,* Beginning of the sixth week, showing the midgut loop partially within the umbilical cord. Note the elongated, double-layered dorsal mesentery containing the superior mesenteric artery. *A₁,* Transverse section through the midgut loop, illustrating the initial relationship of the limbs of the midgut to the artery. *B,* Later stage showing the beginning of midgut rotation. *B₁,* illustrates the 90-degree counterclockwise rotation which carries the cranial limb to the right. *C,* About 10 weeks, showing the intestines returning to the abdomen. *C₁,* illustrates a further rotation of 90 degrees. *D,* Slightly later, following return of intestines to the abdomen. *D₁,* shows there has been a further 90-degree rotation of the gut, making a total of 270 degrees. *E,* Late fetal period, after rotation of the cecum to its normal position and fixation of the gut.

elongation of the colon occurs during childhood; hence, a subhepatic cecum is not common in adults.

Mobile Cecum. In about 10 per cent of people the cecum has an unusual amount of freedom. It may herniate through the right inguinal canal. This condition results from incomplete fixation of the ascending colon.

Midgut Volvulus (Fig. 13–8F). In this condition, the small bowel fails to enter the abdominal cavity normally. As a result, the mesenteries fail to undergo normal fixation. Twisting of the intestine commonly occurs with incomplete rotation of the midgut loop. Because of the twisting of the intestines, *intestinal obstruction* and occlusion of the superior mesenteric artery frequently occur.

Intestinal Stenosis and Atresia (see Fig. 13–4). Narrowing, or stenosis, and complete obstruction, or atresia, of the intestinal lumen occur most often in the duodenum and the ileum. The length of the area affected varies. Failure of an adequate number of vacuoles to form during recanalization leaves a transverse membrane or diaphragm, producing a so-called diaphragmatic atresia.

Most jejunoileal atresias are probably caused by infarction of the fetal bowel as the result of impairment of its blood supply. This probably occurs during the tenth week, when the intestines are returning to the abdomen. Malfixation of the gut predisposes it to strangulation and impairment of its blood supply, owing to *volvulus* (twisting of the gut).

Meckel's Diverticulum (Fig. 13–9). This ileal diverticulum is one of the most common malformations of the digestive tract. It occurs in 2 to 4 per cent of people. This malformation is three to five times more prevalent in males than in females.

A Meckel's diverticulum is of clinical significance

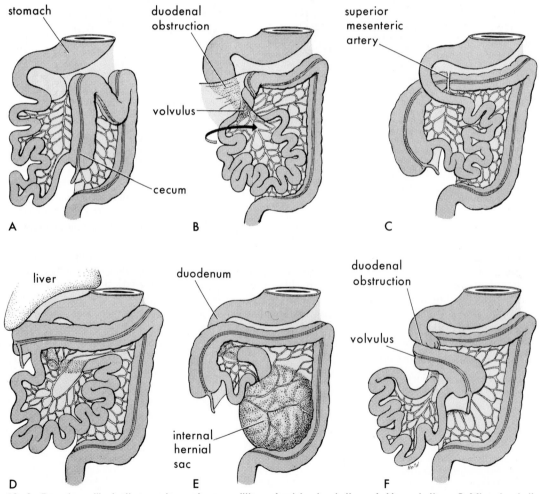

Figure 13–8. Drawings illustrating various abnormalities of midgut rotation. *A*, Nonrotation. *B*, Mixed rotation and volvulus (twisting of the intestines). *C*, Reversed rotation. *D*, Subhepatic cecum. *E*, Paraduodenal hernia. *F*, Midgut volvulus.

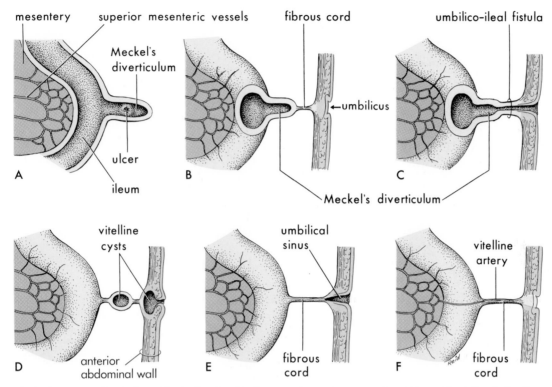

Figure 13–9. Drawings illustrating Meckel's diverticulum and other remnants of the yolk stalk. *A*, Section of the ileum and a Meckel's diverticulum with an ulcer. *B*, Meckel's diverticulum connected to the umbilicus by a fibrous cord. *C*, Umbilico-ileal fistula resulting from persistence of the entire intra-abdominal portion of the yolk stalk. *D*, Vitelline cysts at the umbilicus and in a fibrous remnant of the yolk stalk. *E*, Umbilical sinus resulting from the persistence of the yolk stalk near the umbilicus. The sinus is not always connected to the ileum by a fibrous cord as illustrated. *F*, The yolk stalk has persisted as a fibrous cord connecting the ileum with the umbilicus. A persistent vitelline artery extends along the fibrous cord to the umbilicus.

because it sometimes becomes inflamed and causes symptoms mimicking appendicitis. The wall of the diverticulum contains all layers of the ileum and *may contain gastric and pancreatic tissues.* The gastric mucosa often secretes acid, producing ulceration.

A Meckel's diverticulum represents the *remnant of the proximal portion of the yolk stalk.* Typically, it appears as a finger-like pouch, about 3 to 6 cm long, arising from the antimesenteric border of the ileum 40 to 50 cm from the ileocecal junction. A Meckel's diverticulum may be connected to the umbilicus by a fibrous cord or a fistula (Fig. 13–9C to F).

THE HINDGUT

The hindgut extends from the midgut to the cloacal membrane. This membrane is composed of endoderm of the *cloaca* and ectoderm of the *proctodeum* or anal pit (Fig. 13–10). The expanded terminal part of the hindgut, the *cloaca*, receives the allantois ventrally.

The cloaca is divided by a coronal sheet of mesenchyme, the *urorectal septum,* which develops in the angle between the allantois and the hindgut (Fig. 13–10B). As this septum grows toward the cloacal membrane, infoldings of the lateral walls of the cloaca form (Fig. 13–10B₁). These folds grow toward each other and fuse, dividing the cloaca into two parts: (1) the *rectum and upper anal canal* dorsally, and (2) the *urogenital sinus* ventrally (Fig. 13–10D and F).

By the end of the sixth week, the urorectal septum has fused with the cloacal membrane, dividing it into a dorsal *anal membrane* and a larger ventral *urogenital membrane* (Fig. 13–10E and F). The anal membranes rupture at the end of the seventh week, thus establishing the *anal canal.*

Imperforate Anus and Related Malformations. Some form of imperforate anus occurs once in about 5000 births. Most anorectal malformations result from

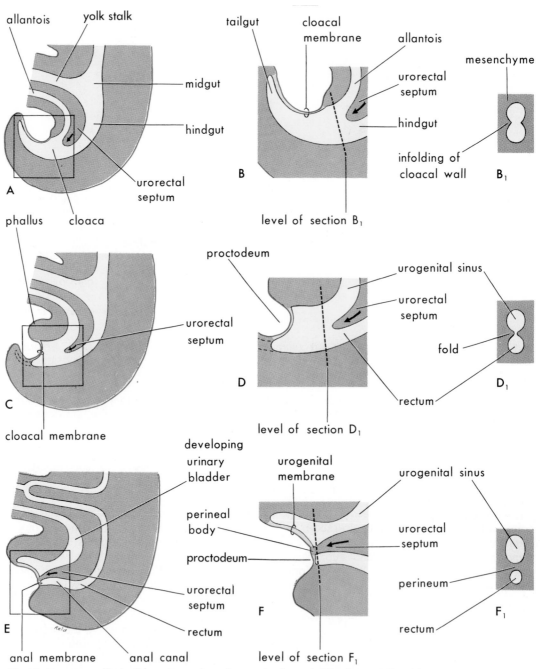

Figure 13–10. Drawings illustrating successive stages in the partitioning of the cloaca into the rectum and urogenital sinus by the urorectal septum. *A, C,* and *E,* Views from the left side at four, six, and seven weeks, respectively. *B, D,* and *F* are enlargements of the cloacal region. *B₁, D₁,* and *F₁* are transverse sections through the cloaca at the levels shown in *B, D,* and *F.*

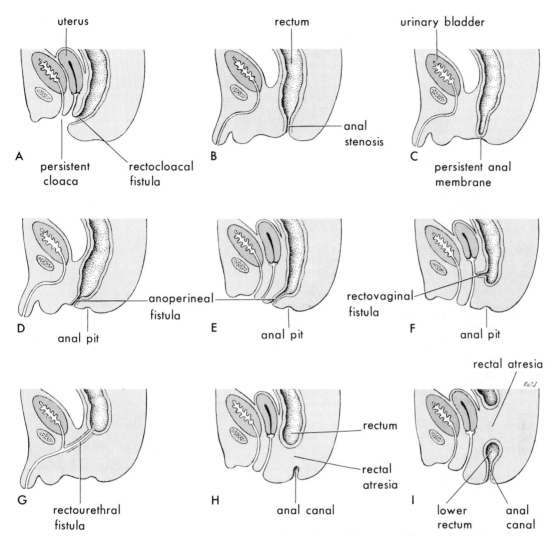

Figure 13–11. Drawings illustrating various anorectal malformations. *A,* Persistent cloaca. Note the common outlet for the intestinal, urinary, and reproductive tracts. This condition usually occurs in females. *B,* Anal stenosis. *C,* Membranous atresia (covered anus). *D* and *E,* Anal agenesis with fistula. *F,* Anorectal agenesis with rectovaginal fistula. *G,* Anorectal agenesis with rectourethral fistula. *F* and *G* are sometimes called persistent cloaca. *H* and *I,* Rectal atresia. Sometimes the two segments of bowel are connected by a fibrous cord.

abnormal development of the urorectal septum, resulting in incomplete separation of the cloaca into urogenital and anorectal portions (Fig. 13–10). If the urorectal septum fails to develop, a *persistent cloaca* results (Fig. 13–11*A*).

Anal Agenesis With or Without Fistula (Fig. 13–11*D* and *E*). The anal canal may end blindly, but more often there is an abnormal opening *(ectopic anus)* or fistula that opens into the perineum. The fistula may, however, open into the vulva in females or into the urethra in males. Anal agenesis with fistula results from incomplete separation of the cloaca by the urorectal septum.

Anal Stenosis (Fig. 13–11*B*). The anus is in the normal position, but the anal canal is narrow. This malformation probably results from a slight dorsal deviation of the urorectal septum as it grows caudally to fuse with the cloacal membrane.

Membranous Atresia of the Anus (Fig. 13–11*C*). The anus is in the normal position, but a thin layer of tissue separates the anal canal from the exterior. This condition results from failure of the anal membrane to perforate at the end of the seventh week.

Anorectal Agenesis With or Without Fistula (Fig. 13–11*F* and *G*). The rectum ends blindly, superior to the anal canal; *this is the most common type of* *anorectal malformation.* Although the rectum may end blindly, there is usually a fistula to the urethra in males or to the vagina in females. Anorectal agenesis has an embryological basis similar to that of anal agenesis, described previously.

Rectal Atresia (Fig. 13–11*H* and *I*). Both the anal canal and rectum are present, but they are separated. Sometimes the atretic segment of rectum is represented by a fibrous cord. The cause of rectal atresia is abnormal recanalization or defective blood supply, as discussed with malformations of the small intestines.

SUMMARY

The *primitive gut* forms during the fourth week by incorporation of the dorsal part of the yolk sac into the embryo. It consists of three parts. The *foregut* gives rise to the pharynx and lower respiratory system, the esophagus, stomach, duodenum (as far as the bile duct), pancreas, liver, and biliary apparatus.

The *midgut* gives rise to the duodenum (distal to the bile duct), jejunum, ileum, cecum, appendix, ascending colon, and right or proximal half to two thirds of the transverse colon.

The midgut herniates into the umbilical cord during the fifth week because of inadequate room in the abdomen. During the tenth week, the intestines return to the abdomen.

Omphalocele, malrotation, and abnormalities of fixation result from failure of or abnormal return of the intestines to the abdomen. Because the gut is normally occluded at one stage, *stenosis* (narrowing), *atresia* (obstruction), and duplications may result if recanalization fails to occur or occurs abnormally. Various remnants of the yolk stalk may persist; *Meckel's diverticulum* is common and is clinically significant.

The *hindgut* gives rise to the left or distal one third to half of the transverse colon, the descending and sigmoid colon, the rectum, and the superior part of the anal canal. The remainder of the anal canal develops from the anal pit or proctodeum. The caudal part of the hindgut is expanded into the *cloaca,* which is divided by the *urorectal septum* into the urogenital sinus and rectum. At first, the rectum is separated from the exterior by the *anal membrane,* but this normally breaks down at the end of the seventh week. Most anorectal malformations arise from abnormal partitioning of the cloaca by the urorectal septum into anorectal and urogenital parts.

Commonly Asked Questions

1. About two weeks after birth, my sister's baby began to vomit shortly after feeding. The unusual thing was that the *vomitus was propelled about two feet.* She was told that the baby had a tumor that resulted in a narrow outlet from its stomach. Is there an embryological basis for this condition, and is the tumor malignant?
2. I have heard that infants with the *Down syndrome* have an increased incidence of *duodenal atresia.* Is this true? Can the condition be corrected?
3. My friend said that his appendix is on his left side. Is this possible, and if so, how could this happen?
4. My father told me about a friend of his who supposedly had two appendices and had had separate operations to remove them. Do people ever have two appendices?
5. What is *Hirschsprung disease?* I have heard that it is a congenital condition resulting from a large bowel obstruction. Is this correct? If so, what is its embryological basis?
6. A nurse friend of mine told me that feces can sometimes be expelled from a baby's umbilicus. She said she has even seen urine dripping from the umbilicus. Was she "pulling my leg"?

Answers

1. Undoubtedly the baby had a condition known as *congenital hypertrophic pyloric stenosis.* There is a diffuse hypertrophy (enlargement) and hyperplasia of the smooth muscle in the pyloric part of the stomach. This produces a mass, sometimes called a tumor. However, it is not a tumor in the usual sense. It is a benign enlargement and is not a malignant tumor. The muscular enlargement causes the exit canal to be narrow, which allows it to become easily obstructed. In response to the outflow obstruction and vigorous peristalsis, the vomiting is projectile, as in the case of your sister's baby. Surgical relief of the pyloric obstruction is the usual treatment. The cause of pyloric stenosis

is not known but is thought to have a *multifactorial inheritance* (see Chapter 9), i.e., genetic and environmental factors are probably involved.

2. It is true that infants with the Down syndrome (see Chapter 9) have an increased incidence of *duodenal atresia*. They are also more likely to have an *imperforate anus* and other congenital malformations (e.g., of the cardiovascular system such

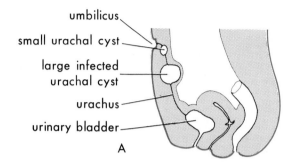

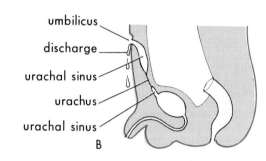

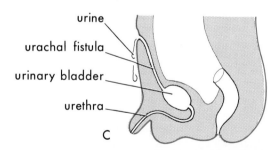

Figure 13–12. Diagrams illustrating malformations of the urachus. *A,* Urachal cysts. The most common site is in the superior end of the urachus, just inferior to the umbilicus. *B,* Two types of urachal sinus are illustrated: one is continuous with the bladder; the other opens at the umbilicus, *C,* Patent urachus or urachal fistula, connecting the bladder and umbilicus.

as *atrial septal defect; see* Chapter 15). These malformations are likely caused by the abnormal chromosome constitution of the infants (i.e., three instead of two chromosomes 21). The atresia can be corrected by bypassing the obstruction through an operation that is called a *duodenoduodenostomy.* Often there are other malformations of the digestive tract such as *anular pancreas,* in which the pancreas surrounds and usually obstructs the duodenum.

3. In very uncommon cases when the intestines return to the abdomen, they rotate in a clockwise direction rather than in the usual counterclockwise manner. As a result, the cecum and appendix are located on the left side. This is called *situs inversus abdominis.* Left-sided cecum and appendix could also result from a condition known as *mobile cecum.* If the cecum does not become fixed to the posterior abdominal wall, it is freely movable and the cecum and appendix could migrate to the left side.

4. Undoubtedly your father's friend had a *Meckel's diverticulum,* a finger-like outpouching of the ileum (see Fig. 13–9). This common malformation is sometimes referred to as a "second appendix," which is a misnomer. Meckel's diverticulum produces symptoms that are similar to those produced by appendicitis. It is also possible that the person had a *duplication of the cecum,* which would result in two appendices.

5. Hirschsprung disease, also known as *congenital megacolon* (Gr. *megas,* big) is the most common cause of obstruction of the colon in newborn infants. The cause of the condition is thought to be *failure of migration of neural crest cells* (see Fig. 17–8) into the wall of the intestine. As these cells form neurons, there is a deficiency of the nerve cells to innervate the muscles in the wall of the bowel. When the wall collapses, obstruction occurs and constipation results in the older child. In newborn infants, signs may be noted early—e.g., failure to pass *meconium* (fetal feces).

6. No, she was not. If the baby had an *umbilical-ileal fistula* (see Fig. 13–9C), the abnormal canal connecting the ileum and the umbilicus could permit the passage of feces from the umbilicus. This occurrence would be an important diagnostic clue to the presence of such a fistula. Urine could also drip from the umbilicus if a *urachal fistula was present* (Fig. 13–12).

14

The Urogenital System

Development of the urinary (excretory) and genital (reproductive) systems is closely associated and parts of one system are used by the other and vice versa.

Both the urinary and genital systems develop from the intermediate mesoderm (see Fig. 5–5B), which extends along the entire length of the dorsal body wall of the embryo. During folding of the embryo in the horizontal plane, the intermediate mesoderm is carried ventrally and loses its connection with the somites. This longitudinal ridge of mesoderm on each side of the primitive aorta in the trunk region is called the *urogenital ridge* (Fig. 14–1D). It gives rise to parts of both the urinary and genital systems. The part of the urogenital ridge giving rise to the urinary system is known as the *nephrogenic cord* (Fig. 14–1D) or nephrogenic ridge, and the part that gives rise to the genital system is known as the *gonadal ridge* or genital ridge (see Fig. 14–9).

Development of the urogenital system is easier to understand if the urinary and genital systems are described separately. Development of the urinary system begins first.

THE URINARY SYSTEM

The urinary system consists of the following structures: (1) the kidneys which excrete urine; (2) the ureters which convey urine to (3) the urinary bladder where it is stored temporarily, and (4) the *urethra* through which the urine is discharged to the exterior.

The Kidney and Ureter

Three successive sets of excretory organs develop in human embryos: the *pronephros,* the *mesonephros,* and the *metanephros.* The third set remains as the permanent kidneys.

The pronephros is a transitory, nonfunctional structure that appears early in the fourth week (Fig. 14–1A). The pronephros soon degenerates, but most of its duct is utilized by the next kidney (Fig. 14–1B).

The mesonephros appears later in the fourth week caudal to the rudimentary pronephros (Fig. 14–1). It may function while the permanent kidney is developing. By the end of the embryonic period, the mesonephros has degenerated and disappeared, except for its duct and a few tubules which persist as genital ducts in males or vestigial remnants in females.

The metanephros becomes the permanent kidney. It appears in the fifth week and begins to function about six weeks later. Urine formation continues actively throughout fetal life. The urine mixes with the amniotic fluid that the fetus drinks. This fluid is absorbed by the intestine, and the waste products pass to the placenta for transfer to the mother's blood and elimination by her kidneys.

The metanephros develops from two sources: the *metanephric diverticulum,* or ureteric bud, and a mass of *metanephric mesoderm* (Fig. 14–2A and B). Both primordia of the permanent kidney are of mesodermal origin.

The metanephric diverticulum is a dorsal bud from the mesonephric duct that grows into the mass of

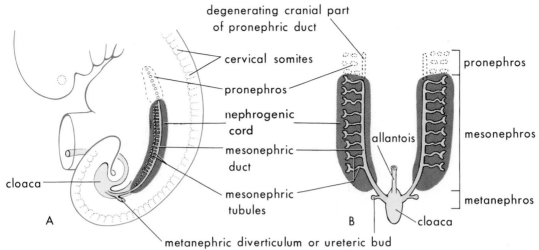

Figure 14–1. Diagrammatic sketches illustrating the three sets of excretory structures present in an embryo during the fifth week. *A,* Lateral view. *B,* Ventral view. The metanephros becomes the permanent kidney. For simplicity, the mesonephric tubules have been pulled out to the sides of the mesonephric ducts. Actually, the tubules lie medial to ducts.

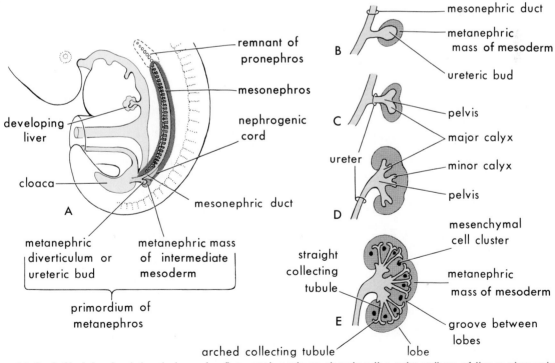

Figure 14–2. *A,* Sketch of a lateral view of a five-week embyro showing the primordium of the metanephros or permanent kidney. *B* to *E,* Sketches showing successive stages in the development of the metanephric diverticulum (fifth to eighth weeks) into the ureter, renal pelvis, calyces, and collecting tubules. The renal lobes illustrated in *E* are visible in the kidneys of newborn infants. The external evidence of the lobes normally disappears by the end of the first year.

metanephric mesoderm (Fig. 14–2B). The stalk of the metanephric diverticulum becomes the ureter, and its expanded cranial end forms the renal pelvis. The pelvis divides into *major* and *minor calyces,* from which collecting tubules soon grow (Fig. 14–2C to E).

Each collecting tubule undergoes repeated branching, forming successive generations of collecting tubules. Near the blind end of each arched collecting tubule (Fig. 14–3A), clusters of mesenchymal cells develop into *metanephric tubules* (Fig. 14–3C). The ends of these tubules are invaginated by an ingrowth of the fine blood vessels, the *glomerulus,* to form a double-layered cup, the *glomerular capsule* (Bowman's capsule). The renal corpuscle (glomerulus and capsule) and its associated tubules form a *nephron.* The distal convoluted tubule of the nephron contacts an arched collecting tubule, and the two tubules become confluent (Fig. 14–3D).

Positional Changes of the Kidney (Fig. 14–4). Initially, the kidneys are in the pelvis, but they gradually come to lie in the abdomen. This migration results mainly from growth of the embryo's body caudal to the kidneys. In effect, the caudal part of the embryo grows away from the kidneys so that they occupy progressively higher levels. Eventually, they come to lie retroperitoneal or exterior to the peritoneum on the posterior abdominal wall.

As the kidneys move out of the pelvis, they are supplied by arteries at successively higher levels. The caudal arteries normally degenerate as the kidneys ascend and new vessels form.

Abnormalities of the Kidneys and Ureters. These abnormalities occur in 3 to 4 per cent of the population and include variations in blood supply, abnormal positions, and urinary tract duplications.

Renal Agenesis (Fig. 14–5A). Unilateral absence of a kidney is relatively common, occurring about once in every 1000 births. *Unilateral renal agenesis* causes no symptoms and is usually not discovered during infancy because the other kidney is able to perform the function of the missing kidney.

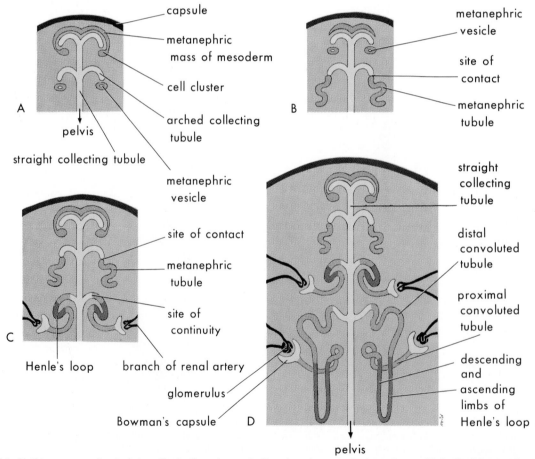

Figure 14–3. Diagrammatic sketches illustrating stages in the development of nephrons. Note that the metanephric tubules, the primordia of the nephrons, become continuous with the collecting tubules to form uriniferous tubules.

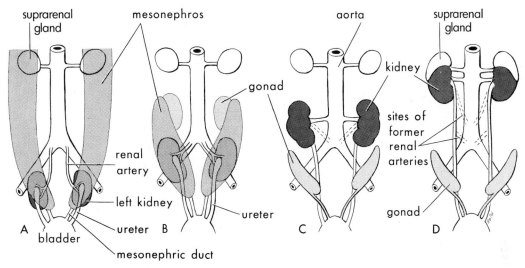

Figure 14–4. Diagrams of ventral views of the abdominopelvic region of embryos and fetuses (sixth to ninth weeks) showing the medial rotation and ascent of the kidneys from the pelvis to the abdomen. Note that as the kidneys ascend, they are supplied by arteries at successively higher levels.

Bilateral renal agenesis is uncommon and is incompatible with postnatal life. Most infants afflicted with this malformation die at birth or a few hours later. Because no urine is excreted into the amniotic fluid, *bilateral renal agenesis is associated with oligohydramnios* (a deficiency in the amount of amniotic fluid).

Renal agenesis results when the metanephric diverticulum fails to develop, or when early degeneration of this ureteric bud occurs. Failure of the metanephric diverticulum to penetrate the metanephric mesoderm results in absence of kidney development because no nephrons are induced by the collecting tubules to develop from the metanephric mesoderm.

Ectopic Kidneys (Fig. 14–5*B* and *E*). One or both kidneys may be in an abnormal position. They are lower than usual and malrotated. Most ectopic kidneys are located in the pelvis, but some are in the inferior part of the abdomen.

Pelvic kidney and other forms of ectopic kidney result from failure of the kidneys to "ascend." Pelvic kidneys may fuse to form a round mass known as a *discoid or pancake kidney* (Fig. 14–5*E*). Ectopic kidneys receive their blood supply from blood vessels near them; they are often supplied by multiple vessels.

An unusual type of ectopic kidney is a *unilateral fused kidney* (Fig. 14–5*D*). The developing kidneys fuse while in the pelvis, and one kidney "ascends" to its normal position, carrying the other one with it across the median plane.

Horseshoe Kidney (Fig. 14–6). In 1 in about 600 persons, the kidneys are fused in the median plane; usually it is the inferior poles that are fused.

The large U-shaped kidney usually lies in the hypogastrium at the level of the inferior lumbar vertebrae, because normal ascent was prevented by the root of the inferior mesenteric artery.

Horseshoe kidney usually produces no symptoms because the collecting system commonly develops normally and the ureters enter the bladder normally. If urinary outflow is impeded, signs and symptoms of obstruction and/or infection may appear.

Multiple Renal Vessels. Variations in the number of renal arteries and in their position with respect to the renal veins are common. About 25 per cent of kidneys have two or more renal arteries. Supernumerary arteries, usually two or three, are about twice as common as supernumerary veins, and they usually arise at the level of the kidney.

Accessory vessels may arise from the suprarenal artery and pass to the superior pole of the kidney. Polar vessels may also arise from the aorta and pass to the inferior pole of the kidney. Sometimes an accessory renal artery supplying the inferior pole of the kidney compresses and obstructs the ureter at the ureteropelvic junction.

Variations in the blood supply of the kidneys are most common in ectopic kidneys. As the kidney moves out of the pelvis, it is supplied by successively higher vessels, and the lower vessels normally degenerate (see Fig. 14–4).

Vascular variations result from persistence of embryonic vessels that normally disappear when the definitive renal arteries form.

Duplications of the Upper Urinary Tract (Fig. 14–5). Duplications of the abdominal part of the ureter and renal pelvis are common, but a supernumerary kidney is uncommon. These abnormalities result from division of the metanephric diverticulum

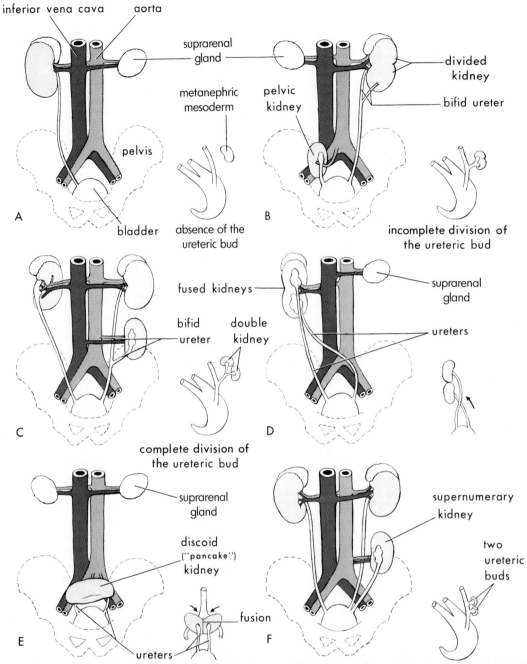

Figure 14–5. Drawings illustrating various congenital abnormalities of the urinary system. The small sketch to the lower right of each drawing illustrates the probable embryological basis of the malformation. *A*, Unilateral renal agenesis. *B*, Right side, pelvic kidney; left side, bifid ureter. *C*, Right side, malrotation of the kidney; left side, bifid ureter and two kidneys. *D*, Crossed renal ectopia. The left kidney crossed to the right side and fused with the right kidney. *E*, "Pancake" or discoid kidney resulting from fusion of the unascended kidneys. *F*, Supernumerary left kidney resulting from the development of two ureteric buds.

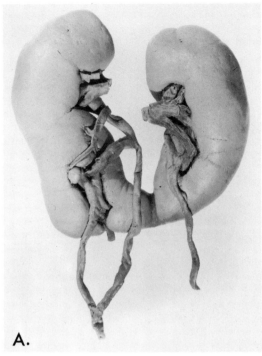
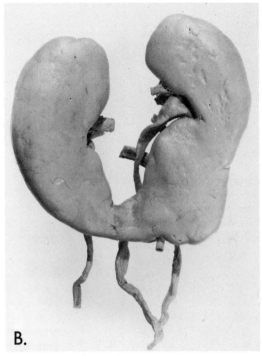

Figure 14–6. Photographs of a horseshoe kidney resulting from fusion of the inferior poles of the kidneys early in development. *A,* Anterior view. *B,* Posterior view. *Half actual size.* The larger right kidney has a bifid ureter. Horseshoe kidney develops in one of 600 persons and is asymptomatic unless urinary outflow is obstructed.

(ureteric bud). The extent of ureteral duplication depends on how complete the division of the diverticulum is. Incomplete division of the diverticulum results in a divided kidney with a bifid ureter (Fig. 14–5*B*). Complete division of the diverticulum results in a supernumerary, or double, kidney with a bifid ureter (Fig. 14–5) or with separate ureters. A supernumerary kidney with its own ureter probably results from the formation of an extra ureteric bud (Fig. 14–5*F*).

The Bladder and Urethra

Division of the cloaca by the *urorectal septum* into a dorsal rectum and a ventral urogenital sinus is described in Chapter 13 and illustrated in Figure 14–7.

The urinary bladder and urethra are derived from the urogenital sinus and from the adjacent splanchnic mesenchyme. As the bladder enlarges, the caudal portions of the mesonephric ducts are incorporated into its dorsal wall (Fig. 14–7*D*). As the mesonephric ducts are absorbed, the ureters come to open separately into the urinary bladder (Fig. 14–7*F*).

Exstrophy of the Bladder (Fig. 14–8). Fortunately, this severe malformation occurs only about once in every 50,000 births.

Exposure and protrusion of the posterior wall of the urinary bladder characterize this congenital mal-

formation, which occurs chiefly in males. The trigone of the bladder and the ureteric orifices are exposed, and urine dribbles intermittently from the everted bladder.

Epispadias (see Fig. 14–16*D*) and wide separation of the pubic bones are associated with complete exstrophy of the bladder. In some cases, the penis or clitoris is divided and the halves of the scrotum or labia majora are widely separated.

Exstrophy of the bladder is caused by incomplete median closure of the inferior part of the anterior abdominal wall. The fissure involves not only the anterior abdominal wall but also the anterior wall of the urinary bladder. The defective closure results from failure of mesenchymal cells to migrate between the surface ectoderm and the urogenital sinus during the fourth week. As a result, no muscle and connective tissue form in the anterior abdominal wall over the urinary bladder. Later, the thin epidermis and the anterior wall of the bladder rupture, causing a wide communication between the exterior and the mucous membrane of the bladder, as shown in Figure 14–8.

THE SUPRARENAL GLANDS

The cortex and medulla of the suprarenal glands (adrenal glands) have different origins. The *cortex*

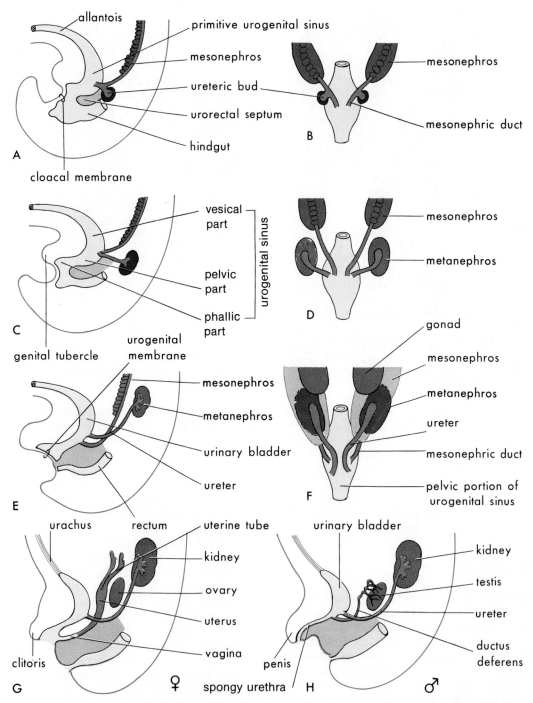

Figure 14–7. Diagrams showing (1) division of the cloaca into the urogenital sinus and rectum, (2) absorption of the mesonephric ducts, (3) development of the urinary bladder, urethra, and urachus, and (4) changes in the location of the ureters. *A,* Lateral view of the caudal half of a five-week embryo. *B, D,* and *F,* Dorsal views. *C, E, G,* and *H,* Lateral views. The stages shown in *G* and *H* are reached by 12 weeks.

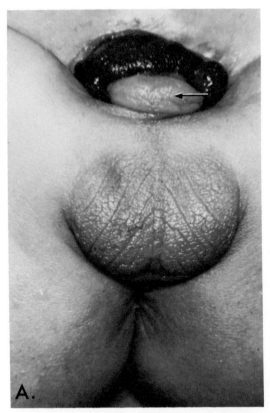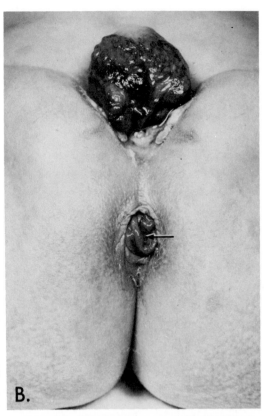

Figure 14–8. Photographs of infants with exstrophy of the urinary bladder. Because of defective closure of the inferior portion of the anterior abdominal wall and the anterior wall of the bladder, the bladder appears as an everted bulging mass inferior to the umbilicus. *A*, Male. Epispadias is also present and the penis (arrow) is small and flattened. (Courtesy of Dr. Colin C. Ferguson, Children's Centre, Winnipeg, Canada.) *B*, Female. The arrow indicates a slight prolapse of the rectum. (Courtesy of Mr. Innes Williams, Genitourinary Surgeon, The Hospital for Sick Children, Great Ormond Street, London, England.)

develops from mesoderm and the medulla from neural crest cells. The cells that form the medulla are derived from the neural crest which appears as the neural tube forms (see Chapters 5 and 17). The cells that form the *suprarenal cortex* are derived from the coelomic epithelium lining the posterior abdominal wall: During the fifth week, cells migrate from adjacent sympathetic ganglia and form a mass on the medial side of the fetal cortex (Fig. 14–9C). These cells are gradually encapsulated by the fetal cortex as they differentiate into the *secretory cells* of the suprarenal medulla (Fig. 14–9D). Differentiation of the characteristic suprarenal cortical zones begins during the late fetal period but is not complete until the end of the third year.

Hyperplasia of the fetal suprarenal cortex during the fetal period usually results in female pseudohermaphroditism (see Fig. 14–15). The adrenogenital syndrome associated with congenital suprarenal or adrenal hyperplasia manifests itself in various clinical forms. *Congenital hyperplasia of the suprarenal glands* is caused by a genetically determined deficiency of suprarenal cortical enzymes that are necessary for the synthesis of various steroid hormones. The reduced hormone output results in an increased release of ACTH, which causes suprarenal hyperplasia and overproduction of androgens by the hyperplastic suprarenal glands. In females, this causes masculinization. In males, the excess androgens may cause precocious sexual development.

THE GENITAL SYSTEM

Although the genetic sex of an embryo is determined at fertilization by the kind of sperm that fertilizes the ovum (see Chapter 3), there is no morphological indication of a sex difference until the seventh week, when the *gonads* (future ovaries or testes) begin to acquire sexual characteristics.

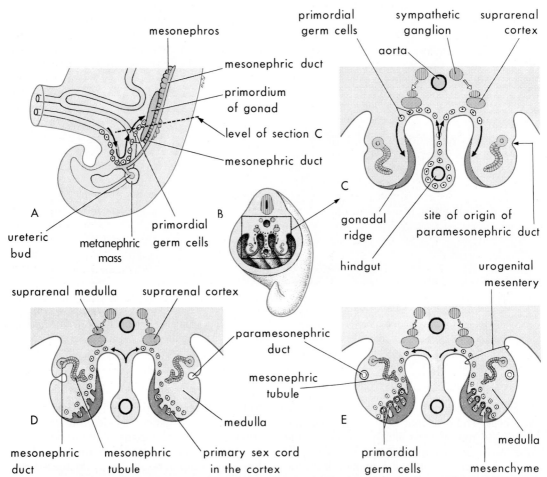

Figure 14–9. *A,* Sketch of five-week embryo illustrating the migration of primordial germ cells from the yolk sac. *B,* Three-dimensional sketch of the caudal region of a five-week embryo showing the location and extent of the gonadal ridges on the medial aspect of the urogenital ridges. *C,* Transverse section showing the primordium of the suprarenal glands, the gonadal ridges, and the migration of primordial germ cells into the developing gonads (ovaries or testes). *D,* Transverse section through a six-week embryo showing the primary sex cords and the developing paramesonephric ducts. *E,* Similar section at later stage showing the indifferent gonads and the mesonephric and paramesonephric ducts.

The early genital system is similar in both sexes.
This period of early genital development is referred
to as the *indifferent stage* of the reproductive organs.

Development of Testes and Ovaries

The gonads (testes and ovaries) are derived from
three sources: the *coelomic epithelium,* the underlying
mesenchyme, and the *primordial germ cells.*

The Indifferent Gonads (Figs. 14–9 and 14–10A).
The gonads are first indicated during the fifth week,
when a thickened area of coelomic epithelium develops on the medial aspect of the mesonephros. Proliferation of these epithelial cells soon produces a bulge
on the medial side of each mesonephros known as
the *gonadal ridge.*

Finger-like epithelial cords, called *primary sex cords,*
soon grow from the gonadal ridges into the underlying
mesenchyme (Fig. 14–9D). The indifferent gonad
now consists of an outer *cortex* and an inner *medulla.*

In embryos with an XX sex chromosome complex,
the cortex normally differentiates into an ovary, and
the medulla regresses. In embryos with an XY sex
chromosome complex, the medulla normally differentiates into a testis, and the cortex regresses.

Large spherical primitive sex cells, called *primordial
germ cells,* are visible early in the fourth week on the
wall of the yolk sac. These cells later migrate along
the dorsal mesentery of the hindgut to the gonadal
ridges (Fig. 14–9), and become incorporated in the
primary sex cords.

Sex Determination. *Genetic sex* is established at
fertilization and depends upon whether an X-bearing
sperm or a Y-bearing sperm fertilizes the ovum.
Gonadal sex is determined by the sex chromosome
complex (XX or XY) that is present.

*The Y chromosome has a strong testis-determining
effect on the medulla of the indifferent gonad.* It is
the presence of the *H-Y antigen gene* on the Y
chromosome that determines testicular differentiation.
Under its influence, the primary sex cords differentiate
into seminiferous tubules (Fig. 14–10B and D).

The absence of a Y chromosome results in formation of an ovary (Fig. 14–10C and E). Thus, the type
of sex chromosome complex established at fertilization
determines the type of gonad that develops from the
indifferent gonad.

Development of Testes (Fig. 14–10B, D, and F).
In embryos with a Y chromosome, the primary sex
cords condense and branch. Their ends anastomose
to form the *rete testis.* The sex cords, now called
seminiferous cords, lose their connections with the
germinal epithelium as the thick fibrous capsule called
the *tunica albuginea* develops (Fig. 14–10B and D).

The seminiferous cords develop into the *seminiferous tubules, tubuli recti,* and *rete testis.* The walls of
the seminiferous tubules are composed of two kinds
of cells (Fig. 14–10F): supporting or *sustentacular
cells* (of Sertoli), derived from the surface epithelium,
and *spermatogonia,* derived from the primordial germ
cells.

The seminiferous tubules become separated by
mesenchyme that gives rise to the *interstitial cells* (of
Leydig). These cells produce the male sex hormone
testosterone, which induces masculine differentiation
of the external genitalia. In addition to testosterone,
genital duct inducer and suppressor substances are
produced by the interstitial cells. As described subsequently, these substances induce development of the
mesonephric ducts and suppress development of the
paramesonephric ducts (see Fig. 14–11).

Development of Ovaries (Fig. 14–10C, E and G).
In embryos lacking a Y chromosome, gonadal development occurs very slowly. The ovary is not identifiable until about the tenth week. Thereafter the characteristic cortex begins to develop. The primary sex
cords do not become prominent in the gonads of
female embryos. The rete ovarii, comparable to the
rete testis, is a transitory remnant of these cords.

During the fetal period, secondary sex cords, called
cortical cords, extend from the surface epithelium into
the underlying mesenchyme (Fig. 14–10C). As these
cords increase in size, *primordial germ cells* are incorporated into them. The cords break up into isolated
cell clusters called *primordial follicles,* consisting of
oogonia derived from primordial germ cells, surrounded by a layer of follicular cells (Fig. 14–10E and
G). Active mitosis of oogonia occurs during fetal life,
producing thousands of these primitive germ cells.

No oogonia form postnatally. All oogonia enlarge
and become *primary oocytes* before birth (see Fig.
2–5).

Development of the Genital Ducts

The Indifferent Stage (Figs. 14–9 and 14–11).
Two pairs of genital ducts develop in both sexes:
mesonephric ducts and *paramesonephric ducts.* The
paramesonephric ducts come together in the median
plane in both sexes and fuse into a Y-shaped *uterovaginal primordium* or canal (Fig. 14–11A). The
funnel-shaped openings of the ducts open into the
coelomic cavity (future peritoneal cavity). The uterovaginal primordium projects into the dorsal wall of
the urogenital sinus and produces an elevation, called
the *sinus tubercle* (Fig. 14–11B).

The fetal testes produce two hormones: a *masculinizing hormone* (testosterone) and a *müllerian inhibit-*

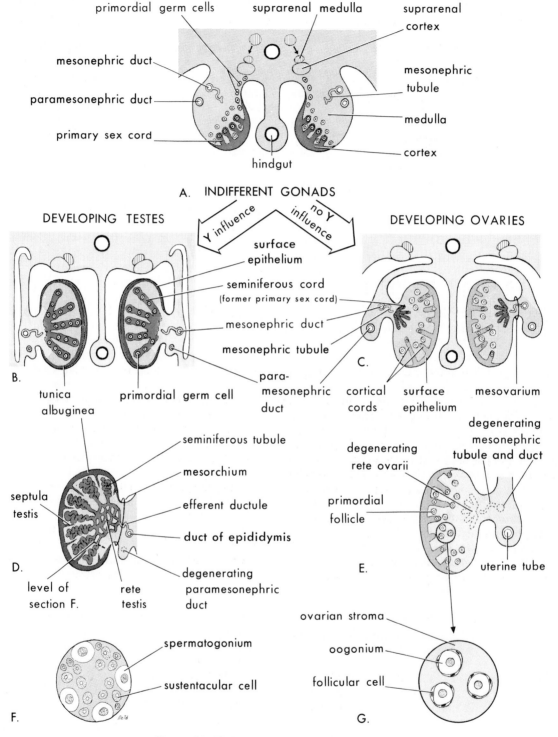

primordial germ cells

suprarenal medulla

suprarenal cortex

mesonephric duct

paramesonephric duct

primary sex cord

mesonephric tubule

medulla

cortex

hindgut

A. INDIFFERENT GONADS

Y influence

no Y influence

DEVELOPING TESTES

DEVELOPING OVARIES

surface epithelium

seminiferous cord (former primary sex cord)

mesonephric duct

mesonephric tubule

para-mesonephric duct

B.

tunica albuginea

primordial germ cell

C.

cortical cords

surface epithelium

mesovarium

seminiferous tubule

mesorchium

efferent ductule

duct of epididymis

degenerating paramesonephric duct

septula testis

degenerating rete ovarii

primordial follicle

degenerating mesonephric tubule and duct

D.

level of section F.

rete testis

E.

uterine tube

spermatogonium

sustentacular cell

ovarian stroma

oogonium

follicular cell

F.

G.

Figure 14–10 *See legend on opposite page*

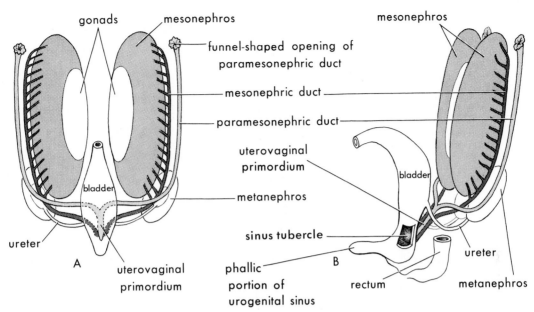

Figure 14–11. *A,* Sketch of a frontal view of the posterior abdominal wall of a seven-week embryo showing the two pairs of genital ducts present during the indifferent stage. *B,* Lateral view of a nine-week fetus showing the sinus tubercle on the posterior wall of the urogenital sinus. It becomes the hymen in females and the seminal colliculus, or urethral crest, in males. This colliculus (L. mound) is an elevated area on the posterior wall of the prostatic portion of the urethra upon which open the ejaculatory ducts.

ing substance. The testosterone, produced by the interstitial cells, stimulates development of the mesonephric ducts into the male genital tract, and the müllerian inhibiting substance, produced by the sustentacular cells, suppresses development of the paramesonephric ducts (formerly called müllerian ducts) which develop into female ducts in female fetuses.

Development of the Male Genital Ducts. When the mesonephros degenerates, some mesonephric tubules near the testis persist and are transformed into *efferent ductules* (Fig. 14–12A). These ductules open into the mesonephric duct which becomes the *ductus epididymidis* or *duct of the epididymis* in this region. Beyond the *epididymis* (coiled duct of the epididymis), the mesonephric duct acquires a thick investment of smooth muscle and becomes the *ductus deferens* (vas deferens).

A lateral outgrowth from the caudal end of each mesonephric duct gives rise to a *seminal vesicle.* The part of the mesonephric duct between the duct of this gland and the urethra becomes the *ejaculatory duct.* The remainder of the male genital duct system is formed by the urethra.

The Prostate Gland (Fig. 14–12A). Multiple endodermal outgrowths arise from the prostatic portion of the urethra and grow into the surrounding mesenchyme. The glandular epithelium of the prostate differentiates from the endodermal cells, and the associated mesenchyme differentiates into the stroma and smooth muscle fibers of the prostate.

Figure 14–10. Schematic sections illustrating differentiation of the indifferent gonads into testes or ovaries. *A,* Six weeks, showing the indifferent gonads composed of an outer cortex and an inner medulla. *B,* Seven weeks, showing testes developing under the influence of a Y chromosome. Note that the primary sex cords have become seminiferous cords. *C,* 12 weeks, showing ovaries beginning to develop. Cortical cords have extended from the surface epithelium, displacing the primary sex cords centrally into the mesovarium, where they form the rudimentary rete ovarii. *D,* Testis at 20 weeks, showing the rete testis and the seminiferous tubules derived from the seminiferous cords. An efferent ductule has developed from a mesonephric tubule, and the mesonephric duct has become the ductus epididymidis (duct of the epididymis). *E,* Ovary at 20 weeks, showing the primordial follicles formed from the cortical cords. *F,* Section of a seminiferous tubule from a 20-week fetus. Note that no lumen is present at this stage and that the seminiferous epithelium is composed of two kinds of cells. *G,* Section from the ovarian cortex of a 20-week fetus showing three primordial follicles.

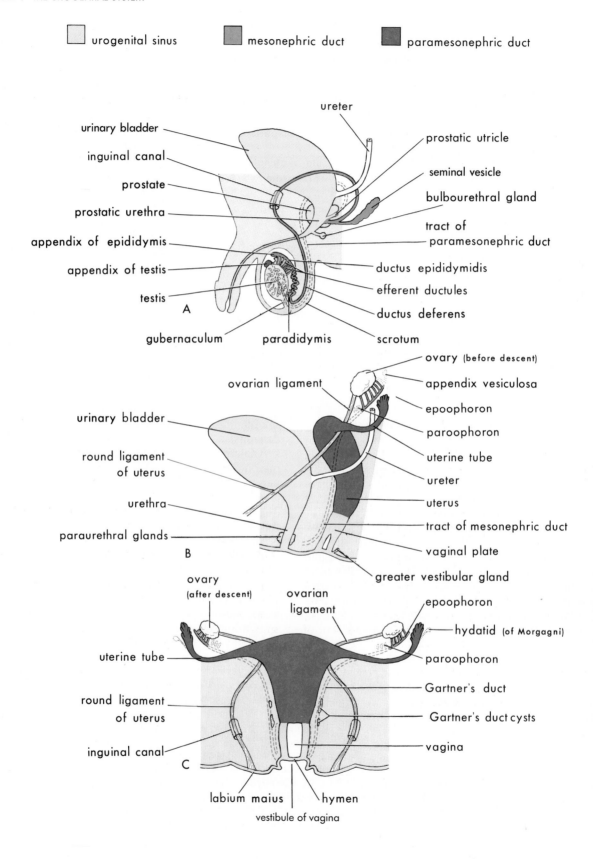

☐ urogenital sinus   ■ mesonephric duct   ■ paramesonephric duct

urinary bladder
inguinal canal
prostate
prostatic urethra
appendix of epididymis
appendix of testis
testis

ureter
prostatic utricle
seminal vesicle
bulbourethral gland
tract of paramesonephric duct
ductus epididymidis
efferent ductules
ductus deferens

gubernaculum   paradidymis   scrotum

A

ovarian ligament

urinary bladder
round ligament of uterus
urethra
paraurethral glands

ovary (before descent)
appendix vesiculosa
epoophoron
paroophoron
uterine tube
ureter
uterus
tract of mesonephric duct
vaginal plate
greater vestibular gland

B

ovary (after descent)   ovarian ligament   epoophoron

uterine tube
round ligament of uterus
inguinal canal

hydatid (of Morgagni)
paroophoron
Gartner's duct
Gartner's duct cysts
vagina

labium maius   hymen

vestibule of vagina

C

The Bulbourethral Glands (Fig. 14–12A). These pea-sized structures develop from paired endodermal outgrowths from the spongy portion of the urethra. Their smooth muscle fibers and stroma differentiate from the adjacent mesenchyme.

Development of the Female Genital Ducts. In female embryos, the mesonephric ducts regress and the paramesonephric ducts develop into the female genital tract. The cranial unfused portions of the paramesonephric ducts develop into the uterine tubes, and the fused portions, called the *uterovaginal primordium,* or uterovaginal canal, give rise to the epithelium and glands of the uterus (Fig. 14–12B and C). The endometrial stroma and the myometrium are derived from the adjacent mesenchyme.

Although testes are essential for the stimulation of male sexual development, female sexual development does not depend on the presence of ovaries. Hence, embryos without gonads (ovaries or testes) develop as females.

Development of the Vagina. The vaginal epithelium is derived from the endoderm of the urogenital sinus (see Fig. 11–7). The fibromuscular wall of the vagina develops from the surrounding mesenchyme. A solid cord of endodermal cells called the *vaginal plate* forms, and then the central cells break down, forming the lumen of the vagina. The peripheral cells remain as the vaginal epithelium (Fig. 14–12C).

Until late fetal life, the lumen of the vagina is separated from the vestibule of the vagina by a membrane called the *hymen* (Figs. 14–12C and 14–13H). The hymen usually ruptures during the perinatal period and remains as a thin fold of mucous membrane around the entrance to the vagina.

Vestigial Structures Derived From the Embryonic Genital Ducts (Fig. 14–12). During conversion of the mesonephric and paramesonephric ducts into adult structures, some parts of them may remain as vestigial structures (e.g., the appendix of the testis and the epoophoron). These vestiges are rarely seen unless pathological changes develop in them.

Auxiliary Female Genital Glands. Buds grow out from the urethra into the surrounding mesenchyme and form the *urethral glands* and the *paraurethral glands.* These glands correspond to the prostate gland in the male. Similar outgrowths from the urogenital sinus form the *greater vestibular glands,* which are homologous with the bulbourethral glands in the male.

Descent of the Testes. Inguinal canals develop and later form pathways for the testes to descend through the abdominal wall into the scrotum. Inguinal canals also develop in female embryos even though the ovaries do not descend through them. Descent of the testes through the inguinal canals usually begins during the twenty-eighth week and takes about three days. About four weeks later, the testes enter the scrotum and the inguinal canals contract.

Undescended Testes. This condition occurs in about 3 per cent of full-term male infants. A cryptorchid or undescended testis may be located in the abdominal cavity or anywhere along the usual path of descent of the testis; usually it lies in the inguinal canal. The cause of most cases of cryptorchidism is unknown, but failure of normal androgen production appears to be a factor.

Development of the External Genitalia

The Indifferent Stage (Fig. 14–13A and B). The external genitalia also pass through a stage that is not distinguishable as male or female. Early in the fourth week, a *genital tubercle* develops ventral to the cloacal membrane, and *labioscrotal swellings* and *urogenital folds* develop on each side of the cloacal membrane. The genital tubercle soon elongates and is called a *phallus;* initially it is as large in females as in males. A *urethral groove* forms on the ventral surface of the phallus (Fig. 14–13C and D).

Although external sexual characteristics begin to appear during the early fetal period, the external genitalia of males and females appear somewhat similar until the end of the ninth week. The final form is not established until the twelfth week (Fig. 14–13G and H).

Development of Male External Genitalia (Fig. 14–13C, E, and G). Masculinization of the indifferent external genitalia is caused by androgens produced by the fetal testes.

As the phallus elongates to form a *penis,* the urogenital folds fuse with each other along the ventral surface of the penis to form the *spongy urethra* (penile urethra). As a result, the external urethral orifice moves to the *glans penis.*

The *labioscrotal swellings* grow toward each other and fuse to form the *scrotum.*

Figure 14–12. Schematic drawings illustrating development of the male and female reproductive systems from the primitive genital ducts. Vestigial structures (paradidymis, paroophoron, appendix of testis, appendix of epididymis, Gartner's duct, hydatid of Morgagni) are also shown. A, Reproductive system in a newborn male. B, Female reproductive system in a 12-week fetus. C, Reproductive system in a newborn female.

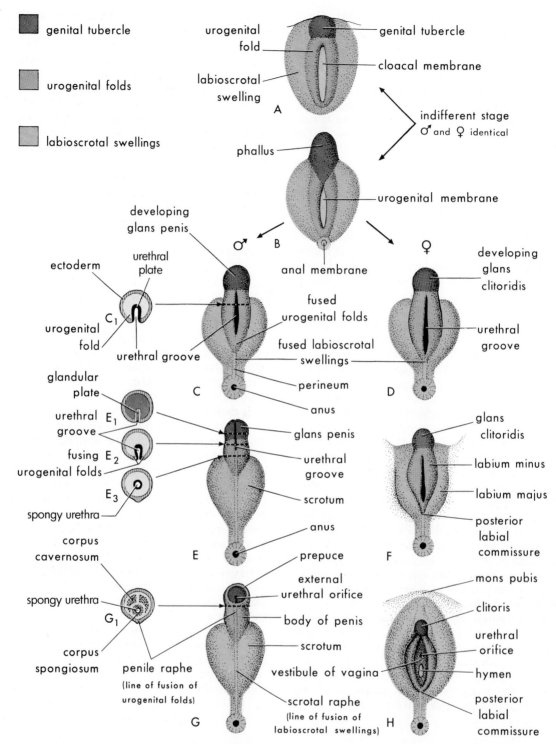

Figure 14–13. *A* and *B,* Diagrams illustrating development of the external genitalia during the indifferent stage (four to seven weeks). *C, E,* and *G,* Stages in the development of male external genitalia at about 9, 11, and 12 weeks, respectively. To the left are schematic transverse sections (*C₁, E₁* to *E₃,* and *G₁*) through the developing penis illustrating formation of the spongy urethra. *D, F,* and *H,* Stages in the development of female external genitalia at 9, 11, and 12 weeks, respectively.

Development of Female External Genitalia (Fig. 14–13D, F, and H). Feminization of the indifferent external genitalia occurs in the absence of hormones. The phallus becomes a relatively small *clitoris* which develops like the penis except that the urogenital folds do not fuse. The unfused urogenital folds form the *labia minora* and the unfused labioscrotal folds form the *labia majora*.

Intersexuality

Because an early embryo has the potential to develop as either a male or a female, errors in sex development may result in various degrees of intermediate sex, a condition known as *intersexuality* or *hermaphroditism*. A person with ambiguous external genitalia is called a hermaphrodite or *intersex*.

Intersexual conditions are classified according to the histological appearance of the gonads. *True hermaphrodites* have both ovarian and testicular tissue. Some *pseudohermaphrodites* have testes and are called male pseudohermaphrodites; others have ovaries and are known as female pseudohermaphrodites.

True Hermaphrodites. Persons with this *extremely rare condition* usually have a 46,XX chromosome constitution. Both ovarian and testicular tissues are present, either in the same or in opposite gonads. The physical appearance may be male or female but the external genitalia are usually ambiguous. This condition results from an error in sex determination.

Male Pseudohermaphrodites. These persons have a 46,XY chromosome constitution. The external and internal genitalia are intersexual and variable, resulting from varying degrees of development of the external genitalia and genital ducts. Either an inadequate amount of androgenic hormones is produced, or they are formed after the period of maximum tissue sensitivity of the sexual structures has passed.

Testicular Feminization (Fig. 14–14). Persons with this uncommon condition, related to intersexuality, appear as normal females despite the presence of testes and XY sex chromosomes. Normal breast development occurs at puberty. The vagina usually ends blindly and the other internal genitalia are absent or rudimentary. The testes are usually in the inguinal canals, but they may descend into the labia majora. *The psychosexual orientation of these women is entirely female.* Medically, legally, and socially, these persons are females.

Embryologically, these females represent an extreme form of male pseudohermaphroditism, but they are not regarded as intersexes because they have normal feminine external genitalia. Although testes develop and secrete androgens, masculinization of the genitalia fails to occur apparently because the indifferent external genitalia were insensitive to androgens.

Female Pseudohermaphrodites. These persons have a 46,XX chromosome constitution. The most common cause of female pseudohermaphroditism is the *adrenogenital syndrome,* resulting from congenital virilizing suprarenal hyperplasia (Fig. 14–15). There is no ovarian abnormality, but the excessive production of androgens by the fetal suprarenal glands causes masculinization of the external genitalia, varying from enlargement of the clitoris to almost masculine genitalia (Fig. 14–15C). Commonly, there is clitoral hypertrophy and partial fusion of the labia majora.

Persons with this virilizing syndrome are the most frequently encountered group of intersexes, accounting for about half of all cases of ambiguous external genitalia.

Prompt recognition and treatment of the associated suprarenal or adrenal imbalance are most important. Congenital virilizing suprarenal hyperplasia is caused by recessive mutant genes.

Female pseudohermaphrodites who do not have congenital virilizing suprarenal hyperplasia are uncommon. The administration of androgenic hormones to a mother during pregnancy can cause these abnormalities of the female external genitalia (see Fig. 9–14).

Hypospadias (Fig. 14–16A to C). Once in about every 300 male infants, the external urethral orifice is on the ventral surface of the penis instead of at the tip of the glans. Usually the penis is curved downward or ventrally, a condition known as *chordee.*

There are four types of hypospadias: *glandular, penile, penoscrotal,* and *perineal.* The glandular and penile types constitute about 80 per cent of cases.

Hypospadias results from an inadequate production of androgens by the fetal testes; this causes failure of fusion of the urogenital folds. Differences in the timing and degree of hormonal failure account for the various types of hypospadias.

Epispadias (Fig. 14–16D). Once in about 30,000 male infants, the urethra opens on the dorsal surface of the penis. Although epispadias may occur as a separate entity, it is *often associated with exstrophy of the bladder* (see Fig. 14–8) and has a similar cause.

Uterovaginal Malformations (Fig. 14–17). Various types of uterine duplication result from failure of the paramesonephric ducts to fuse normally.

Double uterus results from failure of fusion of the caudal parts of the paramesonephric ducts and may be associated with a double or a single vagina (Fig. 14–17A and B). If the doubling involves only the superior portion of the body of the uterus, the condition is called *bicornuate (double-horned) uterus* (Fig. 14–17C and D). In some cases, the uterus is divided internally by a thin septum (Fig. 14–17E).

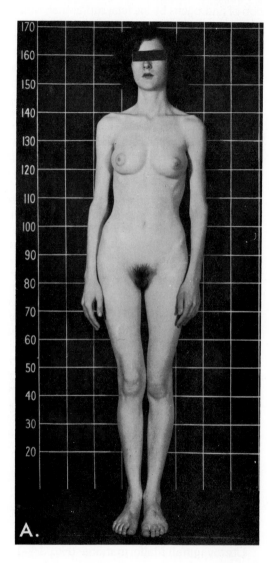

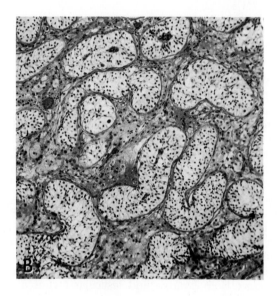

Figure 14–14. *A,* Photograph of a 17-year-old female with testicular feminization. *B,* Photomicrograph of a section through a testis removed from the inguinal region of this woman showing seminiferous tubules. There are no germ cells. (From Jones, W. W., and Scott, W. W.: *Hermaphroditism, Genital Anomalies* and *Related Endocrine Disorders.* Baltimore, Williams & Wilkins Company, 1958.)

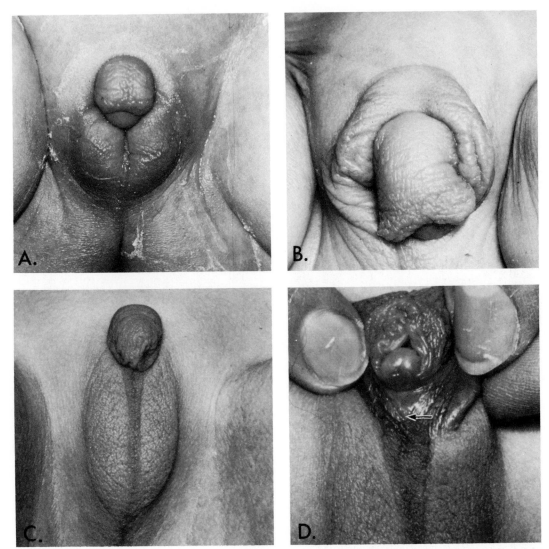

Figure 14–15. Photographs of the external genitalia of female pseudohermaphrodites resulting from congenital virilizing suprarenal or adrenal hyperplasia. *A,* External genitalia of a newborn female, exhibiting enlargement of the clitoris and fusion of the labia majora. *B,* External genitalia of a female infant, showing considerable enlargement of the clitoris. The labia majora have partially fused to form a scrotum-like structure. *C* and *D,* External genitalia of this six-year-old girl showing the enlarged clitoris and fused labia majora. In *D,* note the glans clitoridis and the opening of the urogenital sinus (arrow).

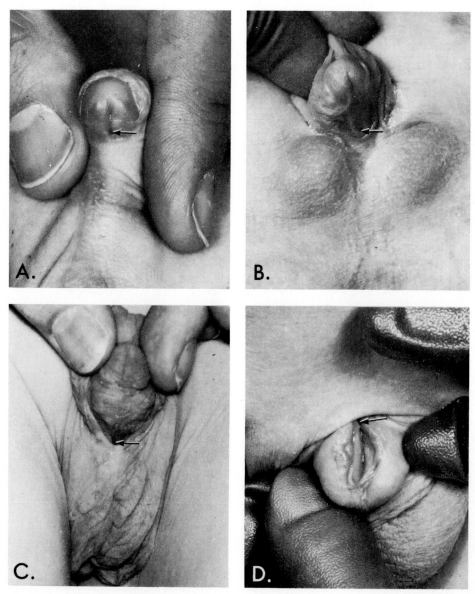

Figure 14–16. Photographs of penile malformations. *A*, Glandular hypospadias. This is the most common form of hypospadias. The external urethral orifice is indicated by the arrow. There is a shallow pit at the usual site of the orifice. Note the moderate degree of chordee causing the penis to curve ventrally. (From Jolly, H.: *Diseases of Children, 2nd ed.* Oxford, Blackwell Scientific Publications, 1968.) *B*, Penile hypospadias. The penis is short and curved (chordee). The external urethral orifice (arrow) is near the penoscrotal junction. *C*, Penoscrotal hypospadias. The external urethral orifice (arrow) is located at the penoscrotal junction. *D*, Epispadias. The external urethral orifice (arrow) is on the dorsal (upper) surface of the penis near its origin. (Courtesy of Mr. Innes Williams, Genitourinary Surgeon, The Hospital for Sick Children, Great Ormond Street, London, England.)

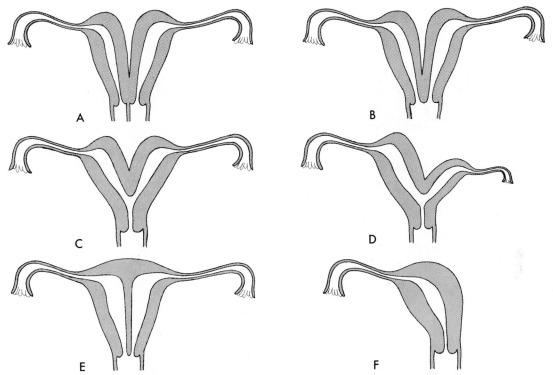

Figure 14–17. Drawings illustrating various types of congenital uterine abnormalities. *A,* Double uterus (uterus didelphys) and double vagina. *B,* Double uterus with single vagina. *C,* Bicornuate uterus. *D,* Bicornuate uterus with a rudimentary left horn. *E,* Septate uterus. *F,* Unicornuate uterus.

Uncommonly, one paramesonephric duct degenerates or fails to form; this results in a *unicornuate (single-horned) uterus* (Fig. 14–17*F*).

Once in about every 4000 females *absence of the vagina* occurs. This results from failure of the vaginal plate to develop (see Fig. 14–12*B*). When the vagina is absent, the uterus is usually also absent. Failure of canalization of the vaginal plate results in *vaginal atresia*. Failure of the hymen to rupture results in a condition known as *imperforate hymen*.

SUMMARY

The urogenital system develops from the intermediate mesoderm, the mesodermal epithelium of the peritoneal cavity, and the endoderm of the urogenital sinus.

Three successive sets of kidneys develop: (1) the transitory vestigial and nonfunctional *pronephros,* (2) the *mesonephros,* which may serve as a temporary excretory organ, and (3) the functional *metanephros* or permanent kidney.

The metanephros develops from two sources: (1) the metanephric diverticulum or ureteric bud, which gives rise to the ureter, renal pelvis, calyces, and collecting tubules, and (2) a mass of metanephric mesoderm, which gives rise to the nephrons.

At first the kidneys are located in the pelvis, but they gradually "ascend" to the abdomen. This apparent migration results from a disproportionate growth of the lumbar and sacral regions of the embryo.

The *urinary bladder* develops from the urogenital sinus and the surrounding splanchnic mesenchyme. The female urethra and almost all of the male urethra have a similar origin.

Developmental abnormalities of the kidney and excretory passages are common. Incomplete division of the metanephric diverticulum or ureteric bud results in bifid or double ureter and a supernumerary kidney. Failure of the kidney to ascend from its embryonic position in the pelvis results in an *ectopic kidney.*

The genital or reproductive system develops in close association with the urinary or excretory system. *Genetic sex* is established at fertilization, but the gonads do not acquire sexual characteristics until the seventh week, and the external genitalia do not become distinctly masculine or feminine until the twelfth week.

The genital or reproductive organs in both sexes develop from primordia which appear identical at first. During this *indifferent stage,* an embryo has the potential to develop into a male or female.

Gonadal sex is controlled by the Y chromosome, which exerts a positive testis-determining action on the *indifferent gonad.* It is the presence of the H-Y antigen on the Y chromosome that causes the testes to develop and produce hormomes. These testicular hormones stimulate development of the mesonephric ducts into the male genital ducts, and the indifferent external genitalia into the penis and scrotum. These hormones also suppress development of the paramesonephric ducts.

In the absence of a Y chromosome and in the presence of two X chromosomes, ovaries develop, the mesonephric ducts regress, the paramesonephric ducts develop into the uterus and uterine tubes, the vagina develops from the urogenital sinus, and the indifferent external genitalia develop into the clitoris and labia minora and majora.

Errors of the sex-determining mechanism produce *true hermaphroditism,* an uncommon condition. These persons have both ovarian and testicular tissue and variable internal and external genitalia.

Errors in sexual differentiation cause *pseudo-hermaphroditism.* In the male, this results from failure of the fetal testes to produce adequate amounts of masculinizing hormones. In the female, pseudohermaphroditism usually results from a disorder of the fetal suprarenal glands which causes an excessive production of androgens.

Commonly Asked Questions

1. Does a *horseshoe kidney* usually function normally? What sort of problems may occur with this malformation and how can they be corrected?
2. My uncle has *two kidneys on one side* and none on the other side. How did this probably happen? Are there any problems associated with this condition?
3. Do *true hermaphrodites* ever marry? Are they ever fertile?
4. When a baby is born with *ambiguous external genitalia,* how long does it take to assign the appropriate sex? What does the doctor tell the parents? How is the appropriate sex determined?
5. What is the most common type of disorder producing ambiguity of the external genitalia? Will masculinizing or *androgenic hormones* given after the twelfth week of development cause ambiguity of genitalia?

Answers

1. Most people with a horseshoe kidney have no urinary problems, and most of these abnormal kidneys are discovered only at autopsy or in the dissecting room. Nothing needs to be done with this abnormal kidney unless infection of the urinary tract occurs that cannot be controlled. In some of these cases, the urologist may divide the kidney into two parts and fix them in positions that do not result in urinary stagnation.
2. Probably the developing kidneys fused during early gestation. The fused kidneys then ascended toward the normal position on one side or the other. Usually there are no problems associated with fused kidneys, but surgeons have to be conscious of the possibility of this condition and recognize it for what it is. Removal of fused kidneys would be a catastrophic error because they represent the only kidneys the person has.
3. Some true hermaphrodites have married, but most of them do not. These people have both ovarian and testicular tissue. Although spermatogenesis is uncommon, ovulation is not and pregnancy and childbirth have been observed in a few patients with an XX sex chromosome complex.
4. By 72 hours after birth a definite gender assignment can be made in most cases. The parents are told that their infant's genital development has not been completed by birth, and that tests are needed to determine whether the baby is a boy or a girl. They are usually advised against announcing their infant's birth to their friends until the sex has been assigned. The buccal smear test for the identification of sex chromatin is done as soon as possible. Chromatin-positive cells (those with sex chromatin) almost always indicate a female. Chromatin-negative cells usually indicate a male, but study of the baby's chromosomes may be required before sex can be assigned. Hormone studies may also be required.

5. Virilization or masculinization of the female fetus is the most common cause of ambiguous external genitalia resulting in intersexuality. Androgens enter the maternal and fetal circulations following maternal ingestion of androgenic hormones. In unusual cases the hormones are produced by a tumor on the mother's suprarenal gland. The female fetus may also produce excessive amounts of androgen owing to hyperplasia of its suprarenal cortices. Partial or complete fusion of the urogenital folds or labioscrotal swellings is the result of exposure to androgens prior to the twelfth week of development. Clitoral enlargement will occur after this period, but androgens will not cause sexual ambiguity because the other external genitalia are fully formed by this time.

15

The Cardiovascular System

The cardiovascular system is the first system to function in the embryo. Blood begins to circulate at the end of the third week. This early development is necessary because the rapidly growing embryo needs an efficient method of acquiring nutrients and disposing of waste products.

EARLY HEART DEVELOPMENT

Heart development is first indicated toward the end of the third week in the *cardiogenic area* (Fig. 15–1A). A pair of *cardiogenic cords* appears and soon become canalized to form *endocardial heart tubes*

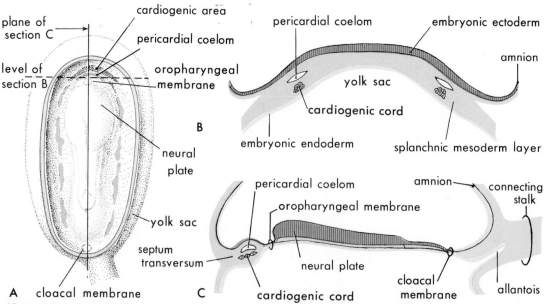

Figure 15–1. *A,* Diagrammatic dorsal view of an embryo of about 18 days showing the cardiogenic area. *B,* Transverse section of an embryo demonstrating the cardiogenic cords. *C,* Longitudinal section of the embryo illustrating the relationship of the developing heart to the oropharyngeal membrane, the pericardial coelom (cavity), and the septum transversum (future central part of the diaphragm).

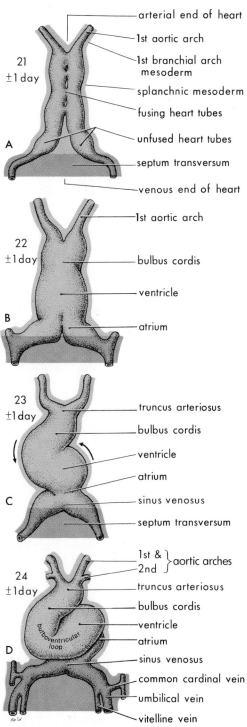

Figure 15–3. Sketches of ventral views of the developing heart during the fourth week, showing fusion of the heart tubes and bending of the single heart tube. Because the primitive heart grows within a confined space (see Figs. 15–2 and 15–4), it folds on itself and forms a bulboventricular loop.

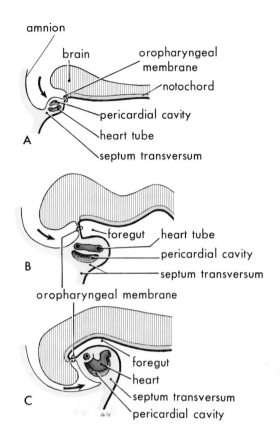

amnion

brain

oropharyngeal membrane

notochord

pericardial cavity

heart tube

septum transversum

A

foregut heart tube

pericardial cavity

septum transversum

B

oropharyngeal membrane

foregut

heart

septum transversum

pericardial cavity

C

Figure 15–4. Schematic drawings of longitudinal sections through the cranial half of human embryos during the fourth week, showing the effect of the head fold (arrow) on the heart tube and other structures. As the head fold develops, the heart and pericardial cavity come to lie ventral to the foregut and caudal to the oropharyngeal membrane.

Fate of Sinus Venosus and Formation of Adult Right Atrium. Initially the sinus venosus is a separate chamber of the heart and opens into the caudal wall of the right atrium (see Figs. 15–5 and 15–6). The *left horn* of the sinus venosus forms the **coronary sinus** (Fig. 15–9B), and the *right horn* becomes part of the wall of the *right atrium* (Fig. 15–9B and C). The remnant of the right part of the primitive atrium is represented by the rough portion of the atrium and the *right auricle* (Fig. 15–9).

Formation of the Adult Left Atrium. The smooth part of the wall of the left atrium is derived from the *primitive pulmonary vein.* As the atrium expands, the terminal portion of this vein and its main branches are gradually incorporated into the wall of the left atrium. The remnant of the left part of the primitive atrium is the *left auricle,* an appendage of the atrium.

Partitioning of Primitive Ventricle. Division of the primitive ventricle into right and left ventricles is indicated at the end of the fourth week by a muscular ridge, the *interventricular septum,* in the floor of the ventricle near its apex (see Figs. 15–6D and 15–7B).

An *interventricular foramen* between the free edge of the interventricular septum and the fused endocardial cushions permits communication between the right and left ventricles.

The interventricular foramen normally closes around the end of the seventh week as the result of fusion of tissue from three sources (see Fig. 15–11). After closure of the interventricular foramen, the pulmonary trunk is in communication with the right ventricle and the aorta with the left ventricle.

Partitioning and Fate of the Bulbus Cordis and Truncus Arteriosus. During the fifth week, bulges form in the walls of the bulbus cordis (Fig. 15–10B and C). These bulges, called *bulbar ridges,* are first filled with cardiac jelly but are later invaded by mesenchymal cells. Similar *truncal ridges* form in the truncus arteriosus, which are continuous with the bulbar ridges.

The spiral orientation of the ridges, possibly caused by the streaming of blood from the ventricles, results in a spiral *aorticopulmonary septum* when these ridges fuse (Fig. 15–10D to G). This septum divides the bulbus cordis and truncus arteriosus into two channels, the *aorta* and *pulmonary trunk.*

Text continued on page 214

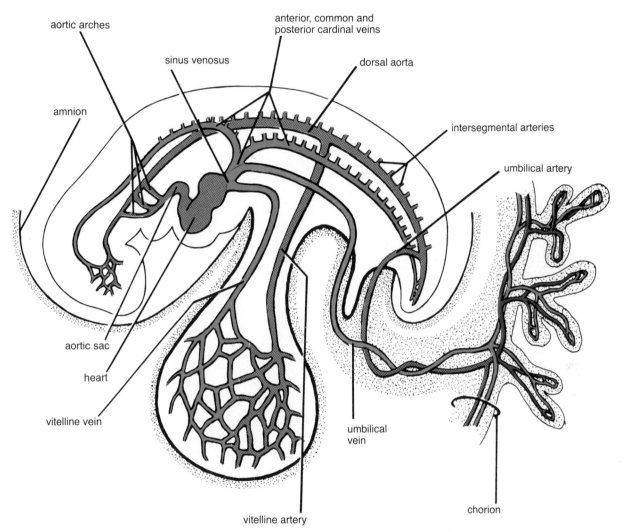

Figure 15–5. Sketch of the cardiovascular system in a 26-day embryo showing vessels of the left side. Although blood circulates to and from the yolk sac, nourishment and oxygen for the embryo come from the chorion (primitive placenta). The umbilical vein is colored red because it carries oxygenated blood. The umbilical arteries are colored medium red to indicate that they are carrying poorly oxygenated blood.

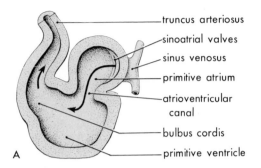

truncus arteriosus
sinoatrial valves
sinus venosus
primitive atrium
atrioventricular
canal
bulbus cordis
primitive ventricle

A

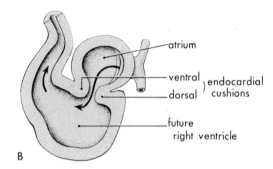

atrium

ventral) endocardial
dorsal) cushions

future
right ventricle

B

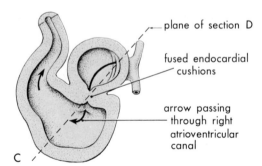

plane of section D

fused endocardial
cushions

arrow passing
through right
atrioventricular
canal

C

Figure 15–6. *A* to *C*, Sketches of sagittal sections of the heart during the fourth and fifth weeks illustrating division of the atrioventricular canal. *D*, Frontal section of the heart at the plane shown in *C*. The interatrial and interventricular septa have also started to develop.

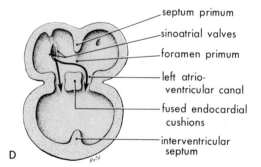

septum primum
sinoatrial valves
foramen primum
left atrio-
ventricular canal
fused endocardial
cushions
interventricular
septum

D

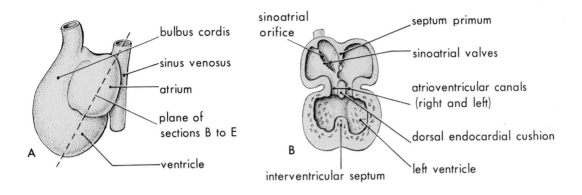

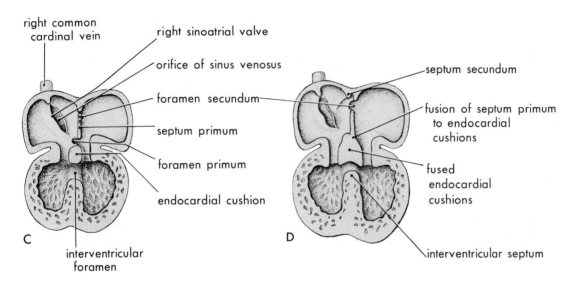

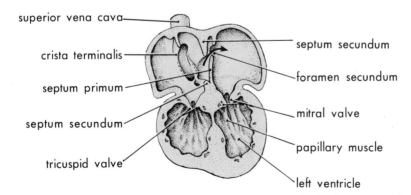

Figure 15–7. Drawings of the developing heart showing partitioning of the atrioventricular canal, atrium, and ventricle. *A,* Sketch showing the plane of frontal sections *B* to *E. B,* About 28 days, showing the early appearance of the septum primum, interventricular septum, and dorsal endocardial cushion. *C,* About 32 days, showing perforations in the dorsal part of the septum. *D,* About 35 days, showing the foramen secundum. *E,* About eight weeks, showing the heart after partitioning into four chambers.

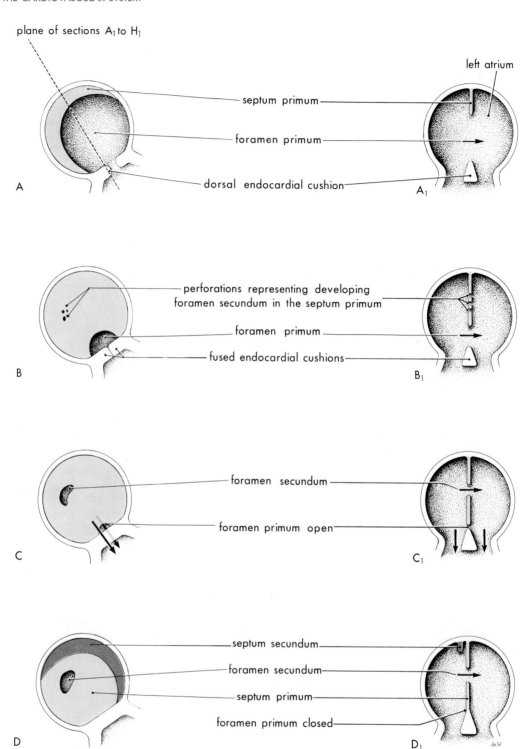

Figure 15–8. Diagrammatic sketches illustrating partitioning of the primitive atrium. *A* to *H* are views of the developing interatrial septum as viewed from the right side. *A₁* to *H₁* are frontal sections of the developing interatrial septum at the plane shown in *A*.

Illustration continued on opposite page

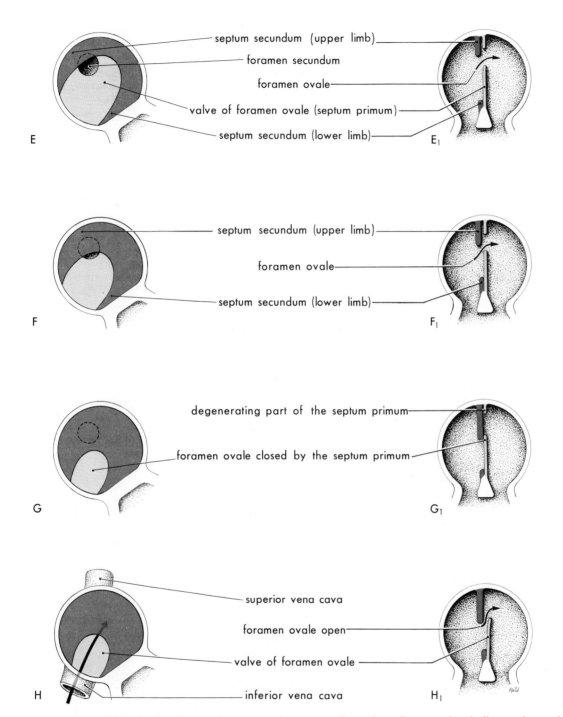

Figure 15–8 *Continued* Note that as the septum secundum grows, it overlaps the opening in the septum primum (foramen secundum). The valvelike nature of the foramen ovale is illustrated in G_1 and H_1. When pressure in the right atrium exceeds that in the left atrium, blood passes from the right to the left side of the heart. When the pressures are equal, the septum primum closes the foramen ovale.

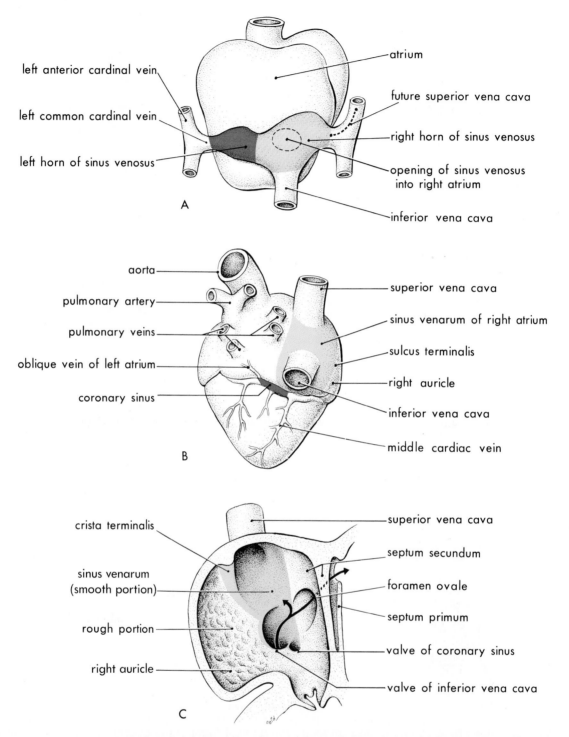

left anterior cardinal vein

left common cardinal vein

left horn of sinus venosus

atrium

future superior vena cava

right horn of sinus venosus

opening of sinus venosus into right atrium

inferior vena cava

A

aorta

pulmonary artery

pulmonary veins

oblique vein of left atrium

coronary sinus

superior vena cava

sinus venarum of right atrium

sulcus terminalis

right auricle

inferior vena cava

middle cardiac vein

B

crista terminalis

sinus venarum (smooth portion)

rough portion

right auricle

superior vena cava

septum secundum

foramen ovale

septum primum

valve of coronary sinus

valve of inferior vena cava

C

Figure 15–9. Diagrams illustrating the fate of the sinus venosus. *A,* Dorsal view of the heart at about 26 days showing the early appearance of the sinus venosus. *B,* Dorsal view at eight weeks after incorporation of the right horn of the sinus venosus into the right atrium. The left horn of the sinus venosus has become the coronary sinus. *C,* Internal view of the fetal right atrium showing (*1*) the smooth part (sinus venarum) of the wall of the right atrium derived from the right horn of the sinus venosus and (*2*) the crista terminalis and the valves of the inferior vena cava and coronary sinus derived from the right sinoatrial valve. The primitive right atrium becomes the right auricle, a conical muscular pouch.

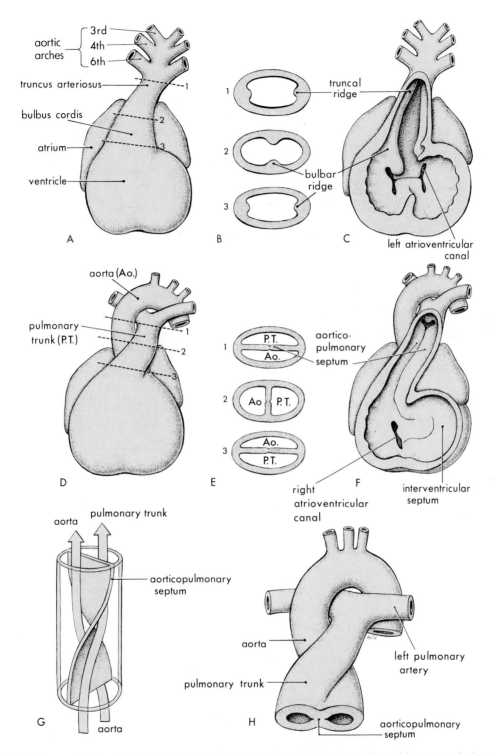

Figure 15-10. Schematic drawings illustrating partitioning of the bulbus cordis and truncus arteriosus. *A*, Ventral aspect of the heart at five weeks. *B*, Transverse sections through the truncus arteriosus and bulbus cordis illustrating the truncal and bulbar ridges. *C*, The ventral wall of the heart has been removed to demonstrate the ridges. *D*, Ventral aspect of the heart after partitioning of the truncus arteriosus. *E*, Sections through the newly formed aorta (Ao.) and pulmonary trunk (P.T.) showing the aorticopulmonary septum. *F*, Six weeks. The ventral wall of the heart and pulmonary trunk have been removed to show the aorticopulmonary septum. *G*, Diagram illustrating the spiral form of the aorticopulmonary septum. *H*, Drawing showing the great arteries twisting around each other as they leave the heart.

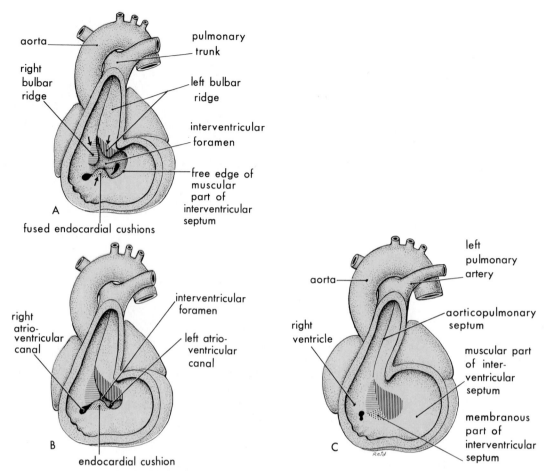

Figure 15–11. Schematic diagrams illustrating closure of the interventricular foramen and formation of the membranous part of the interventricular septum. The walls of the bulbus cordis and the right ventricle have been removed. *A,* Five weeks, showing the bulbar ridges and the fused endocardial cushions. *B,* Six weeks, showing how proliferation of subendocardial tissue diminishes the interventricular foramen. *C,* Seven weeks, showing the fused bulbar ridges and the membranous part of the interventricular septum formed by extensions of tissue from the right side of the endocardial cushions.

Because of the spiral form of the aorticopulmonary septum, the pulmonary trunk twists around the ascending aorta (Figs. 15–10*H* and 15–11).

The bulbus cordis is gradually incorporated into the walls of the ventricles. In the adult right ventricle, it is represented by the *infundibulum* or *conus arteriosus,* which gives origin to the pulmonary trunk. In the adult left ventricle, the bulbus cordis forms the walls of the *aortic vestibule,* the part of the ventricular cavity just inferior to the aortic valve.

CONGENITAL MALFORMATIONS OF THE HEART AND GREAT VESSELS

Because development of the heart and great vessels is complex, congenital heart defects are relatively common. The overall incidence is about 0.7 per cent of live births and 2.7 per cent of stillbirths.

The following malformations are relatively common and many are amenable to surgery.

Atrial Septal Defects (ASD). An atrial septal defect is among the most common of congenital heart defects. There are two main types.

Secundum Type ASD (Fig. 15–12*A* to *D*). The defect is in the area of the foramen ovale and may include defects of the septum primum and septum secundum.

Patent foramen ovale may result from abnormal resorption of the septum primum during the formation of the foramen secundum. If resorption occurs in abnormal locations, the septum primum is fenestrated or netlike (Fig. 15–12*A*). If excessive resorption of the septum primum occurs, the resulting short septum

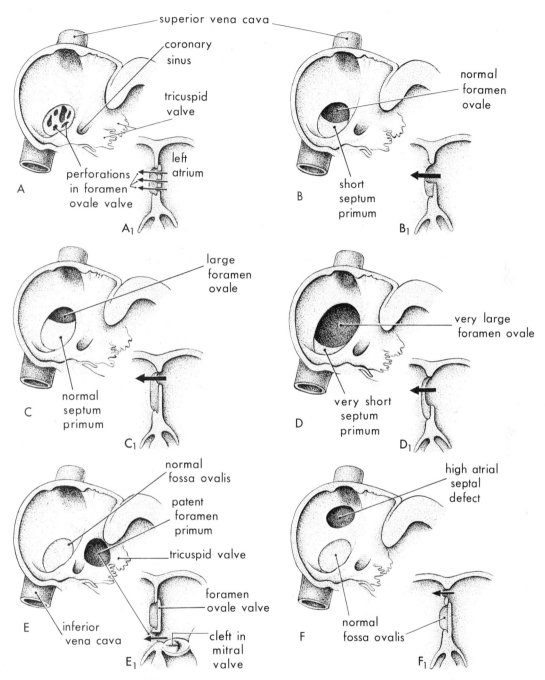

Figure 15–12. Drawings of the right aspect of the interatrial septum (*A* to *F*) and sketches of frontal sections through the septum (*A₁* to *F₁*) illustrating various types of atrial septal defects. *A,* Patent foramen ovale resulting from resorption of the septum primum in abnormal locations. *B,* Patent foramen ovale caused by excessive resorption of the septum primum, sometimes called the "short flap defect." *C,* Patent foramen ovale resulting from an abnormally large foramen ovale. *D,* Patent foramen ovale resulting from an abnormally large foramen ovale and excessive resorption of the septum primum. *E,* Endocardial cushion defect with primum type atrial septal defect. The frontal section *E₁* also shows the cleft in the septal leaflet of the mitral valve. *F,* High septal defect resulting from abnormal absorption of the sinus venosus into the right atrium. This is a very uncommon defect. Note the fossa ovalis in *E* and *F* that forms when the foramen ovale closes normally.

primum does not cover the foramen ovale (Fig. 15–12B). If an abnormally large foramen ovale results from defective development of the septum secundum, a normal septum primum will not close the foramen ovale at birth (Fig. 15–12C).

Large atrial septal defects result from a combination of excessive resorption of the septum primum and a large foramen ovale (Fig. 15–12D). This heart defect is characterized by a *large opening between the left and right atria.* Obviously there is considerable interatrial shunting of blood in these people.

Endocardial Cushion Defect with Primum Type ASD (Fig. 15–12E). The septum primum does not fuse with the endocardial cushions, leaving a *patent foramen primum;* usually there is also a cleft in the mitral valve of the heart.

Ventricular Septal Defects (VSD). *This congenital malformation ranks first in frequency on all lists of cardiac defects.* Membranous septal defect is the commonest type of VSD (Fig. 15–13B). Incomplete closure of the interventricular foramen and failure of the membranous part of the interventricular septum to develop result from failure of tissue to grow from the right side of the fused endocardial cushions and fuse with the aorticopulmonary septum and the muscular part of the interventricular septum (see Fig. 15–11C).

Persistent Truncus Arteriosus. This malformation *results from failure of development of the aorticopul-* *monary septum.* As a result, the truncus arteriosus does not divide into the aorta and pulmonary trunk. The most common type is a single arterial vessel which gives rise to the pulmonary trunk and ascending aorta (Fig. 15–14A and B). The next most common type is for the right and left pulmonary arteries to arise close together from the dorsal wall of the persistent truncus arteriosus.

Transposition of the Great Arteries (TGA). In typical cases, the aorta lies anterior to the pulmonary trunk and arises from the right ventricle, and the pulmonary trunk arises from the left ventricle. For survival there must be a septal defect (ASD or VSD), or a patent ductus arteriosus (see Fig. 15–19B), to permit some interchange of blood between the pulmonary and systemic circulations.

During partitioning of the truncus arteriosus, the aorticopulmonary septum fails to pursue a spiral course. As a result the origins of the great arteries are reversed.

Tetralogy of Fallot (Fig. 15–15B). This is a combination of four cardiac defects consisting of (1) pulmonary stenosis or narrowing of the region of the right ventricular outflow, (2) ventricular septal defect, (3) overriding aorta, and (4) hypertrophy of the right ventricle. This condition results in cyanosis (blueness) of the lips and fingernails; consequently, these infants are sometimes referred to as "blue babies."

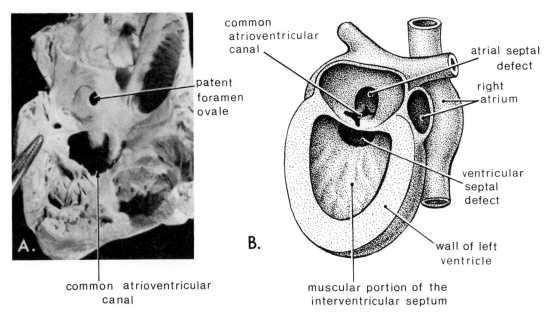

Figure 15–13. *A,* Photograph of an infant's heart, sectioned and viewed from the right side, showing a patent foramen ovale and a common atrioventricular canal. (From Lev, M.: *Autopsy Diagnosis of Congenitally Malformed Hearts.* Springfield, IL, Charles C Thomas, 1953.) *B,* Schematic drawing of a heart illustrating various defects of the cardiac septa.

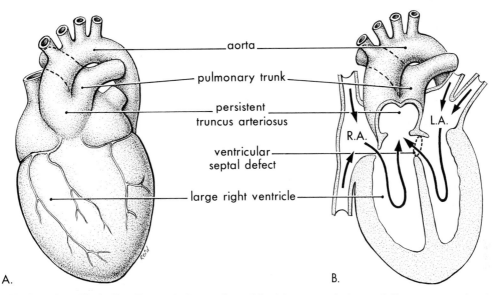

Figure 15–14. Drawings illustrating the main type of persistent truncus arteriosus. *A,* The common trunk divides into an aorta and short pulmonary trunk. *B,* Sketch showing circulation in this heart and a ventricular septal defect.

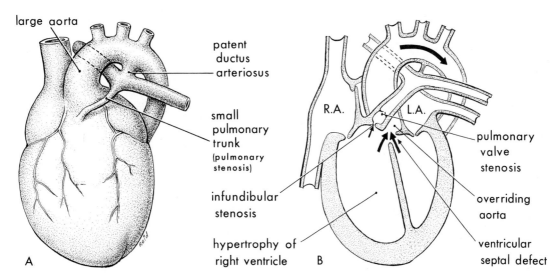

Figure 15–15. *A,* Drawing of an infant's heart showing a small pulmonary trunk (pulmonary stenosis) and a large aorta resulting from unequal partitioning of the truncus arteriosus. There is also hypertrophy of the right ventricle and a patent ductus arteriosus. *B,* Frontal section of a heart illustrating the tetralogy of Fallot. Note that the large aorta lies over the VSD and receives blood from both ventricles. There are two types of pulmonary stenosis. In *pulmonary valve stenosis,* the pulmonary valve cusps are fused, and a narrow opening remains. In *infundibular pulmonary stenosis,* the conus arteriosus (infundibulum) of the right ventricle is underdeveloped.

THE AORTIC ARCHES

As the branchial arches develop during the fourth week (Fig. 15–16), they receive arteries from the heart. These aortic arches (arteries) arise from the truncus arteriosus and terminate in the dorsal aorta of the corresponding side (Fig. 15–16*B*).

Although six pairs of aortic arches develop, they are not all present at the same time, e.g., by the time the sixth pair of aortic arches forms, the first two pairs have disappeared (Fig. 15–16*C*).

Derivatives of the Aortic Arches (Figs. 15–16 and 15–17). During the sixth to eighth weeks, the primitive aortic arch pattern of arteries is transformed into the basic adult arterial arrangement.

The first and second pairs of aortic arches largely disappear.

The proximal parts of the third pair of aortic arches form the *common carotid arteries,* and distal portions join with the dorsal aortae to form the *internal carotid arteries.*

The left fourth aortic arch forms part of the *arch of the aorta.* The right fourth aortic arch becomes the proximal portion of the *right subclavian artery.* The distal part of this artery forms from the right dorsal aorta and the right seventh intersegmental artery (Fig. 15–17*B*).

The fifth pair of aortic arches have no derivatives.

The *left sixth aortic arch* develops as follows: the proximal part persists as the proximal part of the *left pulmonary artery,* and the distal part persists as a shunt or passageway between the pulmonary artery and the aorta, called the **ductus arteriosus** (Figs. 15–17*C* and 15–18).

The right sixth aortic arch develops as follows: the proximal part persists as the proximal part of the *right pulmonary artery,* and the distal part degenerates.

Malformations Resulting From Abnormal Transformation of the Aortic Arches

Because of the many changes involved in transformation of the embryonic aortic arch system into the adult arterial pattern, it is understandable that malformations may occur. Abnormalities result from the persistence of parts of aortic arches that normally disappear, from disappearance of other parts that normally persist, or from both.

Coarctation of the Aorta (Fig. 15–18). This relatively common malformation is characterized by a narrowing of the aorta, just superior or inferior to the ductus arteriosus.

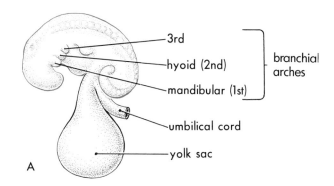

A

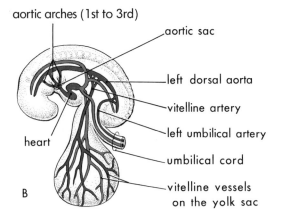

B

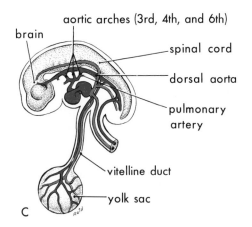

C

Figure 15–16. Drawings illustrating the aortic arches and the primitive cardiovascular system. *A,* Left side of a 26-day embryo. *B,* Schematic drawing of this embryo showing the left aortic arches arising from the aortic sac of the truncus arteriosus, running through the branchial arches, and terminating in the left dorsal aorta. *C,* 37-day embryo showing the single dorsal aorta and that the first two pairs of aortic arches have largely degenerated.

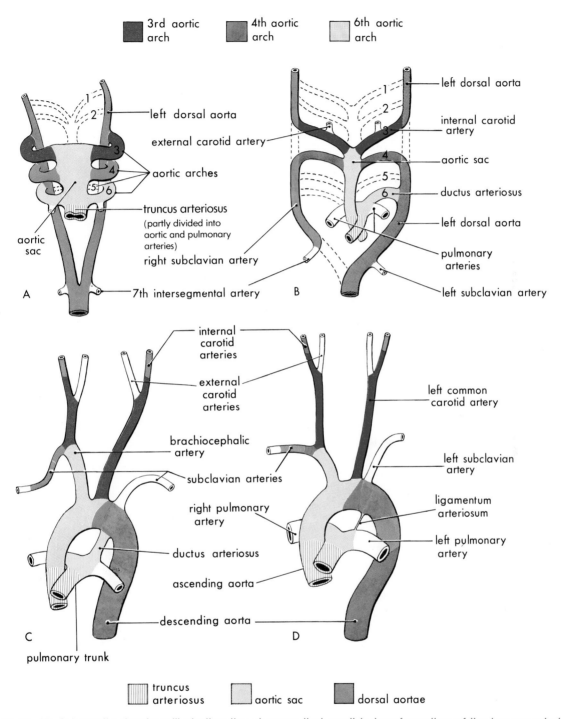

3rd aortic arch 4th aortic arch 6th aortic arch

A

left dorsal aorta
external carotid artery
aortic arches
truncus arteriosus (partly divided into aortic and pulmonary arteries)
aortic sac
right subclavian artery
7th intersegmental artery

B

left dorsal aorta
internal carotid artery
aortic sac
ductus arteriosus
left dorsal aorta
pulmonary arteries
left subclavian artery

C

internal carotid arteries
external carotid arteries
brachiocephalic artery
subclavian arteries
ductus arteriosus
ascending aorta
descending aorta
pulmonary trunk

D

left common carotid artery
left subclavian artery
ligamentum arteriosum
left pulmonary artery
right pulmonary artery

truncus arteriosus   aortic sac   dorsal aortae

Figure 15–17. Schematic drawings illustrating the changes that result in transformation of the truncus arteriosus, aortic sac, aortic arches, and dorsal aortae into the adult arterial pattern. The vessels which are not shaded or colored are not derived from these structures. *A*, Aortic arches at six weeks; by this stage the first two pairs of aortic arches have largely disappeared. *B*, Aortic arches at seven weeks; the parts of the dorsal aortae and aortic arches that normally disappear are indicated with broken lines. *C*, Arterial arrangement at eight weeks. *D*, Sketch of the arterial vessels of a six-month infant. The ductus arteriosus normally becomes functionally closed 10 to 15 hours after birth. Eventually the ductus arteriosus becomes the ligamentum arteriosum.

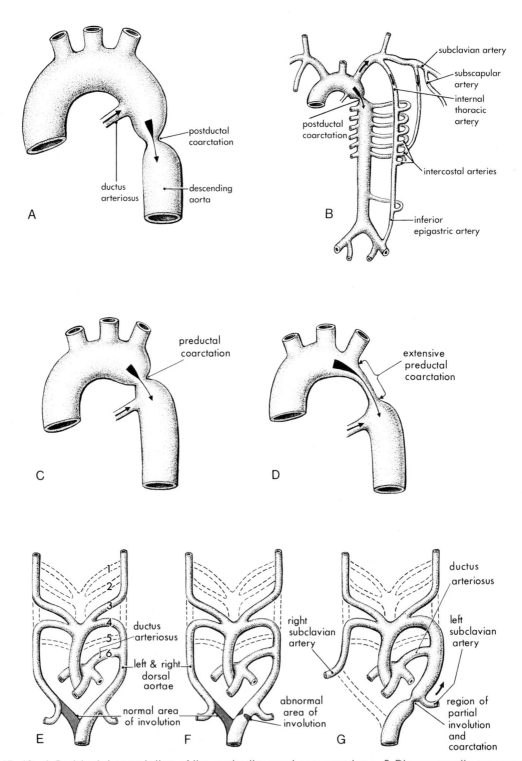

Figure 15–18. *A,* Postductal coarctation of the aorta, the most common type. *B,* Diagrammatic representation of the common routes of collateral circulation that develop with postductal coarctation of the aorta. *C* and *D,* Preductal coarctation. The type illustrated in *D* is usually associated with major cardiac defects. *E,* Sketch of the aortic arch pattern in a seven-week embryo showing the areas that normally involute. Note that the distal segment of the right dorsal aorta normally involves as the right subclavian artery develops. *F,* Localized abnormal involution of a small distal segment of the left dorsal aorta. *G,* Later stage showing the abnormally involuted segment appearing as a coarctation of the aorta. This moves (arrow) to the region of the ductus arteriosus with the left subclavian artery.

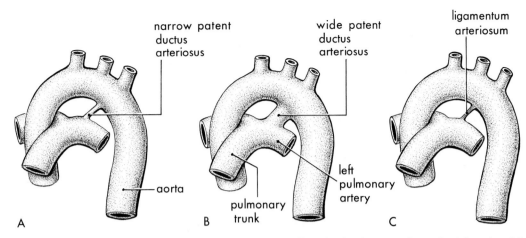

Figure 15–19. *A,* The ductus arteriosus of a newborn infant. The ductus is normally patent for about two weeks after birth. *B,* Abnormal patent ductus arteriosus in a six-month infant. In this case, some of the blood that should go through the aorta to the inferior part of the body goes back to the lungs via the ductus arteriosus and the pulmonary arteries. The ductus is nearly the same size as the left pulmonary artery. *C,* The ligamentum arteriosum, the normal remnant of the ductus arteriosus, in a six-month infant.

The embryological basis of coarctation of the aorta is unclear. One explanation is illustrated (Fig. 15–18*E* to *G*). There is abnormal involution of a small segment of the left dorsal aorta. Later this constricted segment (area of coarctation) moves cranially with the left subclavian artery to the region of the ductus arteriosus.

In the common type of coarctation, the constriction is inferior to the level of the ductus arteriosus (Fig. 15–18*A*). A collateral circulation develops during the fetal period, assisting with passage of blood to inferior parts of the body (Fig. 15–18*B*).

Patent Ductus Arteriosus (Fig. 15–19*B*). This malformation is two to three times *more common in females* than in males. The embryological basis of patent ductus arteriosus is failure of the ductus arteriosus to involute after birth and form the ligamentum arteriosum.

Patent ductus arteriosus is the most common cardiac malformation associated with maternal rubella infection during early pregnancy (see Chapter 9).

PRENATAL CIRCULATION

The fetal cardiovascular system is designed to serve prenatal needs and to permit modifications at birth that establish the postnatal circulatory pattern.

Course of the Fetal Circulation (Fig. 15–20). Well-oxygenated blood returns from the placenta in the *umbilical vein.* About half of this blood bypasses the liver, going through the *ductus venosus.* After a short course in the *inferior vena cava,* the blood enters the right atrium.

Because the inferior vena cava also contains deoxygenated blood from the lower limbs, abdomen, and pelvis, the blood entering the right atrium is not so well oxygenated as that in the umbilical vein. The blood from the inferior vena cava is largely directed by the inferior border of the septum secundum through the *foramen ovale* into the left atrium. Here it mixes with a relatively small amount of deoxygenated blood returning from the lungs via the pulmonary veins. The blood passes into the left ventricle and leaves via the ascending aorta. Consequently, the vessels to the heart, head and neck, and upper limbs receive well-oxygenated blood.

A small amount of oxygenated blood from the inferior vena cava remains in the right atrium. This blood mixes with deoxygenated blood from the superior vena cava and coronary sinus and passes into the right ventricle. The blood leaves by the pulmonary trunk and most of it passes through the ductus arteriosus into the aorta.

Very little blood goes to the lungs before birth because they are nonfunctional and so require little blood. Most of the mixed blood in the descending aorta passes into the umbilical arteries and is returned to the placenta for reoxygenation. The blood remaining in the aorta circulates through the inferior part of the body and eventually enters the inferior vena cava.

POSTNATAL CIRCULATION

Changes in the Cardiovascular System at Birth (Fig. 15–21). Important circulatory adjustments occur

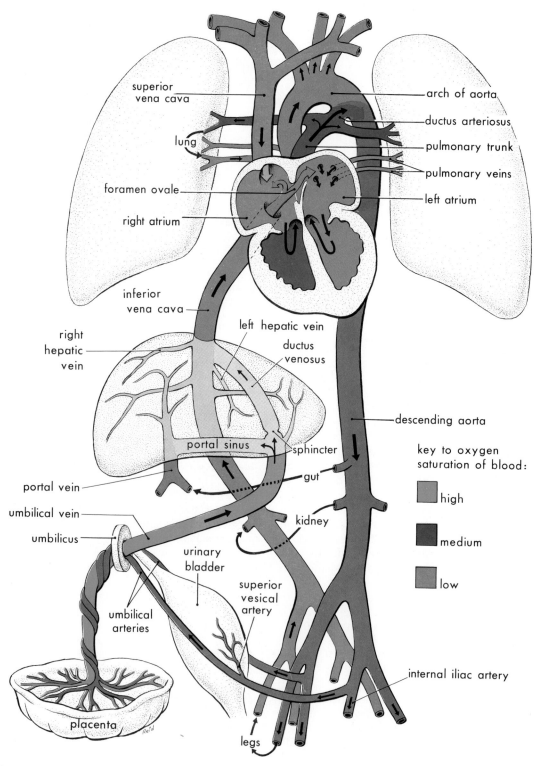

Figure 15–20. A simplified scheme of the fetal circulation. The colors indicate the oxygen saturation of the blood, and the arrows show the course of the fetal circulation. The organs are not drawn to scale. Observe that there are three shunts that permit most of the blood to bypass the liver and the lungs: (1) the *ductus venosus*, (2) the *foramen ovale*, and (3) the *ductus arteriosus*.

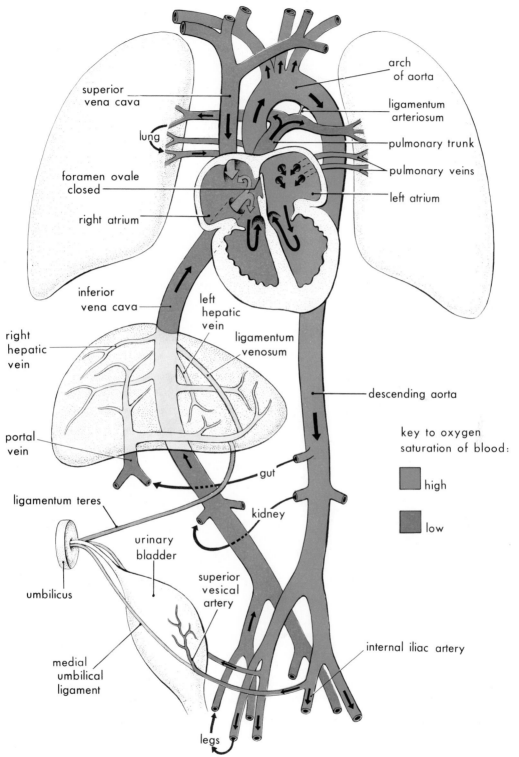

Figure 15-21. A simplified representation of the circulation after birth. The adult derivatives of the fetal vessels and structures that become nonfunctional at birth are also shown. The arrows indicate the course of the neonatal circulation. The organs are not drawn to scale. After birth, the three shunts that short-circuited the blood during fetal life cease to function, and the pulmonary and systemic circulations become separated.

at birth when the circulation of fetal blood through the placenta ceases and the lungs begin to function. The foramen ovale, ductus arteriosus, ductus venosus, and umbilical vessels are no longer needed.

Occlusion of the placental circulation causes an immediate fall of blood pressure in the inferior vena cava and right atrium. Aeration of the lungs is associated with a dramatic fall in pulmonary vascular resistance, a marked increase in pulmonary blood flow, and a progressive thinning of the walls of the pulmonary arteries. As a result of this increased pulmonary blood flow, the pressure in the left atrium rises above that in the right atrium. This closes the foramen ovale by pressing its valve, the septum primum, against the septum secundum.

Because of the changes in the cardiovascular system at birth, the vessels and structures that are no longer required are transformed as follows (Fig. 15–21).

The intra-abdominal portion of the umbilical vein becomes the *ligamentum teres,* which passes from the umbilicus to the left branch of the portal vein.

The ductus venosus eventually becomes the *ligamentum venosum,* which passes through the liver from the left branch of the portal vein to the inferior vena cava.

Most of the intra-abdominal portions of the umbilical arteries form the *medial umbilical ligaments.* The proximal parts of these vessels persist as the *superior vesical arteries,* which supply the superior part of the urinary bladder.

The *foramen ovale normally closes* functionally at birth. Later anatomical closure results from tissue proliferation and adhesion of the septum primum (valve of foramen ovale) to the left margin of the septum secundum.

The ductus arteriosus eventually becomes the *ligamentum arteriosum,* which passes from the left pulmonary artery to the arch of the aorta. Anatomical closure of the ductus normally occurs by the end of the third postnatal month.

The change from the fetal to the adult pattern of circulation is not sudden. It takes place over a period of days and weeks. During the transitional stage, there may be a right-to-left flow through the foramen ovale, and the ductus arteriosus usually remains patent for two or three months.

SUMMARY

The cardiovascular system begins to develop during the third week from splanchnic mesoderm in the cardiogenic area. Paired heart tubes form and fuse into a single heart tube.

By the end of the third week, a functional cardiovascular system is present. As the heart tube grows, it bends to the right and soon acquires the general external appearance of the adult heart. The heart becomes partitioned into four chambers between the fourth and seventh weeks.

The critical period of heart development is from about day 20 to day 50 after fertilization. Because partitioning of the heart is complex, defects of the cardiac septa are relatively common, particularly ventricular septal defects. Some congenital malformations result from abnormal transformation of the aortic arches into the adult arterial pattern.

Because the lungs are nonfunctional during prenatal life, the fetal cardiovascular system is structurally designed so that blood is oxygenated in the placenta and largely bypasses the lungs. The modifications that establish the postnatal circulatory pattern at birth are not abrupt, but extend into infancy. Failure of the normal changes in the circulatory system to occur at birth results in a *patent foramen ovale or a patent ductus arteriosus* or both.

Commonly Asked Questions

1. The pediatrician said that our newborn baby had a *heart murmur.* What causes this condition and what does it indicate?
2. Are congenital malformations of the heart common? What is the most common *congenital cardiac defect* in children?
3. What are the causes of congenital malformations of the cardiovascular system? Can drugs cause congenital cardiac defects? A friend of mine who drank heavily during her pregnancy had a child with a heart defect. Could her drinking have caused her infant's heart malformation?
4. Can viral infections cause congenital heart disease? I have heard that if a mother has *measles during pregnancy,* her baby will have an abnormality of the cardiovascular system. Is this true? I have also heard that women can be given a *vaccine* that will protect their babies against the rubella syndrome. Is this true?
5. My sister's baby had its *aorta arising from the right*

ventricle and its pulmonary artery arising from the left ventricle. The baby died during the first week. What is this malformation called and how common is this disorder? Can the condition be corrected surgically?

6. I know a set of healthy identical twin sisters in their forties. It was found during a routine examination that one of them had a *reversed heart*. How common is this among identical twins, and what causes this condition to develop?

Answers

1. Heart murmurs are sounds transmitted to the thoracic wall that result from turbulence of the blood within the heart or great arteries. Loud murmurs often represent narrowing or *stenosis of one of the semilunar valves* (aortic or pulmonary valves). A ventricular septal defect or a patent foramen ovale may also produce a loud murmur.

2. Yes, congenital heart defects are common. They occur in about 8 of every 1000 newborns and represent about 10 per cent of all congenital malformations. *Ventricular septal defects are the most common type of heart malformation.*

3. *The cause of most congenital malformations of the cardiovascular system is unknown.* In about 8 per cent of children with heart disease, there is a clear genetic basis. Most of these are associated with obvious chromosomal abnormalities (e.g., trisomy 21, or the Down syndrome) and deletion of parts of chromosomes. *The Down syndrome is associated with congenital heart disease in 50 per cent of cases.* The maternal ingestion of drugs, such as antimetabolites and Coumadin (an anticoagulant), has been shown to be associated with a high incidence of cardiac malformations. There is suggestive evidence that a high consumption of alcohol during pregnancy may cause heart defects, but it is impossible to say whether the excessive use of alcohol by your friend caused her baby's heart disease. I doubt it.

4. Several viral infections have been shown to be associated with congenital cardiac malformations, but only the *rubella virus* is known to cause cardiovascular disease (e.g., patent ductus arteriosus). *Measles* is a general term that is used for two different viral diseases. Rubeola (common

measles) does not cause congenital cardiovascular defects, but *rubella* (German measles) does. *Rubella virus vaccine* is now available and is effective in preventing the development of rubella infection in a woman who has not had the disease and is planning to have a baby. Subsequently it will prevent the rubella syndrome in her baby as well. The vaccine is given only if there is assurance that there is no likelihood of pregnancy for the next two months, because of potential hazard to the embryo.

5. This condition is called *transposition of the great arteries (TGA)* because the position of the great vessels (aorta and pulmonary arteries) is reversed. Survival after birth depends on mixing between the pulmonary and systemic circulations (e.g., via an atrial septal defect or patent foramen ovale). TGA occurs in slightly more than 1 per 5000 live births and is more common in male infants (almost 2:1). Most infants with this severe cardiac malformation die during the first months of life, but corrective surgery can be done in those who survive for several months. Initially an atrial septal defect may be created to increase mixing between the systemic and pulmonary circulations. Later an arterial switch operation (reversing the aorta and pulmonary artery) can be performed, but more commonly a baffle is inserted in the atrium to divert systemic venous blood through the mitral valve, left ventricle, and pulmonary artery to the lungs, and pulmonary venous blood through the tricuspid valve and right ventricle to the aorta. This physiologically corrects the circulation.

6. Very likely the one twin has a condition known as *dextrocardia* (L. *dexter,* right). In some cases the heart is simply displaced to the right, and in others there is a complete transposition of the right and left chambers. In the condition represented by your friend, the heart presents a mirror picture of the normal cardiac structure. This results during the fourth week of development when the heart tube rotates to the left, rather than to the right. Similar evidence of asymmetry often occurs in the direction of the hair whorl at the back of the head. Usually it is clockwise, but it may be counterclockwise in one of the twins. The cause of these types of asymmetry is unknown, but the differences arise very early in development.

16

The Articular, Skeletal, and Muscular Systems

The articular, skeletal, and muscular systems develop from mesoderm, the formation of which is described in Chapter 5. As the notochord and neural tube form, the *intraembryonic mesoderm* lateral to these structures thickens to form two longitudinal columns of *paraxial mesoderm* (Fig. 16–1A). The somites arise from the paraxial mesoderm, beginning around 20 days, as the columns of paraxial mesoderm are divided into short segments. Externally, the somites appear as pairs of beadlike elevations along the dorsolateral surface of the embryo (see Fig. 6–3). The development and early differentiation of the somites are illustrated in Figure 16–1.

Initially the somites are composed of *compact aggregates of mesenchymal cells*. Each somite soon becomes differentiated into a ventromedial part called the *sclerotome* and a dorsolateral part called the *dermomyotome* (Fig. 16–1C). Sclerotomal cells soon surround the notochord and neural tube, and give rise to the vertebral column, ribs, and the ligaments associated with them. The *dermomyotome* gives rise to the dermis of the skin and the intrinsic back muscles.

THE ARTICULAR SYSTEM

Most junctions between bones are constructed to allow movement of parts of the body (e.g., the knee joint).

Development of Joints

The terms *articulation* and *joint* are used synonymously to refer to the structural arrangements that join two or more bones together at their place of meeting.

Joints may be classified in several ways. Those with little or no movement are classified according to the type of material holding the bones together, e.g., the bones involved in *fibrous joints* are joined by fibrous tissue (Fig. 16–2D).

Joints begin to develop during the sixth week and by the end of the eighth week, they closely resemble adult joints.

Synovial Joints (Fig. 16–2B). The mesenchyme between the developing bones, known as *interzonal mesenchyme*, differentiates as follows: (1) peripherally, it gives rise to the capsular and other ligaments; (2) centrally, it disappears and the resulting space becomes the joint cavity; (3) where it lines the capsule and the articular surfaces, it forms the synovial membrane. Probably as a result of joint movement, the mesenchymal cells subsequently disappear from the surfaces of the articular cartilages. Examples of this type of joint are the knee and elbow joints.

Cartilaginous Joints (Fig. 16–2C). The interzonal mesenchyme between the developing bones differentiates into hyaline cartilage (e.g., the costochondral joints) or fibrocartilage (e.g., the symphysis pubis).

Fibrous Joints (Fig. 16–2D). The interzonal mesenchyme between the developing bones differentiates into dense fibrous connective tissue, e.g., the sutures of the skull (see Fig. 16–7).

THE SKELETAL SYSTEM

The skeletal system develops from mesoderm, the formation of which is described in Chapter 5. Bones

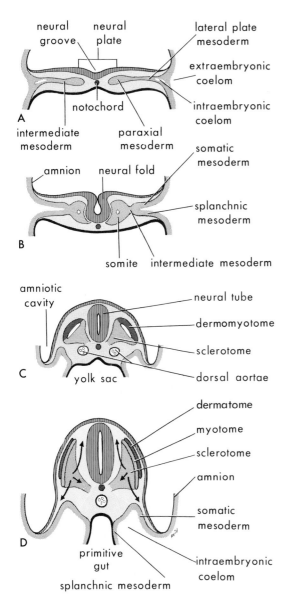

Figure 16–1. Transverse sections through embryos of various ages illustrating the formation and early differentiation of somites. See Figure 6–3 for the external appearance of these embryos. *A,* Embryo of about 18 days, showing the paraxial mesoderm from which the somites are derived. *B,* Embryo of about 22 days. *C,* Embryo of about 26 days. The dermomyotome region of the somite gives rise to a myotome and a skin plate (future dermis). *D,* Embryo of about 28 days. The arrows indicate the migration of cells from the sclerotome regions of the somites.

first appear as mesenchymal models. Some bones develop in mesenchyme by *intramembranous bone formation.* In other cases, the mesenchymal or membranous bone models are transformed into cartilage

models of the bones that later become ossified by *endochondral bone formation.*

Development of the Vertebral Column

Precartilaginous Stage. During the fourth week, mesenchymal cells from the somites migrate in three main directions (Figs. 16–1D and 16–3A):

1. Cells move ventromedially to surround the notochord. The body of each vertebra develops from the caudal part of one somite together with the cranial portion of the next somite. The notochord eventually degenerates and disappears where it is surrounded by the developing vertebral body. Between the vertebrae, the **notochord** expands to form the gelatinous center of the intervertebral disc, called the *nucleus pulposus.*

2. Cells migrate dorsally to cover the neural tube.

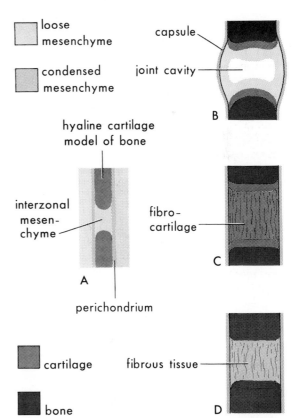

Figure 16–2. Schematic drawings illustrating the development of different types of joints. *A,* Condensed mesenchyme continues across the gap, or interzone, between the developing bones, enclosing some loose mesenchyme (the interzonal mesenchyme) between them. This primitive joint may differentiate into *B,* a synovial joint, *C,* a cartilaginous joint, or *D,* a fibrous joint.

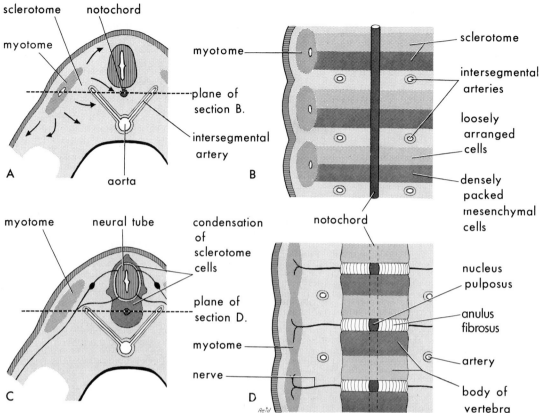

Figure 16–3. *A,* Partial transverse section through a four-week embryo. The arrows indicate the spread of mesenchymal cells from the sclerotome region of the somite on the right. *B,* Diagrammatic frontal section of this embryo, showing that the condensation of sclerotome cells around the notochord consists of a cranial area of loosely packed cells and a caudal area of densely packed cells. *C,* Partial transverse section through a five-week embryo showing the condensation of sclerotome cells around the notochord and the neural tube, forming a mesenchymal vertebra. *D,* Diagrammatic frontal section illustrating that the vertebral body forms from the cranial and caudal halves of two successive sclerotome masses. The intersegmental arteries now cross the bodies of the vertebrae, and the spinal nerves lie between the vertebrae. The notochord is degenerating except in the region of the intervertebral disc, where it forms the nucleus pulposus.

These mesenchymal cells give rise to the *vertebral arch* of the vertebra.

3. Cells pass ventrolaterally into the body wall and form the costal processes, which develop into ribs in the thoracic region.

Chondrification of Typical Vertebrae (Fig. 16–4). During the sixth week, chondrification centers appear in each mesenchymal vertebra. The two centers in each centrum fuse at the end of the embryonic period to form the cartilaginous centrum. Concomitantly the centers in the vertebral arches fuse with each other and with the centrum. The spinous and transverse processes develop from extensions of chondrification centers in the vertebral arch. Chondrification spreads until a *cartilaginous vertebral column* is formed.

Ossification of Typical Vertebrae (Fig. 16–4C to *F*). Ossification begins during the embryonic period and ends around the 25th year.

Prenatal Period (Fig. 16–4C to *F*). At first there are two *primary ossification centers,* ventral and dorsal, for the centrum. The two **primary ossification centers** soon fuse to form one center. Three primary centers are present by the end of the embryonic period: one in the centrum and one in each half of the vertebral arch (Fig. 16–4C).

Ossification becomes evident in the vertebral arches around the eighth week. At birth, each vertebra consists of three bony parts connected by cartilage (Fig. 16–4D).

Postnatal Period. The halves of the vertebral arch usually fuse during the first three to five years. The laminae of the arches first unite in the lumbar region, and subsequent union progresses cranially.

The vertebral arch articulates with the centrum at cartilaginous *neurocentral joints,* which permit the vertebral arches to grow as the spinal cord enlarges.

These joints disappear when the vertebral arch fuses with the centrum during the third to sixth years.

After puberty, five **secondary ossification centers** appear: one for the tip of the spinous process, one for the tip of each transverse process, and two rim epiphyses *(anular epiphyses),* one on the superior and one on the inferior rim of the vertebral body (Fig. 16–4E).

The vertebral body is a composite of the superior and inferior anular epiphyses and the mass of bone between them. It includes the centrum, parts of the vertebral arch, and the facets for the heads of the ribs. All secondary centers unite with the rest of the vertebra at about 25 years.

Malformations of Vertebrae

Variation in the Number of Vertebrae. About 95 per cent of normal people have 7 cervical, 12 thoracic, 5 lumbar, and 5 sacral vertebrae. About 3 per cent of people have one or two more vertebrae, and about 2 per cent have one less.

To determine the number of vertebrae, it is necessary to examine the entire vertebral column, because an apparent extra (or absent) vertebra in one segment of the column may be compensated for by an absent (or extra) vertebra in an adjacent segment, e.g., 11 thoracic-type vertebrae with 6 lumbar-type vertebrae.

Spina Bifida Occulta (see Fig. 17–10A). This defect of the vertebral arch results from failure of development and fusion of the halves of the vertebral arch. It is commonly observed in radiographs of the cervical, lumbar, and sacral regions. Frequently, only one vertebra is affected.

Spina bifida occulta of the first sacral vertebra occurs in about 20 per cent of people, and usually they are unaware of the defect. The spinal cord and spinal nerves are usually normal and neurological symptoms are commonly absent. The skin over the defect is intact and there may be no external evidence of the abnormality. Sometimes the malformation is indicated by a dimple or a tuft of hair.

Rachischisis (see Fig. 16–8). The term *rachischisis* (cleft of vertebral column) refers to the vertebral abnormalities encountered in a complex group of developmental malformations that affect primarily the axial structures of the body. In these cases, the neural folds fail to fuse, either because of faulty induction by the underlying notochord and its associated mesen-

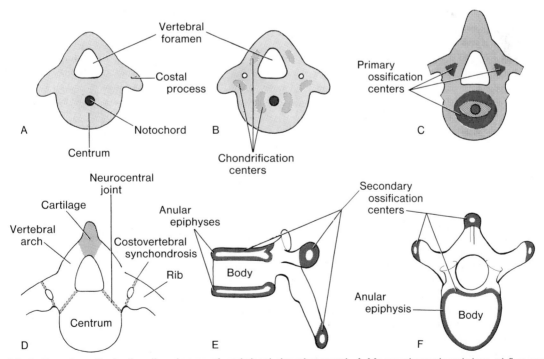

Figure 16–4. Drawings illustrating the stages of vertebral development. *A,* Mesenchymal vertebra at five weeks. *B,* Chondrification centers in a mesenchymal vertebra at six weeks. *C,* Primary ossification centers in a cartilaginous vertebra at seven weeks. *D,* A thoracic vertebra at birth, consisting of three bony parts. Note the cartilage between the halves of the vertebral arch and between the arch and the centrum (the neurocentral joint). *E* and *F,* Two views of a typical thoracic vertebra at puberty, showing the location of the secondary centers of ossification.

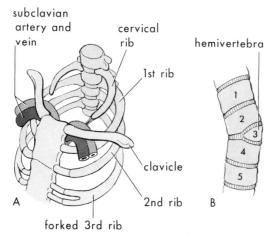

Figure 16–5. Drawings of vertebral and rib abnormalities. A, Cervical and forked ribs. Observe that the left cervical rib has a fibrous band passing posterior to the subclavian vessels and attaching to the sternum. Very likely this condition produced neurovascular changes in the left upper limb. B, Anterior view of the vertebral column showing a hemivertebra (half vertebra). The right half of the third thoracic vertebra is absent. Note the associated lateral curvature, or scoliosis, of the vertebral column.

chyme, or because of the action of teratogenic agents on the neuroepithelial cells making up the neural folds. The neural and vertebral defects may be extensive, or they may be restricted to a small area.

Hemivertebra (Fig. 16–5B). The developing vertebral bodies have two chondrification centers that soon unite (Fig. 16–4B). A hemivertebra results from failure of one of the chondrification centers to appear and subsequent failure of half of the vertebra to form. These defective vertebrae produce *scoliosis* (lateral curvature of the vertebral column). There are other causes of scoliosis, such as weakness of the spinal muscles.

Development of Ribs

The ribs develop from the mesenchymal costal processes of the thoracic vertebrae (Fig. 16–4A). They become cartilaginous during the embryonic period and later ossify. The original union of the costal processes with the vertebra is replaced by synovial joints, the *costovertebral joints* (Fig. 16–4D).

Malformations of Ribs

Accessory Ribs (Fig. 16–5A). Accessory ribs, which may be rudimentary or well developed, result

from the development of the costal processes of cervical or lumbar vertebrae. These processes form ribs in the thoracic region. The most common type of accessory rib is a *lumbar rib*, but it causes no problems.

Cervical ribs are less common but are present in 0.5 to 1 per cent of people. A cervical rib is attached to the seventh cervical vertebra and may be unilateral or bilateral. Pressure of a cervical rib on the brachial plexus or the subclavian vessels may produce neurovascular symptoms.

Fused Ribs. Fusion of ribs occasionally occurs posteriorly when two or more ribs arise from a single vertebra. Fused ribs are often associated with a hemivertebra.

Forked Ribs (Fig. 16–5A). Forking of a rib at its anterior end is not uncommon. Usually the abnormality is unilateral and of no significance. Rib anomalies are often seen in combination with vertebral abnormalities and scoliosis (Fig. 16–5B).

Development of the Skull

The skull develops from mesenchyme around the developing brain. It consists of the *neurocranium*, a protective case for the brain, and the *viscerocranium*, the skeleton of the face.

Cartilaginous Neurocranium (Fig. 16–6). Initially, the cartilaginous neurocranium or *chondrocranium* consists of the cartilaginous base of the developing skull which forms by fusion of several cartilages (Fig. 16–6A). Later, endochondral ossification of this chondrocranium forms various bones in the base of the skull.

Membranous Neurocranium (Figs. 16–6D and 16–7). Intramembranous ossification occurs in the mesenchyme investing the brain and forms the bones of the cranial vault that form the *calvaria*.

During fetal life and infancy, the flat bones of the skull are separated by dense connective tissue membranes that constitute fibrous joints called *sutures* (Fig. 16–7). Six large fibrous areas, or "soft spots," called *fontanelles* are present where several sutures meet. The softness of the bones and their loose connections at the sutures enable the cranial vault or calvaria to undergo changes of shape during birth, called *molding* (e.g., the forehead becomes flattened and the occiput [back of the head] drawn out as the bones overlap). Within a day or so after birth, the shape of the calvaria returns to normal. This construction of the skull also enables the skull to enlarge rapidly with the brain during infancy and childhood.

Cartilaginous Viscerocranium (see Fig. 16–6D). This consists of the cartilaginous skeleton of the first two pairs of *branchial arches* (see Chapter 11). During

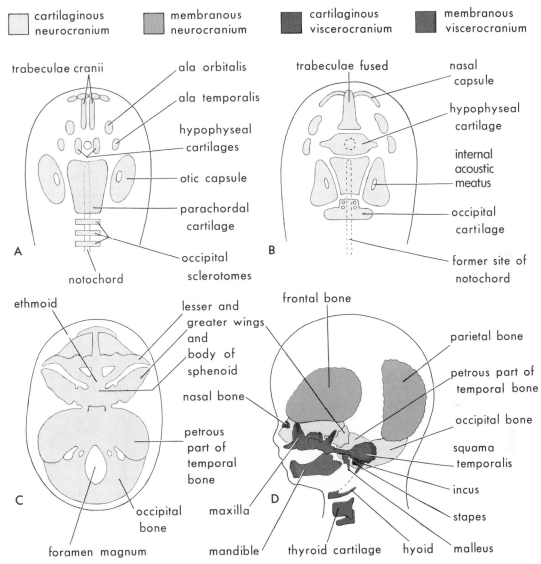

Figure 16–6. Diagrams illustrating stages in the development of the skull. *A* to *C* are of the base of the developing skull as viewed superiorly; *D* is a lateral view. *A,* Six weeks, showing the various cartilages that will fuse to form the chondrocranium. *B,* Seven weeks, after fusion of some of the paired cartilages. *C,* 12 weeks, showing the cartilaginous base of the skull or chondrocranium formed by the fusion of various cartilages. *D,* 20 weeks, indicating the derivation of the bones of the fetal skull. The sides and roof of the skull (cranial vault or calvaria) develop from the mesenchyme investing the brain that undergoes intramembranous ossification.

endochondral ossification, the dorsal end of the *first arch cartilage* (Meckel's cartilage) forms two middle ear bones, the malleus and incus. The dorsal end of the *second arch cartilage* (Reichert's cartilage) forms the stapes of the middle ear and the styloid process of the temporal bone. The ventral end ossifies to form the lesser cornu and superior part of the body of the hyoid bone. The ventral end of the *third arch cartilage* gives rise to the greater cornu and inferior part of the body of the hyoid bone.

Membranous Viscerocranium (Fig. 16–6D). Intramembranous ossification occurs within the maxillary prominence of the first branchial arch (see Fig. 11–4) and forms the premaxilla, maxilla, zygomatic, and squamous temporal bones. The mesenchyme of the mandibular prominence of this arch condenses around the first arch cartilage (Meckel's cartilage) and undergoes intramembranous ossification to form the mandible. This cartilage disappears ventral to the portion that forms the sphenomandibular ligament.

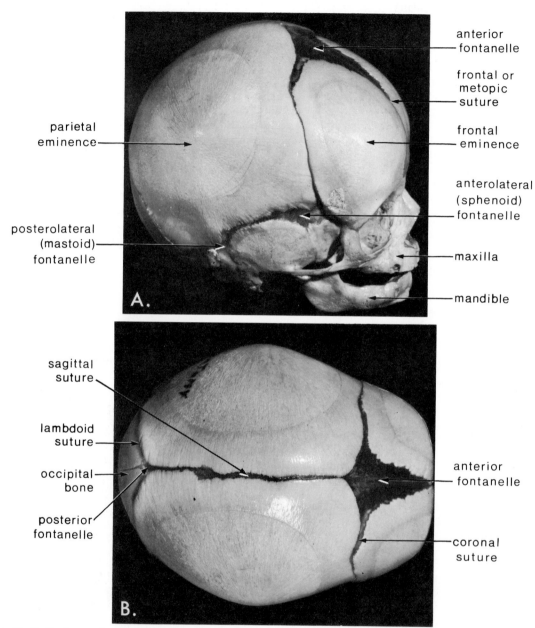

Figure 16–7. Photographs of a fetal skull showing the fontanelles, bones, and connecting sutures. *A,* Lateral view. *B,* Superior view. The posterior and anterolateral fontanelles close within two to three months after birth by growth of the surrounding bones. The posterolateral fontanelles close similarly by the end of the first year, and the anterior fontanelle closes about the middle of the second year. The two halves of the frontal bone normally begin to fuse during the second year, and the frontal or metopic suture is often obliterated by the eighth year. The other sutures begin to disappear during adult life, but the times when the sutures close are subject to wide variation.

The Newborn Skull (Fig. 16–7). The skull of a newborn infant is large in proportion to the rest of the skeleton, and the face is relatively small compared with the cranial vault or calvaria. The small facial region results from the small size of the jaws, the virtual absence of paranasal sinuses, and the general underdevelopment of the facial bones.

Postnatal Growth of the Skull. The fibrous sutures of the newborn calvaria (cranial vault) permit it and the brain to enlarge during infancy and childhood. The increase in the size of the calvaria is greatest during the first two years, the period of most rapid postnatal growth of the brain.

A person's calvaria normally increases in capacity until 15 to 16 years of age. This growth is also related to growth and development of the brain. There is also rapid growth of the face and jaws, coinciding with the eruption of the primary or deciduous teeth; these changes are still more marked after the permanent teeth erupt (see Chapter 19). There is concurrent enlargement of the frontal and facial regions associated with the increase in the size of the paranasal sinuses.

Most of the paranasal sinuses are rudimentary or absent at birth. Growth of these sinuses is important in altering the shape of the face and in adding resonance to the voice.

Malformations of the Skull

Acrania (Fig. 16–8). In this condition, the cranial vault or calvaria is absent and a large defect of the vertebral column is usually present. Acrania is associated with *anencephaly* or *meroanencephaly* (absence of most of the brain); this severe brain malformation is further discussed in Chapter 17.

Craniosynostosis. Several rare skull deformities result from premature closure of the skull sutures. Prenatal closure results in the most severe abnormalities. The cause of craniosynostosis is unknown, but genetic factors appear to be important. These abnormalities are much more common in males than in females, and they are often associated with other skeletal malformations. The type of deformed skull produced depends upon which sutures close prema-

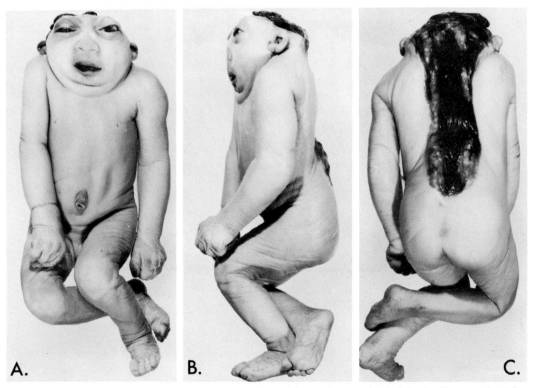

Figure 16–8. Photographs of anterior, lateral, and posterior views of a newborn infant with acrania (absence of cranial vault), meroanencephaly (partial absence of the brain), rachischisis (extensive cleft in vertebral column), and myeloschisis (severe malformation of the spinal cord). Infants with these severe craniovertebral malformations usually die within a few days after birth.

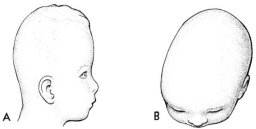

Figure 16-9. Drawing illustrating skull malformations. *A,* Oxycephaly, or turricephaly, showing the tower-like skull resulting from premature closure of the coronal suture. *B,* Plagiocephaly, illustrating a type of asymmetrical skull resulting from premature closure of the coronal and lambdoid sutures on the left side.

turely. If the sagittal suture closes early, the skull becomes long, narrow, and wedge-shaped *(scaphocephaly)*; this type constitutes about half the cases of craniosynostosis. Another 30 per cent of cases involve premature closure of the coronal suture. This results in high, tower-like skull *(oxycephaly,* or *turricephaly,* Fig. 16–9A). If the coronal or the lambdoid suture closes prematurely on one side only, the skull is twisted and asymmetrical *(plagiocephaly;* Fig. 16–9B).

THE APPENDICULAR SKELETON

The appendicular skeleton consists of the pectoral (shoulder) and pelvic girdles and the limb bones. The general features of early limb development are described and illustrated in Chapter 6.

The limb buds first appear as small elevations of the ventrolateral body wall toward the end of the fourth week (Fig. 16–10A). The early stages of limb development are alike for the upper and lower limbs (Fig. 16–11), except that development of the *upper limb buds* precedes that of the *lower limb buds* by a

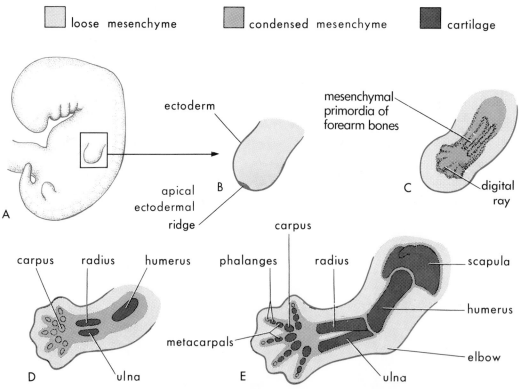

Figure 16-10. *A,* An embryo of about 28 days, showing the early appearance of the limb buds. *B,* Schematic drawing of a longitudinal section through an early upper limb bud. The apical ectodermal ridge has an inductive influence on the loose mesenchyme in the limb bud; it promotes growth of the mesenchyme and appears to give it the ability to form specific cartilaginous elements. *C,* Similar sketch of an upper limb bud at 33 days showing the mesenchymal primordium of the limb bones. *D,* Upper limb at six weeks showing the hyaline cartilage models of the various bones. *E,* Later in the sixth week, showing the completed cartilaginous models of the bones of the upper limb.

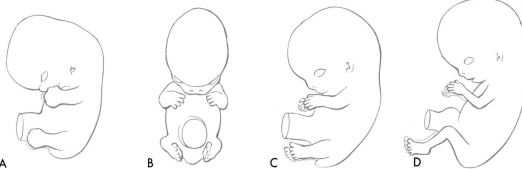

Figure 16–11. Drawing illustrating positional changes of the developing limbs: *A*, About 48 days, showing the limbs extending ventrally and the hand and foot plates facing each other. *B*, About 51 days, showing the upper limbs bent at the elbows and the hands curved over the thorax. *C*, About 54 days, showing the soles of the feet facing each other. *D*, About 56 days. Note that the elbows now point caudally and the knees cranially.

few days. The upper limb buds develop opposite the caudal cervical segments, and the lower limb buds form opposite the lumbar and upper sacral segments. Each limb bud consists of a mass of mesenchyme derived from the somatic mesoderm that is covered by a layer of ectoderm.

The *apical ectodermal ridge* (Fig. 16–10*B*) exerts an inductive influence on the mesenchyme in the limb buds which promotes growth and development of the bones and muscles. The ends of the flipper-like limb buds flatten into paddle-like hand or foot plates; the digits differentiate at the margins of these plates (Fig. 16–12).

As the limbs elongate and the bones form, *myoblasts* (muscle-forming cells) aggregate and develop into a large muscle mass in each limb. In general, this muscle mass separates into dorsal (extensor) and ventral (flexor) components. Initially, the limbs are directed caudally; later they extend ventrally, and then the developing upper and lower limbs rotate in

opposite directions and to different degrees (see Fig. 16–11). Originally, the flexor aspect of the limbs is ventral and the extensor aspect dorsal. The preaxial and postaxial borders are cranial and caudal, respectively (Fig. 16–13). The upper limb buds rotate laterally through 90 degrees on their longitudinal axes; thus the future elbows point backward or dorsally, and the extensor muscles come to lie on the lateral and dorsal aspect of the upper limb.

The lower limb buds rotate medially through almost 90 degrees; thus the future knees point forward or ventrolaterally, and the extensor muscles lie on the ventral aspect of the lower limb. It should also be clear that the radius and tibia and the ulna and fibula are homologous bones, just as the thumb and the big toe are homologous digits.

During the sixth week, the mesenchymal primordia of bones in the limb buds undergo chondrification to form hyaline cartilage models of the future appendicular skeleton (see Fig. 16–10*D* and *E*). The models

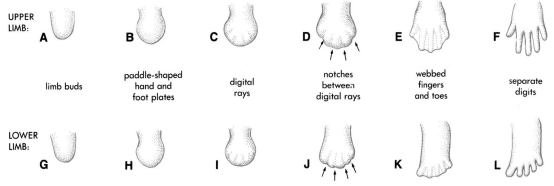

Figure 16–12. Drawings illustrating stages in the development of the hands and feet between the fourth and eighth weeks. The early stages of limb development are alike, except that development of the hands precedes that of the feet by a day or so. *A*, 27 days. *B*, 32 days. *C*, 41 days. *D*, 46 days. *E*, 50 days. *F*, 52 days. *G*, 28 days. *H*, 36 days. *I*, 46 days. *J*, 49 days. *K*, 52 days. *L*, 56 days.

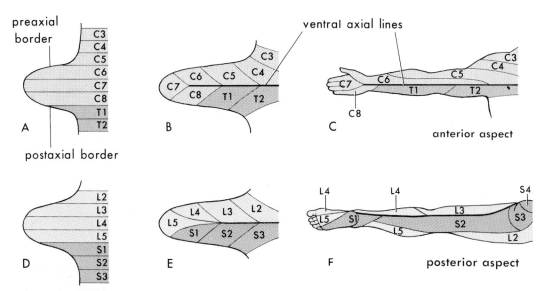

Figure 16–13. Diagrams illustrating development of the dermatomal patterns of the limbs. The *axial lines* indicate where there is no sensory overlap. *A* and *D,* Ventral aspect of the limb buds early in the fifth week. At this stage, the dermatomal patterns show the primitive segmental arrangement. *B* and *E,* Similar views later in the fifth week, showing the modified arrangement of dermatomes. *C* and *F,* The dermatomal patterns in the adult upper and lower limbs. The primitive dermatomal pattern has disappeared, but an orderly sequence of dermatomes can still be recognized. In *F,* note that most of the original ventral surface of the lower limb lies on the posterior aspect of the adult limb. This results from the medial rotation of the lower limb that occurs toward the end of the embryonic period. In the upper limb, the ventral axial line extends along the anterior surface of the arm and forearm. In the lower limb, the ventral axial line extends along the medial side of the thigh and knee to the posteromedial aspect of the leg to the heel.

of the pectoral girdle and the upper limb bones appear slightly before those of the pelvic girdle and lower limbs. The bone models in each limb appear in a proximodistal sequence.

Ossification begins in the long bones by the end of the embryonic period; by 12 weeks primary ossification centers have appeared in nearly all bones of the limbs. Secondary ossification centers usually appear after birth.

Dermatomes and Cutaneous Innervation of the Limbs (Fig. 16–13). Because of its relationship to the growth and rotation of the limbs, the cutaneous segmental nerve supply of the limbs is considered in this chapter rather than in the chapter dealing with the nervous system or the integumentary system.

A *dermatome is defined as the area of skin supplied by a single spinal nerve and its spinal ganglion.* The peripheral nerves grow from the limb plexuses (brachial and lumbosacral) into the mesenchyme of the limb buds during the fifth week.

The spinal nerves are distributed in segmental bands and supply both dorsal and ventral surfaces of the limb buds. As the limbs elongate, the cutaneous distribution of the spinal nerves migrates along the limbs and no longer reaches the surface in the distal part of the limbs. Although the original dermatomal

pattern changes during growth of the limbs, an orderly sequence of distribution can still be recognized in the adult (Fig. 16–13C and F).

A *cutaneous nerve area is the area of skin supplied by a peripheral nerve.* Both cutaneous nerve areas and dermatomes show considerable overlapping. It should be emphasized that the dermatomal patterns indicate only that if the dorsal root of that segment is cut, there may be a slight deficit in the area indicated; however, because there is overlapping of dermatomes, a particular area is not exclusively innervated by a single segmental nerve. The limb dermatomes may be traced progressively down the lateral aspect of the upper limb and back up its medial aspect.

A comparable distribution of dermatomes occurs in the lower limbs, which may be traced down the ventral and up the dorsal aspect of the lower limb. When the limbs descend, they carry their nerves with them; this explains the oblique course of the nerves of the brachial and lumbosacral plexuses.

Malformations of the Limbs

Minor limb defects are relatively common, but major limb malformations are generally uncommon.

An "epidemic" of limb deformities occurred from 1957 to 1962 as a result of maternal ingestion of thalidomide (Fig. 16–14). This drug was withdrawn in 1961.

The critical period of limb development is from 24 to 42 days after fertilization. Hence, a drug or agent that could cause absence of or defects in the limbs would have to act during this period.

Absence of the Hands and Phalanges (Fig. 16–15A to D). Absence of the digits, and often part of the hand, is not common. Often genetic factors cause these abnormalities.

Cleft Hand or Foot (Fig. 16–15E and F). In this uncommon deformity, often called the lobster-claw deformity, there is absence of one or more central digits. Thus the hand or foot is divided into two parts that oppose each other like lobster claws. The remaining digits are partially or completely fused (syndactyly).

Brachydactyly or Short Digits (Fig. 16–16A). Abnormal shortness of the digits (fingers, toes) is uncommon. This results from reduction in the length of the phalanges. It is usually inherited as a dominant trait and is often associated with shortness of stature.

Polydactyly or Supernumerary Digits (Fig. 16–16C and D). Supernumerary (extra) fingers or toes are common. Often the extra digit is incompletely formed and is useless. If the hand is affected, the

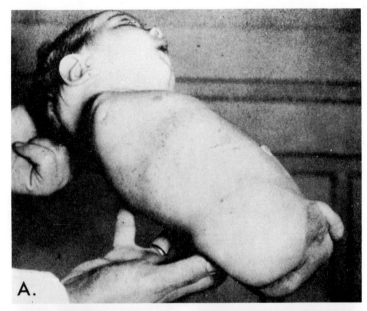

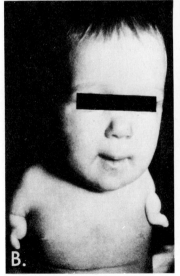

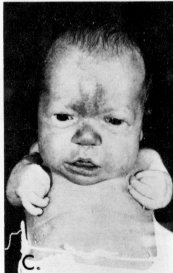

Figure 16–14. Limb malformations caused by thalidomide. *A,* Quadruple amelia. The upper and lower limbs are absent. *B,* Meromelia of the upper limbs. The upper limbs are represented by rudimentary stumps. *C,* Meromelia, with the rudimentary upper limbs attached directly to the trunk. (From Lenz, W., and Knapp, K.: *German Med. Monthly* 7:253, 1962.)

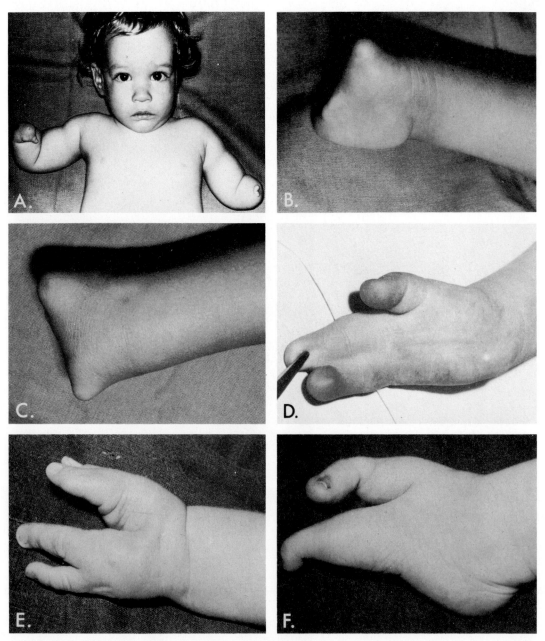

Figure 16–15. Photographs illustrating various types of meromelia. *A*, Absence of the hands and most of the forearms. *B*, Absence of the phalanges. *C*, Absence of the hand. *D*, Absence of the fourth and fifth phalanges and metacarpals. There is also syndactyly. *E*, Absence of the third phalanx, resulting in a cleft hand (lobster claw). *F*, Absence of the second and third toes, resulting in a cleft foot. (*D* from Swenson, O.: *Pediatric Surgery*, 1958. Courtesy of Appleton-Century-Crofts, Publishing Division of Prentice-Hall, Inc., Englewood Cliffs, NJ.)

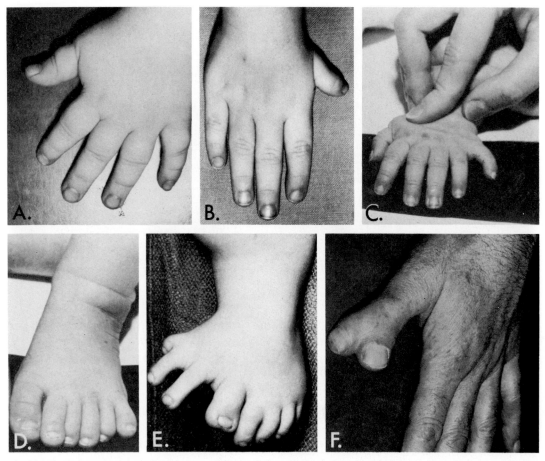

Figure 16–16. Photographs of various types of limb deformities. *A*, Brachydactyly. *B*, Hypoplasia (underdevelopment) of the thumb. *C*, Polydactyly showing a supernumerary finger. *D*, Polydactyly showing a supernumerary toe. *E*, Partial duplication of the foot. *F*, Partial duplication of the thumb. (*C* and *D* from Swenson, O.: *Pediatric Surgery*. 1958. Courtesy of Appleton-Century-Crofts, Publishing Division of Prentice-Hall, Inc., Englewood Cliffs, NJ.)

extra digit is most commonly medial or lateral in position rather than central. In the foot, the extra toe is usually in the lateral position. Polydactyly is inherited as a dominant trait.

Syndactyly or Webbed Digits (Fig. 16–17). Fusion of the fingers or toes is a common limb malformation. Webbing of the skin between fingers or toes results from failure of the tissue to break down between the digits during development (see Fig. 16–12). Syndactyly is most frequently observed between the third and fourth fingers and the second and third toes. It is inherited as a simple dominant or simple recessive trait.

Clubfoot (Fig. 16–17C). *Talipes equinovarus* is the common type of clubfoot. It occurs about once in 1000 births and is about twice as frequent in males. The sole of the foot is turned medially and the foot is inverted.

Flexible types of clubfoot appear to result from abnormal positioning or restricted movement of the lower limbs *in utero*. The feet in these deformities are structurally normal, and the abnormalities usually correct themselves spontaneously. Hereditary and environmental factors appear to be involved in most cases of clubfoot (i.e., *multifactorial inheritance*).

Rigid types of clubfoot result from abnormal development of the ankle and foot joints during the sixth and seventh weeks. In these cases, there are bony deformities, particularly of the talus.

Congenital Dislocation of the Hip. This deformity occurs in about 1 of every 1500 newborn infants and is more common in females than in males. The capsule of the hip joint is very relaxed at birth and there is underdevelopment of the acetabulum of the hip bone and the head of the femur. The actual dislocation almost always occurs after birth. Two causative factors are commonly suggested:

1. *Abnormal development of the acetabulum.* About 15 per cent of infants with congenital dislocation of the hip are breech deliveries, suggesting that

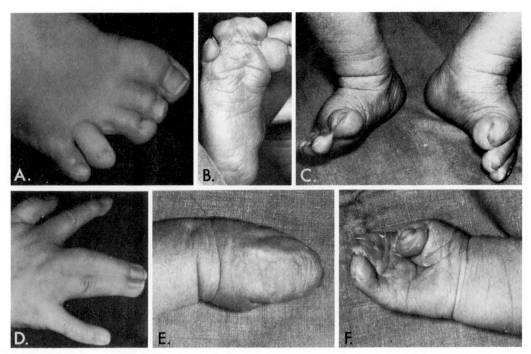

Figure 16–17. Photographs of various types of limb malformations. *A*, Syndactyly showing skin webs between the first and second and second and third toes. *B*, Syndactyly involving fusion of all the toes except the fifth. *C*, Syndactyly associated with clubfoot or talipes equinovarus. *D*, Syndactyly involving webbing of the third and fourth digits. *E* and *F*, Dorsal and palmar views of a child's right hand showing syndactyly or fusion of the second to fifth digits. (*A* and *D* from Swenson, O.: *Pediatric Surgery*. 1958. Courtesy of Appleton-Century-Crofts, Publishing Division of Prentice-Hall, Inc., Englewood Cliffs, NJ.)

breech posture during the terminal months may result in abnormal development of the acetabulum and the head of the femur.

2. *Generalized joint laxity* appears to be associated with congenital dislocation of the hip. Joint laxity is often a dominantly inherited condition. Hence, congenital dislocation of the hip appears to have a multifactorial pattern of inheritance (see Chapter 9).

Causes of Limb Malformations

Abnormalities of the limbs originate at different stages of development. Suppression of limb development during the early part of the fourth week results in absence of the limbs, which is known as *amelia* (see Fig. 16–14*A*). Arrest or disturbance of differentiation or growth of the limbs during the fifth and sixth weeks results in various types of *meromelia* (see Figs. 16–14*B* and *C* and 16–15). Meromelia denotes the partial absence of a limb. This may be terminal, e.g., absence of the hand (see Fig. 16–15*C*).

Like other malformations, some limb defects are caused by genetic factors, e.g., chromosomal abnormalities, as in trisomy 18 (see Fig. 9–5), or mutant genes, as in brachydactyly (see Fig. 16–16*A*); by environmental factors, e.g., thalidomide (see Fig. 16–14*A*); or by a combination of genetic and environmental factors *(multifactorial inheritance)*, e.g., congenital dislocation of the hip.

THE MUSCULAR SYSTEM

Most of the muscular system develops from mesoderm, except for the muscles of the iris (see Chapter 18). Muscle tissue develops from primitive cells called *myoblasts*, which are derived from *mesenchyme*.

Skeletal Musculature

The myoblasts that form the skeletal musculature are derived from the myotome regions of the somites (see Fig. 16–1*D*), the branchial arches, and the somatic mesoderm. The myoblasts elongate, aggregate to form parallel bundles, and then fuse to form multinucleated cells. During early fetal life, myofibrils appear in the cytoplasm and show the characteristic cross-striations by the twelfth week.

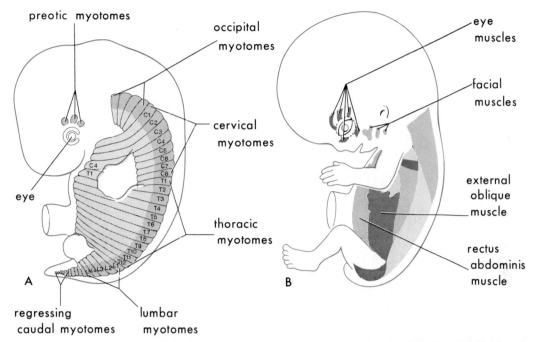

Figure 16–18. Drawings illustrating the developing muscular system. *A,* Six-week embryo, showing the myotome regions of the somites that give rise to most skeletal muscles. *B,* Eight-week embryo, showing the developing superficial trunk musculature. The limb muscles are not shown here because they are derived from the somatic mesoderm not the somites.

The migration of myoblasts from the branchial arches to form the muscles of mastication, facial expression, and of the pharynx and larynx is described in Chapter 11 and is illustrated in Figures 11–5 and 16–18. Myoblasts from the *occipital myotomes* form the tongue muscles.

The musculature of the limbs develops from the mesenchyme in the limb buds (see Fig. 16–10). The mesenchyme in the limbs that gives rise to the muscles is derived from the somatic layer of lateral mesoderm (see Fig. 16–1)

Visceral Musculature

Smooth Muscle. Smooth muscle differentiates from splanchnic mesoderm surrounding the primitive gut and its derivatives (see Chapter 13). Elsewhere, smooth muscle develops from mesenchyme in the area concerned. The myoblasts elongate and develop contractile elements. The muscles of the iris and the myoepithelial cells of mammary and sweat glands appear to be derived from mesenchymal cells that originate from the ectoderm.

Cardiac Muscle. Cardiac muscle develops from splanchnic mesoderm surrounding the heart tube (see Chapter 15). Cardiac myoblasts differentiate from the myoepicardial mantle (see Fig. 15–2C). The myoblasts adhere to each other, as in developing skeletal muscle, but the intervening cell membranes do not disintegrate. These areas of adhesion become the *intercalated discs.* Usually there is a single central nucleus, and myofibrils develop as in skeletal muscle cells.

Late in the embryonic period, special bundles of muscle cells develop with relatively few myofibrils and relatively larger diameters than typical cardiac muscle cells. These atypical cardiac muscle cells, called *Purkinje fibers,* form the conducting system of the heart.

SUMMARY

Most of the articular, skeletal, and muscular systems are derived from mesoderm. The skeleton mainly develops from condensed mesenchyme, which undergoes chondrification to form hyaline cartilage models of the bones. Ossification centers appear in these models by the end of the embryonic period and the bones ossify by *endochondral ossification.* Some bones (e.g., the flat bones of the skull) develop by *intramembranous ossification.*

The vertebral column and ribs develop from

sclerotomal cells that arise from the somites. The developing skull consists of a neurocranium and a viscerocranium, each of which has membranous and cartilaginous components.

The limb buds appear during the fourth week as slight elevations of the ventrolateral body wall. The *apical ectodermal ridge* exerts an inductive influence on the mesenchyme in the limb buds that promotes growth and development of the limbs. The upper limb buds develop slightly before the lower limb buds. The tissues of the limb buds are derived from two main sources, the somatic layer of the lateral mesoderm and the ectoderm. The nerves grow into the limb buds during the fifth week. The upper and lower limbs rotate in opposite directions and to different degrees.

Most skeletal muscle is derived from the myotome regions of the somites, but some head and neck muscles are derived from branchial arch mesoderm, and the limb musculature develops from mesenchyme derived from the somatic layer of lateral mesoderm. Cardiac muscle and smooth muscle are derived from splanchnic mesoderm.

The majority of malformations of the skeletal and muscular systems are caused by genetic factors; however, many congenital malformations result from an interaction of genetic and environmental factors.

Commonly Asked Questions

1. An acquaintance of ours had a baby with very short limbs. His trunk is normally proportioned, but his head is larger than normal. Both parents have normal limbs and these problems have never occurred in either of their families. Could her ingestion of drugs during pregnancy have caused these malformations? If not, what is the probable cause of these skeletal disorders? Could they occur again if they have more children?

2. My sister is interested in marrying a man with very short fingers *(brachydactyly)*. He says that two of his relatives have exhibited short fingers, but none of his brothers or sisters has them. My sister has normal digits and so has everyone else in our family. She asked me what the chances are that her children would have brachydactyly if she were to marry him. I know heredity is involved, but I could not give her an answer. Can you help me?

3. About a year ago I read in the paper about a woman who had a child with no right hand. She started to take a drug called *Bendectin* to alleviate nausea during the tenth week of her pregnancy (eight weeks after fertilization), and is instituting legal proceedings against the drug company that makes the drug. Does this drug cause limb defects and if it does, could it have caused failure of the child's hand to develop?

4. When I was a nurse I saw a baby with *syndactyly* (fused digits) of the left hand, and absence of the left sternal head of the pectoralis major muscle. The baby seemed normal except that the nipple on the left side was about two inches lower than the other one. What is the cause of these malformations? Can they be corrected?

5. Following a routine x-ray examination of my young sister's chest, my parents were told that she had a rib in her neck that was described as a *cervical rib*. They were told that it might eventually cause some pain and tingling in her upper limb. What is the embryological basis of cervical ribs? How common are they? Why may pain and tingling develop in her upper limb as she grows up?

6. I know a fellow who has a long, narrow head. When he was a boy, he was called "peanut head." He had normal intelligence and no apparent disability. What would cause such an abnormally shaped skull? Was it a birth injury?

Answers

1. The ingestion of drugs did not cause the child's short limbs and large head. The infant appears to have a skeletal disorder known as *achondroplasia*. This type of short-limbed dwarfism has an incidence of 1:10,000 and *shows an autosomal dominant inheritance*. About 80 per cent of these infants are born of normal parents, and presumably the condition results from fresh mutations (changes of genetic material) in the parents' germ cells. Most achondroplastics have normal intelligence and lead normal lives within their physical capabilities. If the parents have more children, there is a 50-50 chance that the next child will be an achondroplastic dwarf.

2. Brachydactyly is also an *autosomal dominant trait,* that is, it is determined by a dominant gene. In humans the gene B for brachydactyly is dominant to the gene b for normal digits. If your sister (likely bb) marries the brachydactylous man (likely Bb), there is one chance in four that their first child would have short digits. There is one chance in 16 that other children would be normal. It would

be best for her to discuss her obvious concern with a medical geneticist.

3. *Bendectin, an antinauseant, does not produce limb defects in human embryos.* Several epidemiological studies have failed to show an increased risk of birth defects after exposure to Bendectin or its separate ingredients during early pregnancy. In the case you describe, the mother took the drug two weeks after the end of the critical period of limb development (24 to 42 days after fertilization). Consequently, even a known teratogen, such as *thalidomide,* could not have caused failure of the child's hand to develop if ingested during the fetal period of development. *Most limb reduction defects have a genetic basis.*

4. Congenital absence of a muscle (e.g., the palmaris longis in the forearm or part of a pectoral muscle) is common. When unilateral absence of the sternal head of the pectoralis major muscle is associated with cutaneous *syndactyly of the hand,* the condition is referred to as the *Poland syndrome* or anomaly. It has an incidence of 1 in 20,000, and there may be other associated upper limb defects (e.g., brachydactyly). It has been estimated that 10 per cent of people with syndactyly also have absence of part of the pectoralis major muscle. It has also been suggested that *the Poland syndrome may result from defective development of the subclavian artery,* which results in an early deficit of blood flow to the pectoral region and the upper limb. The cutaneous syndactyly of the hand can be easily corrected surgically, and plastic surgery can be done on the thorax to improve the appearance of the chest. Hence, the defects are not serious and they usually do not cause disabilities.

5. In the thoracic region, the *costal processes* of developing vertebrae give rise to ribs, whereas in the cervical region they usually form part of the transverse processes. In about 0.5 per cent of people, a cervical costal process develops into a *cervical rib,* which is usually several inches long. The cervical rib may compress your sister's subclavian artery and *brachial plexus* on the affected side. This usually causes tingling and/or pain, which begins around puberty when the neck grows. Some people never suffer neurovascular symptoms; others feel numbness and pain when they carry something heavy (e.g., a suitcase). If the symptoms are severe, the rib is usually surgically removed to relieve the pressure on the nerves and vessels of the upper limb.

6. The person has a skull malformation known as *scaphocephaly,* which resulted from premature closure of the sagittal suture of his skull during early childhood. Normally this suture begins to close on the internal aspect of the cranial vault or calvaria during the early twenties, and progresses throughout life. *Scaphocephaly is not a birth injury.* Although the calvaria undergoes changes of shape during birth called *molding,* the calvaria usually returns to its normal shape within a day or so. Scaphocephaly usually does not cause compression of the brain or cranial nerves, and it is usually not associated with complications requiring therapy.

17

The Nervous System

The nervous system develops from the neural plate, a thickened area of embryonic ectoderm that appears around the middle of the third week (Fig. 17–1). Formation of the *neural tube* and *neural crest* from the neural plate is also described and illustrated in Chapter 5.

The neural tube differentiates into the *central nervous system,* consisting of the brain and spinal cord, and the neural crest gives rise to most of the *peripheral nervous system.* Neural crest cells also differentiate into other structures (see Fig. 17–8).

THE CENTRAL NERVOUS SYSTEM

The neural tube begins to form 22 to 23 days after fertilization and is temporarily open both cranially and caudally (Figs. 17–1C and 17–2). These openings, called *neuropores,* normally close during the fourth week. The walls of the neural tube thicken to form the brain and spinal cord (Fig. 17–3). The *neural canal* becomes the ventricular system of the brain and the central canal of the spinal cord.

The Spinal Cord

The neural tube caudal to the fourth pair of somites develops into the spinal cord. The lateral walls of the neural tube thicken until only a minute *central canal* remains at 9 to 10 weeks (Fig. 17–4C).

The wall of the neural tube is composed of a thick neuroepithelium, which gives rise to all neurons and macroglial cells of the spinal cord (Fig. 17–5). The marginal zone of the neuroepithelium gradually becomes the white matter of the cord as axons grow into it and over it from nerve cell bodies in the spinal cord, spinal ganglia, and brain.

Some neuroepithelial cells differentiate into primitive neurons called *neuroblasts.* These cells form an *intermediate zone* between the ventricular and marginal zones (see Fig. 17–4E). When the neuroepithelial cells cease producing neuroblasts and glioblasts, they differentiate into ependymal cells, which give rise to the ependymal epithelium (ependyma) lining the central canal of the spinal cord.

The *microglial cells* (microglia), a smaller type of neuroglial cell, differentiate from mesenchymal cells surrounding the central nervous system (Fig. 17–5). They enter the spinal cord with developing blood vessels.

Thickening of the lateral walls of the spinal cord soon produces a shallow longitudinal groove called the *sulcus limitans* (Figs. 17–4B and 17–6). This groove demarcates the dorsal part or *alar plate* (lamina) from the ventral part or *basal plate* (lamina). The alar and basal plates are later associated with afferent and efferent functions, respectively.

The Alar Plates. Cell bodies in the alar plates form the *dorsal gray matter* in columns that extend the length of the spinal cord. In transverse sections these columns are called *dorsal horns* (Fig. 17–7). As the alar plates enlarge, the *dorsal septum* forms and the central canal becomes small (Figs. 17–4C and 17–7).

The Basal Plates. Cell bodies in the basal plates form the ventral and lateral gray columns, which in cross sections are called *ventral* and *lateral gray horns,* respectively. Axons of ventral horn cells grow out of the spinal cord and form large bundles of nerves called the *ventral roots* of the spinal nerves (see Fig. 17–6). As the basal plates enlarge, they produce the

244

Text continued on page 251

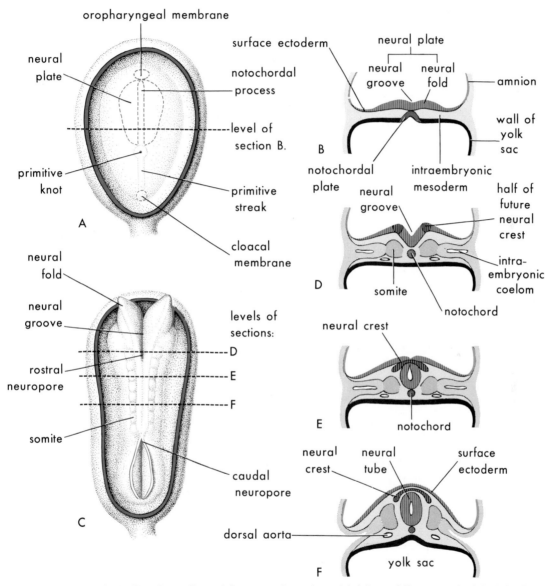

Figure 17–1. Diagrams illustrating formation of the neural crest and folding of the neural plate into the neural tube. *A,* Dorsal view of an embryo of about 18 days, exposed by removing the amnion. *B,* Transverse section of this embryo showing the neural plate and early development of the neural groove. *C,* Dorsal view of an embryo of about 22 days. The neural folds have fused opposite the somites, but are widely spread out at both ends of the embryo. Closure of the neural tube occurs initially in the region corresponding to the future junction of the brain and spinal cord. *D, E,* and *F,* Transverse sections of this embryo at the levels shown in *C,* illustrating formation of the neural tube and its detachment from the surface ectoderm. Note that some neuroectodermal cells are not included in the neural tube but remain between it and the surface ectoderm as the neural crest. (See Figure 17–8 for the derivatives of the neural crest.)

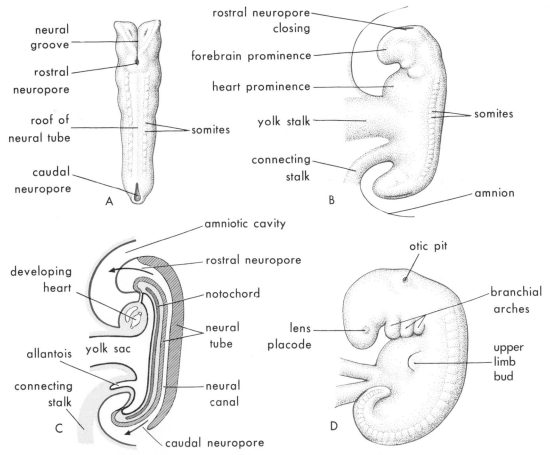

Figure 17–2. *A*, Dorsal view of an embryo of about 23 days showing advanced fusion of the neural folds. *B*, Lateral view of an embryo of about 24 days showing the forebrain prominence and closing of the rostral neuropore. *C*, Sagittal section of this embryo showing the transitory communication of the neural canal with the amniotic cavity (arrows). D, Lateral view of an embryo of 27 days after closure of the neurospores.

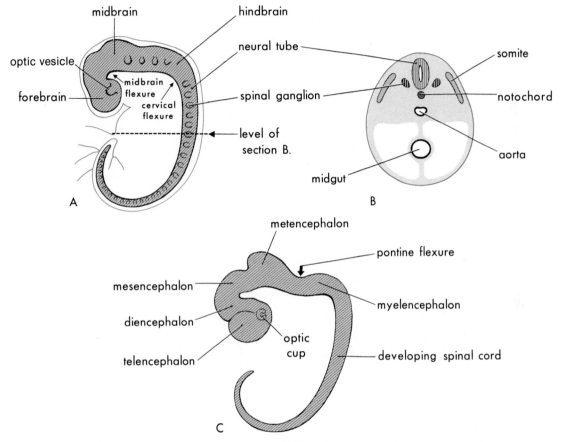

Figure 17–3. *A*, Schematic lateral view of an embryo of about 28 days showing the three primary brain vesicles (forebrain, midbrain, and hindbrain). The two flexures demarcate the primary divisions of the brain. *B*, Transverse section of this embryo showing the neural tube which, in this region, will develop into the spinal cord. The spinal ganglia derived from the neural crest are also shown. *C*, Schematic lateral view of the central nervous system of a six-week embryo, showing the secondary brain vesicles and the pontine flexure. The flexures (bends) occur as the brain grows rapidly. They are important in determining the final shape of the brain.

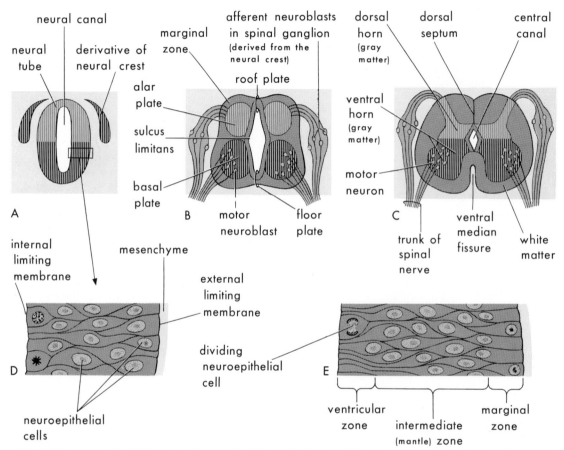

Figure 17–4. Diagrams illustrating development of the spinal cord. *A,* Transverse section through the neural tube of an embryo of about 23 days. *B* and *C,* Similar sections at six and nine weeks, respectively. *D,* Section through the wall of the early neural tube shown in *A. E,* Section through the wall of the developing spinal cord showing the three different zones. Note that the neural canal of the neural tube becomes the central canal of the spinal cord.

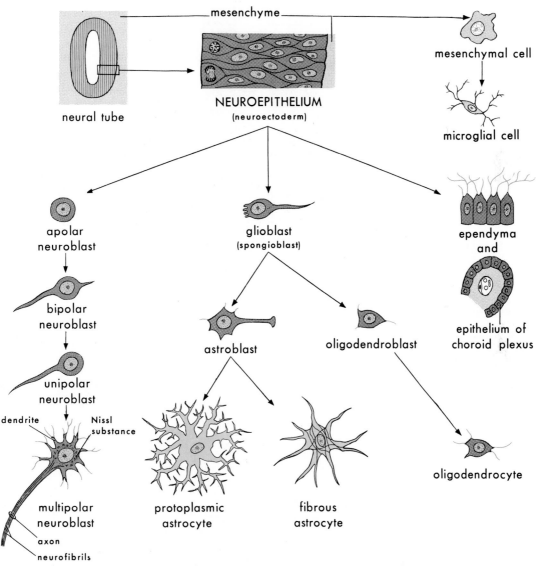

Figure 17–5. Schematic diagram illustrating the histogenesis of cells in the central nervous system. After further development, the multipolar neuroblast (lower left) becomes a nerve cell or neuron. Neuroepithelial cells give rise to all neurons and macroglial cells. Microglial cells are derived from mesenchymal cells which invade the developing nervous system with the developing blood vessels.

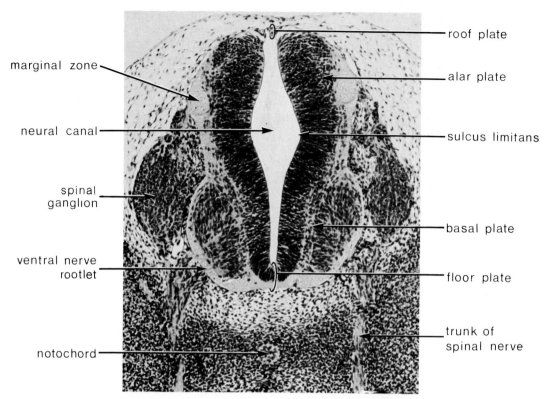

marginal zone

neural canal

spinal ganglion

ventral nerve rootlet

notochord

roof plate

alar plate

sulcus limitans

basal plate

floor plate

trunk of spinal nerve

Figure 17–6. Photomicrograph of a transverse section of the developing spinal cord in a 14-mm human embryo of about 44 days (× 75). The dorsal wall (roof plate) and the ventral wall (floor plate) contain no neuroblasts and are relatively thin. Observe the notochord inside the developing vertebra. (Courtesy of Dr. J. W. A. Duckworth, Professor Emeritus of Anatomy, University of Toronto.)

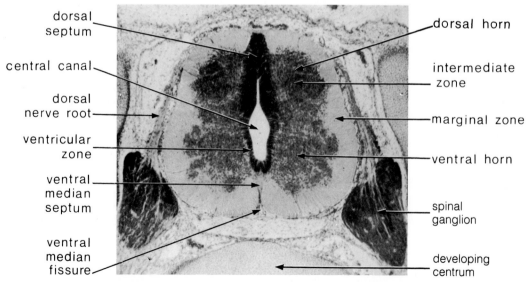

dorsal septum

central canal

dorsal nerve root

ventricular zone

ventral median septum

ventral median fissure

dorsal horn

intermediate zone

marginal zone

ventral horn

spinal ganglion

developing centrum

Figure 17–7. Photomicrograph of a transverse section of the developing spinal cord in a 20-mm human embryo of about 50 days (× 60). (Courtesy of Professor Jean Hay, Department of Anatomy, Faculty of Medicine, University of Manitoba, Winnipeg, Canada.)

ventral median septum and a deep longitudinal groove on the ventral surface of the spinal cord known as the *ventral median fissure* (Figs. 17–4C and 17–7).

Spinal Ganglia (Figs. 17–6 to 17–8). The unipolar neurons in the spinal ganglia (dorsal root ganglia) are *derived from neural crest cells.* Their axons divide in a T-shaped fashion into central and peripheral processes. The central processes enter the spinal cord and constitute the *dorsal roots* of spinal nerves. The peripheral processes pass in the spinal nerves to special sensory endings in somatic or visceral structures.

Positional Changes of the Developing Spinal Cord (Fig. 17–9). The spinal cord initially extends the entire length of the vertebral canal, and the spinal nerves pass through the intervertebral foramina at their levels of origin (Fig. 17–9A). This relationship does not persist because the vertebral column and the dura mater (outer covering of the spinal cord) grow more rapidly than the spinal cord. The caudal end of the spinal cord gradually comes to lie at relatively higher levels. As a result, the spinal roots, especially those of the lumbar and sacral segments, run obliquely from the spinal cord to the corresponding level of the vertebral column (Fig. 17–9B to D).

In the newborn infant, the spinal cord terminates at the level of the second or *third lumbar vertebra* (Fig. 17–9C). *In the adult,* the spinal cord usually termi-

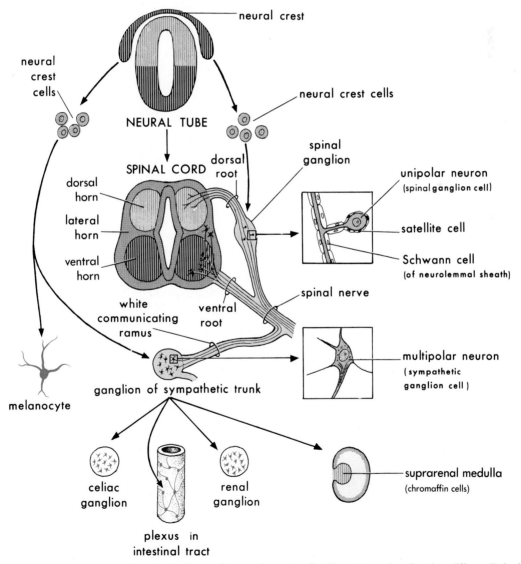

Figure 17–8. Diagram showing the derivatives of neural crest cells. Neural crest cells also differentiate into cells of the afferent ganglia of cranial nerves. Formation of a spinal nerve is also illustrated.

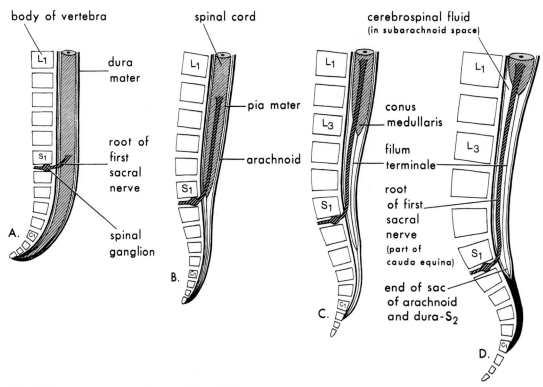

Figure 17–9. Diagram showing the position of the caudal end of the spinal cord in relation to the vertebral column and the meninges at various stages of development. The increasing inclination of the root of the first sacral nerve is also illustrated. *A*, Eight weeks. *B*, 24 weeks. *C*, Newborn. *D*, Adult.

nates at the inferior border of the *first lumbar vertebra* (Fig. 17–9D).

The dorsal and ventral nerve roots inferior to the end of the spinal cord form a sheaf of nerve roots called the *cauda equina* (L. horse's tail). Although the dura extends the length of the vertebral column in the adult, the other layers of the meninges do not. The pia mater inferior to the caudal end of the spinal cord forms a long fibrous thread, the *filum terminale* (Fig. 17–9D). It extends from the *conus medullaris* (conical extremity of the spinal cord) to the periosteum of the first coccygeal vertebra in the adult.

A portion of the subarachnoid space extends inferior to the spinal cord from which cerebrospinal fluid may be removed without damaging the cord. The removal of cerebrospinal fluid is by inserting a needle is between the vertebral arches of the lumbar vertebrae (usually between L3 and L4 or L4 and L5). The procedure in which a needle is inserted into the subarachnoid space is known as *lumbar puncture*.

Myelination. Myelin sheaths begin to form in the spinal cord during midfetal life and continues during the first postnatal year. The myelin sheath is formed around axons or axis cylinders by the plasma mem-

branes of *Schwann cells*. The myelin sheath of axons in the central nervous system is formed in a somewhat similar manner by *oligodendrocytes*. Fiber tracts generally become myelinated at about the time they become functional.

Congenital Malformations of the Spinal Cord and/or Meninges (Figs. 17–10 and 17–11). *Most congenital malformations of the spinal cord result from defective closure of the caudal neuropore* toward the end of the fourth week of development.

Severe neural tube defects also involve the tissues overlying the spinal cord (meninges, vertebral arch, dorsal muscles, and skin).

Malformations involving the caudal end of the neural tube and the vertebral arches are referred to as *spina bifida cystica* (Fig. 17–11). Spina bifida denotes nonfusion of the halves of the vertebral arches, which is common to all types of spina bifida.

Spina Bifida Occulta (Fig. 17–10A). This is a *vertebral defect* resulting from failure of the halves of the vertebral arch to develop fully and fuse, usually in the sacral, lumbar, and cervical regions (see also Chapter 16). *This defect is in L5 or S1 vertebrae in about 20 per cent of people.* In its most minor form,

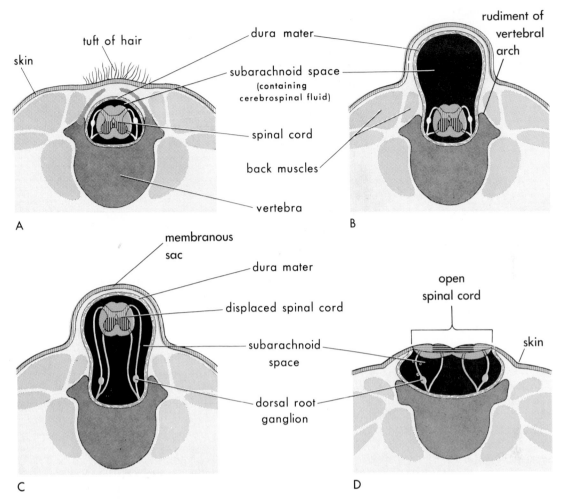

Figure 17–10. Diagrammatic sketches illustrating various types of spina bifida and the commonly associated malformations of the nervous system. *A,* Spina bifida occulta. The halves of the vertebral arch are not fully developed. As a result they are unfused and the spinous process has not formed. About 20 per cent of people have this defect in L5 or S1 vertebra or in both locations. It usually causes no back problems. *B,* Spina bifida with meningocele. *C,* Spina bifida with meningomyelocele. *D,* Spina bifida with myeloschisis. Meningomyelocele is a more common and a very much more severe malformation than meningocele. Meningoceles and meningomyeloceles *(spina bifida cystica)* may occur anywhere along the spinal axis, but they are most common in the lumbar region (Fig. 17–11). The types illustrated in *B* through *D* are often referred to collectively as *spina bifida cystica* because of the cystlike sac associated with them. Of these defects, 75 per cent are meningomyeloceles and 25 per cent are meningoceles.

there is no defect in the skin, and the only evidence of its presence may be a small dimple with a tuft of hair.

Spina bifida occulta produces no clinical symptoms, but a small percentage of affected infants have associated developmental defects of the spinal cord and spinal roots which may produce symptoms.

Spina Bifida Cystica (Figs. 17–10*B* and *C* and 17–11). Severe types of spina bifida, involving protrusion of the spinal cord and/or the meninges through

defects in several vertebral arches, are referred to collectively as *spina bifida cystica* because of the cystlike protrusion, or sac, that is associated with these malformations. *Spina bifida cystica occurs about once in every 1000 births.*

When the sac contains meninges and cerebrospinal fluid, the malformation is called *spina bifida with meningocele* (Fig. 17–10*B*). The spinal cord and spinal roots are in their normal positions, but there may be spinal cord abnormalities.

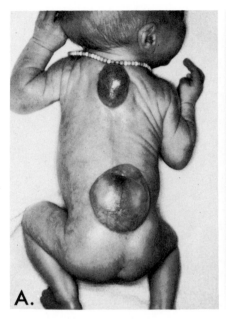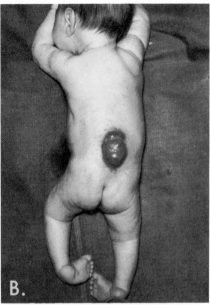

Figure 17–11. Photographs of infants with spina bifida cystica showing the common locations of these defects. *A,* Spina bifida with meningomyelocele in the thoracic and lumbar regions. *B,* Spina bifida with myeloschisis in the lumbar region (see Fig. 17–10*D*). Note the nerve involvement affecting the lower limbs. (Courtesy of Dr. Dwight Parkinson, Children's Centre, Winnipeg.)

When the spinal cord and/or nerve roots are included in the sac, the malformation is called *spina bifida with meningomyelocele* (Fig. 17–10*C*). Of the defects collectively known as *spina bifida cystica,* 75 per cent are meningomyeloceles. Most infants with this defect also have *hydrocephalus* (see Fig. 17–24). In meningomyeloceles, there is often a marked *neurological deficit* inferior to the level of the protruding sac. This deficit occurs because the spinal cord is herniated into the sac and either ends there or continues in an abnormal way farther caudally. Often nervous tissue is incorporated in the wall of the sac, a condition that impairs development of nerve fibers.

Meningomyeloceles may be covered by skin or by a thin, easily ruptured membrane. About 15 to 20 per cent of defects have a covering of intact skin (closed lesions). These tend to cause less neurological disability than open lesions.

The most severe type of spina bifida is called spina bifida with myeloschisis. It is also known as spina bifida with *myelocele* (Figs. 17–10*D* and 17–11*B*). In these cases, the spinal cord is open because the neural folds failed to meet and fuse (Gr. *schisis,* a cleaving). As a result, the spinal cord in the area concerned is represented by a flattened mass of nervous tissue. Extensive *myeloschisis associated with rachischisis,* as shown in Figure 16–8, is uncommon. It is much more usual for a short segment of the neural tube to fail to close (Fig. 17–11*B*).

Spina bifida with myeloschisis in the lumbosacral region probably results from *failure of the caudal neuropore to close* during the fourth week. Another hypothesis, not as well supported, is that the neural tube ruptures after closure, secondary to increased pressure within the neural canal.

The Brain

The neural tube cranial to the fourth pair of somites develops into the brain. The adult brain consists of a number of regions; the relation of these to each other will be understood better after the development of the brain has been considered.

Fusion of the neural folds in the cranial region and closure of the rostral neuropore result in the formation of three primary brain vesicles (Fig. 17–12), from which the brain develops.

The Brain Vesicles (see Figs. 17–3 and 17–12). During the fourth week, the neural folds expand and fuse to form three primary brain vesicles: the *forebrain* or prosencephalon (Gr. *enkephalos,* brain), the *midbrain* or mesencephalon, and the *hindbrain* or rhombencephalon.

During the fifth week, the forebrain partly divides into two vesicles, the *telencephalon* and the *diencephalon,* and the hindbrain partly divides into the *metencephalon* and the *myelencephalon.* As a result, there are five secondary brain vesicles.

The Brain Flexures (see Figs. 17–3 and 17–13). During the fourth week the brain grows rapidly and bends ventrally with the *head fold* (see Fig. 15–4).

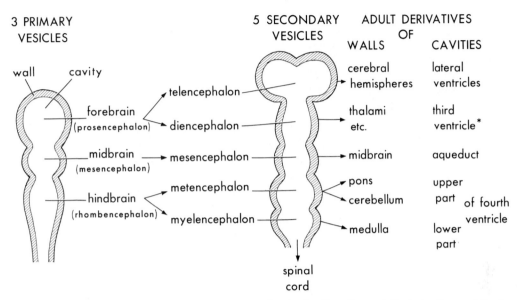

Figure 17–12. Diagrammatic sketches of the brain vesicles indicating the adult derivatives of their walls and cavities. The cerebrum comprises all the derivatives of the forebrain. *The rostral or anterior part of the third ventricle forms from the cavity of the telencephalon.

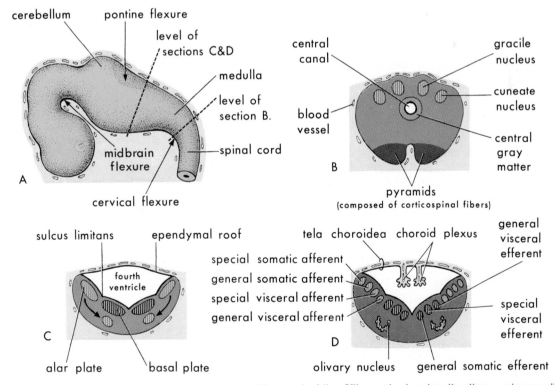

Figure 17–13. *A*, Sketch of the developing brain at the end of the fifth week, showing the three primary divisions of the brain and the brain flexures. *B*, Transverse section through the caudal part of the myelencephalon (developing closed part of the medulla). *C* and *D*, Similar sections through the rostral part of the myelencephalon (developing "open" part of the medulla showing the position and successive stages of differentiation of the alar and basal plates. The arrows show the pathway taken by neuroblasts from the alar plates to form the olivary nuclei.

This produces the *midbrain flexure* in the midbrain region and the *cervical flexure* at the junction of the hindbrain and the spinal cord in the cervical region.

Later, unequal growth in the hindbrain between these flexures produces the *pontine flexure*. This flexure causes thinning of the roof of the hindbrain (Fig. 17–13).

Initially the developing brain has the same basic structure as the developing spinal cord; however, the brain flexures produce considerable variation in the outline of transverse sections at different levels of the brain and in the position of the gray and white matter.

The Hindbrain. The cervical flexure demarcates the hindbrain (rhombencephalon) from the developing spinal cord (Fig. 17–13A). The pontine flexure appears in the future pontine region. The bend of this flexure divides the hindbrain into caudal (myelencephalon) and rostral (metencephalon) parts.

The myelencephalon becomes the *medulla oblongata*, and the metencephalon gives rise to the *pons* and *cerebellum*. The cavity of the hindbrain becomes the fourth ventricle and the central canal in the caudal part of the medulla.

The Myelencephalon (Fig. 17–13). The caudal part of the myelencephalon (closed portion of medulla) resembles the spinal cord both developmentally and structurally. The lumen of the neural tube becomes the small *central canal*.

Unlike the spinal cord, neuroblasts from the alar plates in the myelencephalon migrate into the marginal zone and form the *gracile nucleus* medially and the *cuneate nucleus* laterally (Fig. 17–13B). The ventral area contains a pair of fiber bundles, called the *pyramids,* consisting of nerve fibers from the developing cerebral cortex.

The rostral part of the myelencephalon ("open" portion of the medulla) is wide and rather flat, especially opposite the pontine flexure (Fig. 17–13A and C). The pontine flexure causes the lateral walls of the medulla to move laterally (outward) like the pages of an opening book and the roof plate to become stretched and greatly thinned. The cavity of this part of the myelencephalon becomes the caudal half of the fourth ventricle.

The Metencephalon (Fig. 17–14). The walls of the metencephalon form the pons and the cerebellum, and its cavity forms the superior part of the fourth ventricle.

As in the rostral part of the myelencephalon, the pontine flexure causes divergence of the lateral walls of the medulla and spreading of the gray matter in the floor of the fourth ventricle.

The **cerebellum** develops from thickenings of dorsal parts of the alar plates which enlarge and fuse in the median plane. These cerebellar swellings soon overgrow the rostral half of the fourth ventricle and overlap the pons and medulla (Fig. 17–14D).

Nerve fibers connecting the cerebral and cerebellar cortices with the spinal cord pass through the marginal layer of the ventral region of the metencephalon. This region of the brainstem is called the *pons* (L. *bridge*) because of the band of nerve fibers thus formed.

Choroid Plexuses and Cerebrospinal Fluid (Figs. 17–13D and 17–14C and D). The thin ependymal roof of the fourth ventricle is covered externally by *pia mater*. This internal layer of the meninges, together with the ependymal roof, forms the *tela choroidea,* which invaginates (bulges into) the fourth ventricle, where it differentiates into the *choroid plexus.*

Similar choroid plexuses develop in the roof of the third ventricle and in the medial walls of the lateral ventricles. The *four choroid plexuses secrete cerebrospinal fluid.*

The thin roof of the fourth ventricle bulges outward in three locations. These evaginations rupture to form foramina. The *median and lateral apertures* (foramen of Magendie and foramina of Luschka, respectively) permit the cerebrospinal fluid from the fourth ventricle to enter the *subarachnoid space* (see Fig. 17–9D).

The main site of absorption of cerebrospinal fluid into the venous system is through the *arachnoid villi* (protrusions of the arachnoid) into the *dural venous sinuses*. These villi consist of a thin cellular layer derived from the epithelium of the arachnoid and the endothelium of the venous sinus.

The Midbrain. The midbrain (mesencephalon) undergoes less change than any other part of the developing brain, except the caudal part of the hindbrain. The neural canal narrows to form the cerebral *aqueduct* (Figs. 17–14D and 17–15D), which joins the third and fourth ventricles.

Neuroblasts migrate from the alar plates of the midbrain into the roof or *tectum* and aggregate to form four large groups of neurons, the paired *superior* and *inferior colliculi* (concerned with visual and auditory reflexes, respectively).

The basal plates give rise to the neurons in the *tegmentum* (red nuclei, nuclei of the third and fourth cranial nerves, and neurons of the reticular nuclei). Fibers growing from the cerebrum form the cerebral peduncles.

The *substantia nigra* (black nucleus), a broad layer of gray matter adjacent to the *cerebral peduncle* (Fig. 17–15C), may also differentiate from the basal plate; however, some authorities believe that the substantia nigra is formed by cells from the alar plate.

The Forebrain. Before closure of the rostral neuropore, two lateral outgrowths, or diverticula, called

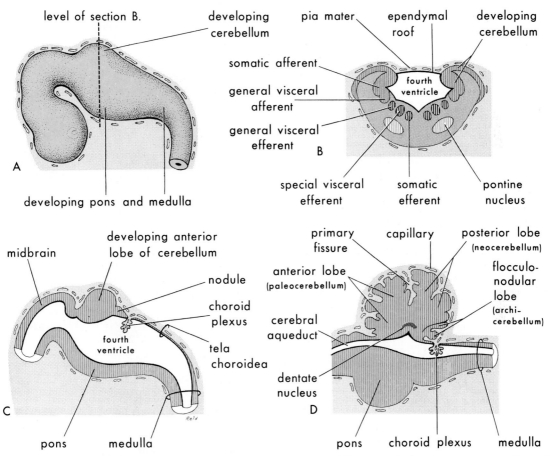

Figure 17–14. *A,* Sketch of the developing brain at the end of the fifth week. *B,* Transverse section through the metencephalon (developing pons and cerebellum) showing the derivatives of the alar and basal plates. *C* and *D,* Sagittal sections of the hindbrain at 6 and 17 weeks, respectively, showing successive stages in the development of the pons and cerebellum.

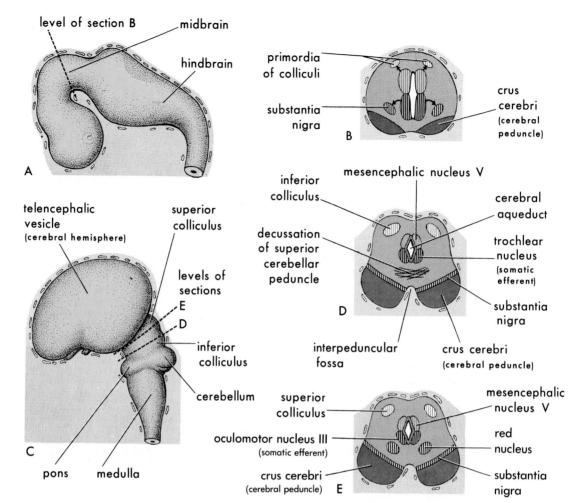

Figure 17–15. *A,* Sketch of the developing brain at the end of the fifth week. *B,* Transverse section through the developing midbrain showing the early migration of cells from the basal and alar plates. *C,* Sketch of the developing brain at 11 weeks. *D* and *E,* Transverse sections of the developing midbrain at the level of the inferior and superior colliculi, respectively.

optic vesicles (Fig. 17–3A) appear, one on each side of the forebrain. The optic vesicles are the primordia of the *retinae* and *optic nerves* (see Chapter 18).

A second pair of larger diverticula soon arise more dorsally and rostrally; these are called the *cerebral vesicles* or *telencephalic vesicles* (Fig. 17–15C). They are the primordia of the **cerebral hemispheres,** and their cavities become the *lateral ventricles.*

The anterior part of the forebrain, including the primordia of the cerebral hemispheres, is known as the *telencephalon.* The posterior part of the forebrain is called the *diencephalon.* The cavities of the telencephalon and diencephalon both contribute to the formation of the *third ventricle* (see Fig. 17–12), although the cavity of the diencephalon contributes more.

The Diencephalon (Fig. 17–16). Three swellings develop in the lateral walls of the third ventricle. Later they become the *epithalamus, thalamus,* and *hypothalamus.* The epithalamus is separated from the thalamus by the epithalamic sulcus.

The *thalamus* on each side develops rapidly and bulges into the cavity of the third ventricle, reducing it to a narrow cleft.

The *hypothalamus* arises by proliferation of neuroblasts in the intermediate zone of the diencephalic walls inferior to the hypothalamic sulcus (Fig. 17–16E).

The *pineal body* (also called the pineal gland or epiphysis) develops as a median diverticulum of the caudal part of the diencephalic roof (Fig. 17–16D).

The Telencephalon (Fig. 17–17). The telence-

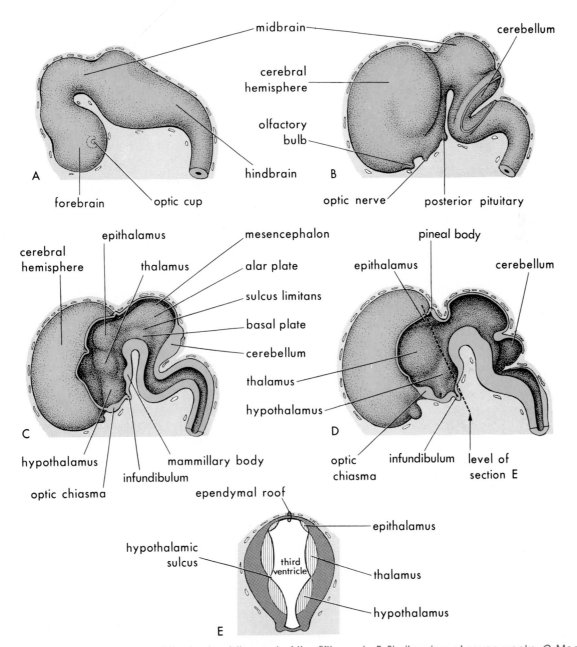

Figure 17–16. *A,* External view of the brain at the end of the fifth week. *B,* Similar view at seven weeks. *C,* Median section of this brain showing the medial surface of the forebrain and midbrain. *D,* Similar section at eight weeks. *E,* Transverse section through the diencephalon showing the epithalamus dorsally, the thalamus laterally, and the hypothalamus ventrally.

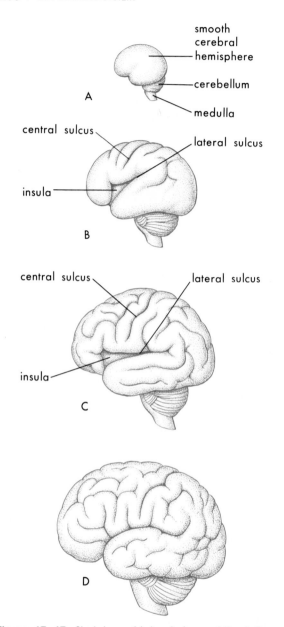

Figure 17–17. Sketches of lateral views of the left cerebral hemisphere showing successive stages in the development of the sulci and gyri. *Half actual size.* Note the gradual narrowing of the lateral sulcus and formation of the insula (L. *island*), an area of cerebral cortex that is concealed from surface view. *A,* 13 weeks. *B,* 26 weeks. *C,* 35 weeks. D, Newborn.

phalon consists of a median part and two cerebral vesicles (the primordia of the *cerebral hemispheres*). The cavity of the median portion forms the anterior part of the *third ventricle*, and the cavities of the cerebral vesicles become the *lateral ventricles.*

At first the cerebral vesicles are in wide communication with the cavity of the third ventricle through the *interventricular foramina* (Fig. 17–18*B*). As the hemispheres expand, they cover the diencephalon, midbrain, and hindbrain. The hemispheres eventually meet each other in the midline, flattening their medial surfaces (Fig. 17–18*A* and *C*).

The **corpus striatum** appears as a prominent swelling in the floor of each hemisphere (Fig. 17–18*B*). The floor of the hemisphere expands more slowly than the thin cortical wall because it contains the rather large corpus striatum. Consequently the cerebral hemispheres become C-shaped (Fig. 17–17). Posterior extension of the hemispheres is limited; thus their caudal ends turn ventrally and rostrally, forming the temporal lobes.

As the cerebral cortex differentiates, fibers passing to and from it go through the corpus striatum and divide it into *caudate* and *lentiform nuclei.* This important fiber pathway is called the *internal capsule* (Fig. 17–18*C*).

The Cerebral Cortex. The walls of the developing cerebral hemispheres initially show the typical zones of the neural tube. Cells of the intermediate zone migrate into the marginal zone and give rise to the cortical layers. Thus, the gray matter is located marginally, and axons from its cell bodies pass centrally and not peripherally as in the spinal cord. These fibers form the large volume of white matter known as the *medullary center.*

Initially the surface of the hemispheres is smooth (Fig. 17–17*A*), but as growth proceeds, sulci (grooves or furrows) and gyri (convolutions or elevations) develop. These permit increase in the surface area of the cerebral cortex without requiring an extensive increase in cranial size.

As hemispheres grow, the cortex covering the external surface of the corpus striatum grows relatively slowly and is soon overgrown (Fig. 17–17*C* and *D*). This buried cortex, hidden from view in the depths of the lateral sulcus of the cerebral hemisphere, is known as the *insula.*

The Pituitary Gland or Hypophysis Cerebri (Fig. 17–19). The pituitary gland *develops entirely from ectoderm,* but the ectoderm is derived from two sources: oral ectoderm of the *stomodeum* (primitive mouth cavity) and neuroectoderm of the *diencephalon* (Table 17–1). This double origin explains why the pituitary gland is composed of two completely different types of tissue. The **adenohypophysis** (glandular portion) arises from the oral ectoderm (ectoderm of the mouth cavity) and the **neurohypophysis** (nervous portion) originates from the neuroectoderm.

During the fourth week, a diverticulum called *Rathke's pouch* arises from the roof of the *stomodeum* (primitive mouth cavity) and grows toward the brain.

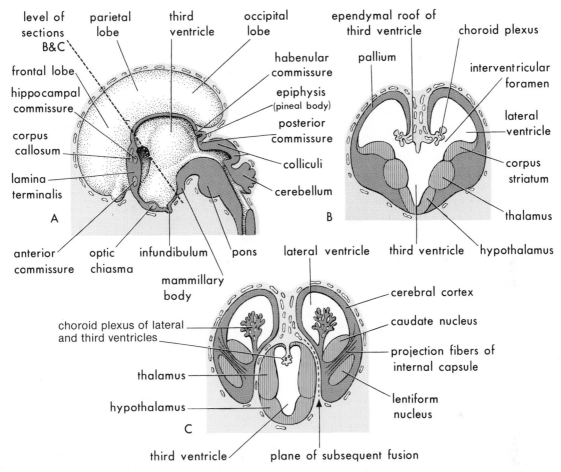

Figure 17–18. *A*, Drawing of medial surface of the forebrain of a 10-week embryo showing the diencephalic derivatives, the main commissures, and the expanding cerebral vesicle. *B*, Transverse section through the forebrain at the level of the interventricular foramen showing the corpus striatum and the choroid plexuses of the lateral ventricle. *C*, Similar section at about 11 weeks showing division of the corpus striatum into caudate and lentiform nuclei by the internal capsule. The developiing relationship of the cerebral hemispheres to the diencephalon is also illustrated.

By the fifth week, this pouch has elongated and come into contact with the *infundibulum*, a ventral diverticulum of the floor of the diencephalon (Figs. 17–18*A* and 17–19*B*).

Adenohypophysis. During the sixth week, the connection of Rathke's pouch with the oral cavity degenerates and disappears (Fig. 17–19*D* and *E*). Cells of the anterior wall of Rathke's pouch proliferate actively and give rise to the *pars distalis* of the pituitary gland. Later a small extension, the *pars tuberalis*, extends around the *infundibular stem*.

Proliferation of the anterior wall of Rathke's pouch reduces its lumen to a narrow cleft (Fig. 17–19*E*). This cleft is usually not recognizable in the adult gland, but it may be represented by a few cysts.

The posterior wall does not proliferate; it remains as the thin, poorly defined *pars intermedia*.

Neurohypophysis. This part of the pituitary gland is derived from the neuroectoderm of the brain (Table 17–1 and Fig. 17–19). The small infundibulum gives rise to the *median eminence*, the *infundibular stem*, and the *pars nervosa* (Fig. 17–19*F*). Nerve fibers grow into the pars nervosa from the hypothalamic area to which the infundibular stem is attached.

Congenital Malformations of the Brain and/or Meninges. *Abnormal development of the brain is not uncommon,* owing to the complexity of its embryological history.

Most major congenital malformations of the brain result from defective closure of the rostral neuropore during the fourth week and involve the overlying tissues (future meninges and calvaria). The factors causing the **neural tube defect** are genetic and/or environmental in nature.

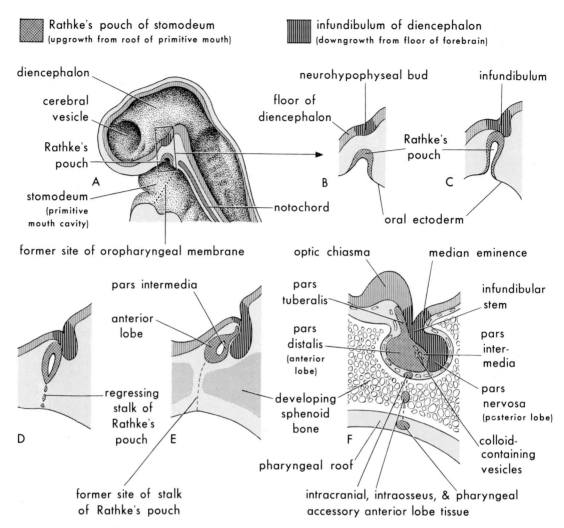

■ Rathke's pouch of stomodeum
(upgrowth from roof of primitive mouth)

▥ infundibulum of diencephalon
(downgrowth from floor of forebrain)

Figure 17–19. Diagrammatic sketches illustrating development of the pituitary gland (hypophysis cerebri). *A,* Sagittal section of the cranial end of an embryo of about 36 days showing Rathke's pouch, an upgrowth from the roof of the primitive mouth cavity, and the neurohypophyseal bud from the floor of the diencephalon. *B to D,* Successive stages of the developing pituitary gland. By eight weeks, Rathke's pouch loses its connection with the oral cavity. *E and F,* Later stages, showing proliferation of the anterior wall of Rathke's pouch and obliteration of its lumen.

Table 17–1. Derivation and Terminology of the Pituitary Gland

Oral Ectoderm (From roof of stomodeum) ⟶	Adenohypophysis (glandular portion)	⎧ Pars distalis ⎨ Pars tuberalis ⎩ Pars intermedia	⎫ Anterior lobe
			⎬
Neuroectoderm (From floor of diencephalon) ⟶	Neurohypophysis (nervous portion)	⎧ Pars nervosa ⎨ Infundibular stem ⎩ Median eminence	⎭ Posterior lobe

Congenital abnormalities of the brain can result from alterations in the morphogenesis or the histogenesis of the nervous tissue, or they can result from developmental failures occurring in associated structures (notochord, somites, mesenchyme, and skull). Faulty development or histogenesis of the cerebral cortex can result in various types of *congenital mental retardation*. Severe mental retardation may result from exposure of the embryo or fetus to viruses *and high levels of radiation during the 8- to 16-week period of development* (see Fig. 9–12).

Defects in the formation of the calvaria or cranium (cranium bifidum) are often associated with congenital malformations of the brain or meninges, or both. These defects are usually in the median plane of the calvaria (cranial vault), often in the squamous part of the occipital bone. They may include the posterior part of the foramen magnum (Fig. 17–20).

When the defect in the cranium is small, usually only the meninges herniate. The malformation is called a *cranial meningocele* or *cranium bifidum with meningocele* (Fig. 17–20B).

When the cranial defect is large, the meninges and part of the brain herniate, forming a *meningoencephalocele* (Fig. 17–20C). If the protruding part of the brain contains part of the ventricular system, the malformation is called a *meningohydroencephalocele* (Figs. 17–20D and 17–21). The part of the brain that is in the meningeal sac is dependent on the location of the cranial defect. Cranium bifidum associated with herniation of the brain and/or its meninges occurs about once in every 2000 births.

Exencephaly, Meroanencephaly, and Anencephaly (see Figs. 16–8 and 17–22). These severe malformations of the brain result from failure of the rostral neuropore to close properly during the fourth week. As a result, the forebrain primordium is abnormal or absent and the calvaria is defective or absent. Most of the embryo's brain is exposed or extruding from the skull, a condition known as *exencephaly.*

Owing to the abnormal structure and vascularization of the embryonic exencephalic brain, the nervous tissue undergoes degeneration. The remains of the brain appear as a spongy, vascular mass consisting

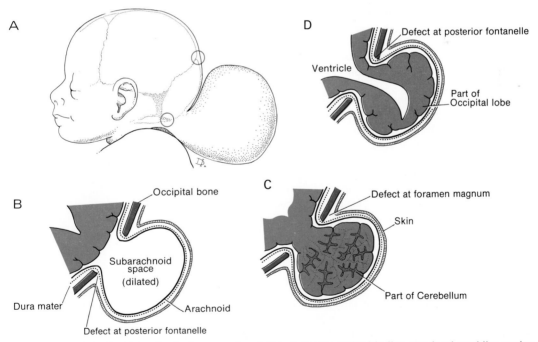

Figure 17–20. Schematic drawings illustrating cranium bifidum (bony defect in the cranium) and the various types of herniation of the brain and/or meninges. *A,* Sketch of the head of a newborn infant with a large protrusion from the occipital region of the skull, similar to that shown in Figure 17–21. The *upper red circle* indicates a cranial defect at the posterior fontanelle, and the *lower red circle* indicates a cranial defect near the foramen magnum. *B, Meningocele* consisting of a protrusion of the cranial meninges that is filled with cerebrospinal fluid. *C, Meningoencephalocele* consisting of a protrusion of part of the cerebellum that is covered by meninges and skin. *D, Meningohydroencephalocele* consisting of a protrusion of part of the occipital lobe that contains part of the posterior horn of a lateral ventricle.

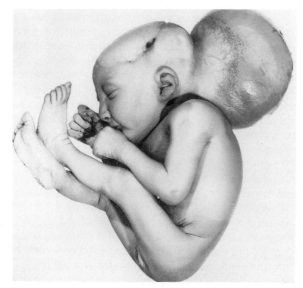

Figure 17–21. Photograph of an infant with a large meningoencephalocele in the *occipital area.* (Courtesy of Dr. Dwight Parkinson, Children's Centre, Winnipeg, Canada.)

mostly of hindbrain structures (Fig. 17–22). Although this condition is usually called *anencephaly* (Gr. *an,* without + *enkephalos,* brain), a rudimentary brain stem and traces of the basal ganglia are usually present. For this reason, the term *meroanencephaly* (Gr. *meros,* part and *enkephalos,* brain) is a better name for this malformation.

Meroanencephaly (anencephaly) is a common malformation, occurring about once in every 1000 births, and it is about four times more common in females than in males. It is always associated with *acrania* and may be associated with *rachischisis* (see Fig. 16–8) when defective neural tube closure is extensive.

Sustained extrauterine life is impossible in infants born with meroanencephaly. Infants afflicted with this defect survive for a few hours after birth, at most.

Prenatal diagnosis of meroanencephaly is possible by a combination of ultrasonography and measurement of alpha fetoprotein in amniotic fluid. These techniques will detect all cases of meroanencephaly.

Microcephaly (Fig. 17–23). In this uncommon condition, the calvaria and brain are small, but the face is normal-sized. These infants are grossly mentally retarded because the brain is underdeveloped, a condition known as *microencephaly.*

Microcephaly (Gr. *mikros,* small + *kephale,* head) results from *microencephaly* (Gr. *mikros,* small + *enkephalos,* brain) because growth of the *calvaria* is largely due to pressure from the growing brain.

The cause of these conditions is often uncertain; some cases appear to be genetic in origin, and others

seem to be associated with environmental factors (e.g., high levels of radiation). Exposure to large amounts of ionizing radiation during the 8- to 16-week period and to infectious agents during this period is a possible contributing factor (see Chapter 9). Microcephaly can be detected in utero by ultrasound (see Chapter 7).

Hydrocephalus (Fig. 17–24). This term is used to describe any condition in which there is *enlargement of the ventricular system of the brain* owing to an imbalance between production and absorption of cerebrospinal fluid (CSF). As a result, there is *an*

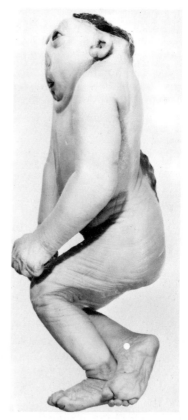

Figure 17–22. Photograph of an infant with acrania (absence of the cranial vault); meroanencephaly (partial absence of the brain), often called anencephaly (absence of the brain); rachischisis (failure of fusion of several vertebral arches); and spina bifida with myeloschisis (failure of closure of the neural folds). (See Figure 16–8 for other views of this malformed baby.) These infants are usually born dead (stillborn) or die shortly after birth. The possibility of preventing the recurrence of neural tube defects such as meroanencephaly by taking a multivitamin preparation has been raised. The results of current research are awaited with interest.

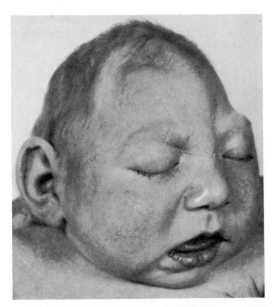

Figure 17–23. Photograph of an infant with microcephaly showing the typical normal-sized face and small calvaria or cranial vault covered with loose, wrinkled skin. (From Laurence, K. M., and Weeks, R.: Abnormalities of the central nervous system. *In* Norman, A. P. (Ed.): *Congenital Abnormalities in Infancy,* 2nd ed. Oxford, Blackwell Scientific Publications, 1971.)

excess of CSF, a condition known as hydrocephalus (Gr. *hydōr,* water + *kephalē,* head).

In *internal or obstructive hydrocephalus* there is interference with the circulation of cerebrospinal fluid *inside the brain.* Obstructive hydrocephalus often results from *congenital aqueductal stenosis,* in which the cerebral aqueduct is narrow or consists of several minute channels.

Blockage of CSF circulation results in dilation of the ventricles superior to the obstruction and in pressure on the cerebral hemispheres. This squeezes the brain between the ventricular fluid and the bones of the calvaria. In infants, the internal pressure results in expansion of the brain and calvaria because the sutures and fontanelles are still open (see Fig. 16–7).

Hydrocephalus usually refers to internal or obstructive hydrocephalus, in which all or part of the ventricular system is enlarged. All ventricles are enlarged if the apertures of the fourth ventricle or the subarachnoid spaces are blocked, whereas the lateral and third ventricles are dilated when only the cerebral aqueduct is obstructed. Although uncommon, obstruction of one interventricular foramen can produce dilation of one ventricle.

In *communicating hydrocephalus* there is an accumulation of CSF outside the brain, between the brain and dura mater (i.e., in the subarachnoid space). This condition results from interference with the absorption of CSF. The CSF pathways inside the brain are open.

Hydrocephalus may be associated with spina bifida cystica, although the hydrocephalus may not be obvious at birth. Hydrocephalus often produces thinning of the bones of the calvaria, prominence of the forehead, atrophy of the cerebral cortex and white matter, and compression of the basal ganglia and diencephalon.

Mental Retardation. Congenital impairment of intelligence may result from various genetically determined conditions. The relation of chromosomal abnormalities to mental retardation is briefly discussed in Chapter 9.

Disorders of metabolism may also cause mental retardation. Maternal and fetal infections (syphilis, German measles, toxoplasmosis, and cytomegalic inclusion disease), high levels of ionizing radiation, and cretinism are commonly associated with mental retardation.

The period of 8 to 16 weeks of human development appears to be the period of greatest sensitivity for

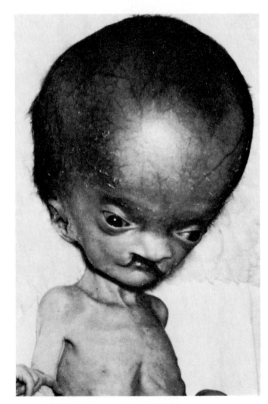

Figure 17–24. Photograph of an infant with hydrocephalus, bilateral cleft lip, and deformed limbs. (Courtesy of Dr. T. V. N. Persaud, Professor and Head of the Anatomy Department, University of Manitoba, Winnipeg, Canada.)

fetal brain damage resulting from high doses of radiation (see Chapter 9). Cell depletion of sufficient degree in the cerebral cortex results in mental retardation.

THE PERIPHERAL NERVOUS SYSTEM

This part of the nervous system consists of the cranial, spinal, and visceral nerves and the cranial, spinal, and autonomic ganglia. Afferent neurons in the spinal ganglia and ganglia of cranial nerves develop from *neural crest cells* (see Figs. 17–1 and 17–

8). Cells of the neural crest also differentiate into multipolar neurons of the *autonomic ganglia,* including ganglia of the sympathetic trunks along the sides of the vertebral bodies, collateral or prevertebral ganglia in plexuses of the thorax and abdomen (e.g., the cardiac, celiac, and mesenteric plexuses), and parasympathetic or terminal ganglia in or near the viscera, e.g., the submucosal plexus (Meissner's plexus).

Chromaffin cells of the paraganglia are also derived from the neural crests. The carotid and aortic bodies also have small islands of chromaffin cells associated with them. These widely scattered groups of chromaffin cells constitute the *chromaffin system.*

SUMMARY

The central nervous system develops from a dorsal thickening of ectoderm known as the *neural plate*. This plate appears around the middle of the third week and soon becomes infolded to form a *neural groove* with *neural folds* on each side. When the neural folds fuse to form the *neural tube,* some neuroectodermal cells are not included in it. They remain between the neural tube and the surface ectoderm as the *neural crest.*

The spinal ganglia and ganglia of the autonomic nervous system are derived from *neural crest cells* as are the sheaths of peripheral nerves (Schwann cells), cells of the suprarenal medulla, melanocytes, and cartilages in the branchial arches.

The cranial end of the neural tube forms the brain, consisting of the *forebrain, midbrain, and hindbrain*. The forebrain gives rise to the cerebral hemispheres and the diencephalon; the *midbrain* becomes the adult midbrain; and the *hindbrain* gives rise to the pons, cerebellum, and medulla (oblongata). The remainder and longest part of the neural tube becomes the *spinal cord.*

The lumen of the neural tube becomes the ventricles of the brain and the central canal of the spinal cord. The walls of the neural tube become thickened by proliferation of its neuroepithelial cells which give rise to all nerve and macroglial cells in the central nervous system. The *microglia* are believed to differentiate from mesenchymal cells which enter the central nervous system with the blood vessels.

Congenital malformations of the central nervous system are common. Defects of closure of the neural tube *(neural tube defects)* account for most abnormalities. The defects may be limited to the nervous system, or they may include overlying tissues (bone, muscle, and connective tissue).

Some malformations are caused by genetic abnormalities; others result from such environmental factors as infectious agents, drugs, and metabolic disease. However, most malformations are probably caused by an interaction of genetic and environmental factors.

Most gross abnormalities (e.g., *meroanencephaly*) are usually incompatible with life. Other severe malformations (e.g., *spina bifida cystica*) often cause functional disability (e.g., muscle paralysis).

There are two main types of *hydrocephalus:* obstructive hydrocephalus (blockage of cerebrospinal fluid flow in the ventricular system) and communicating hydrocephalus (blockage of cerebrospinal fluid in the subarachnoid space).

Mental retardation may result from chromosomal abnormalities, metabolic disorders, maternal and fetal infections, and exposure to high levels of radiation during the period of 8 to 16 weeks of prenatal life.

Commonly Asked Questions

1. Are *neural tube defects* hereditary? The reason I ask is because my mother had a baby with *spina bifida cystica* and my sister had one with *meroanencephaly*. Is my sister likely to have another child with a neural tube defect? Can *meroanencephaly* and spina bifida be detected early in fetal life (e.g., by ultrasound)?

2. I recently read in the paper about a baby born with no cerebral hemispheres, and yet its head appeared normal. However, the baby exhibited

excessive sleepiness, continuous crying when awake, and feeding problems. What is this condition called? What is its embryological basis? Do these children usually survive?

3. I have heard that pregnant women who are heavy drinkers may have babies who exhibit mental and growth retardation. Is this true? I have seen women get drunk during pregnancy and their babies seem to be normal. Is there a safe threshold for alcohol consumption during pregnancy?

4. My aunt told me that my smoking during pregnancy may have caused the slight mental retardation in my baby. Is this true?

5. Do all types of spina bifida cause loss of motor function in the lower limbs? Which type of *spina bifida cystica* is more common and more serious: meningocele or meningomyelocele? How are infants with spina bifida cystica treated?

Answers

1. Neural tube defects such as meroanencephaly and spina bifida cystica have a *multifactorial inheritance*. In other words, both genetic and environmental factors are involved. It is believed that nutritional factors may implicated. Incidently, I prefer the term *meroanencephaly* (partial absence of the brain) over *anencephaly* (absence of the brain) because I have never seen a baby with no brain. Usually most of the hindbrain is present. After the birth of one child with a neural tube defect (as your sister had), whether meroanencephaly or spina bifida cystica, the risk of a subsequent child having a neural tube defect is divided about equally between the two defects. The recurrence risk in the United Kingdom, where neural tube defects are common (e.g., 7.6 per 1000 in South Wales and 8.6 per 1000 in Northern Ireland), the recurrence risk is 1 in 25. It is probably 1 in 50 in North America. Neural tube defects can be detected prenatally by a combination of ultrasound scanning (Fig. 17–25) and measurement of alpha fetoprotein amniotic fluid.

2. The condition you described is called *hydranencephaly*. Most of both cerebral hemispheres are reduced to membranous sacs that contain cerebrospinal fluid. If you hold a bright light against the infant's head in a dark room, it will light up like a lantern. Absence of cerebral hemispheres is fortunately very uncommon; it can result from different developmental disturbances. Most likely the condition resulted from vascular occlusion of both internal carotid arteries owing to a severe intrauterine infection. In some cases hydranencephaly

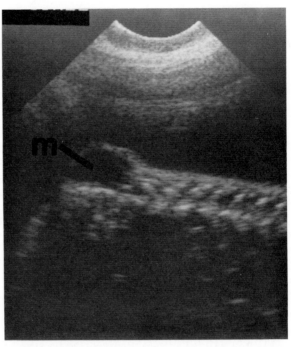

Figure 17–25. Ultrasound scan of a 14-week-old fetus, showing a cystlike protrusion representing a *meningomyelocele (m)* in the sacral region of the vertebral column. The well-formed vertebral arches of the vertebrae superior to the neural tube defect are clearly visible. (Courtesy of Dr. Lyndon M. Hill, Magee–Women's Hospital, Pittsburgh, Pennsylvania.)

appears to be a severe type of intrauterine hydrocephalus (hence the prefix *hydra* in the designation). These infants usually do not survive longer than two or three months.

3. Mental retardation and growth retardation are the most serious aspects of the *fetal alcohol syndrome*. Average IQ scores are 60 to 70. It has been estimated that the incidence of mental retardation resulting from heavy drinking during pregnancy may be as high as one per every 400 live births. *Heavy drinkers are those who consume five or more drinks on occasion,* with a consistent daily average of 45 ml absolute alcohol. At present, there is no safe threshold for alcohol consumption during pregnancy. Some obstetricians recommend complete abstinence from alcohol during pregnancy, but many physicians feel that an occasional beer or glass of wine will not harm the fetus, especially during the third trimester.

4. *There is no conclusive evidence to indicate that maternal smoking affects the mental development of a fetus.* However, maternal smoking compromises oxygen supply to the fetus because blood flow to the placenta is decreased during smoking.

As it is well established that heavy maternal smoking seriously affects physical growth of the fetus, it is not wise for mothers to smoke heavily during pregnancy because the reduced oxygen supply to the brain could affect intellectual development, even though it would probably be undetectable. Again, abstinence gives the fetus the best chance for normal development.

5. Most lay people use the designation "spina bifida" in a general way. Many of them are unaware that the very common type, *spina bifida occulta,* is usually clinically insignificant. It is an isolated finding in up to 20 per cent of vertebral columns examined radiographically. Most people are unaware that they have this vertebral defect, and most doctors would not tell them about it because it produces no symptoms unless it is associated with a *neural tube defect* or an abnormality of the spinal nerve roots. The various types of *spina bifida cystica* are of clinical significance. *Meningomyelocele* is a more severe defect than *meningocele* because neural tissue is included in the lesion. Because of this, the function of abdominal and limb muscles may be affected. Meningoceles are usually covered with skin and motor function in the limbs is usually normal, unless there are associated developmental defects in the spinal cord or brain. Management of infants with spina bifida cystica is complex and involves several medical and surgical specialties. Spinal meningocele is obviously easier to correct surgically than spinal meningomyelocele, and the prognosis is also better.

18

The Eye and Ear

THE EYE AND OPTIC NERVE

The eyes develop from three sources: neuroectoderm of the forebrain, surface ectoderm of the head, and mesoderm between these layers.

Eye development is first evident early in the fourth week when a pair of *optic sulci* appears in the neural folds at the cranial end of the embryo (Fig. 18–1A and B). As the neural folds fuse to form the forebrain, these sulci become a pair of hollow diverticula called *optic vesicles*. They project from the sides of the forebrain into the adjacent mesenchyme. It is this mesenchyme that induces the optic vesicles to form (Fig. 18–1C). As the bulblike optic vesicles grow, their distal ends expand and their connections with the forebrain become constricted to form *optic stalks* (Fig. 18–1D).

As the optic vesicles grow, the surface ectoderm adjacent to them thickens and forms *lens placodes,* the primordia of the *lenses* (Fig. 18–1C). The central region of each lens placode rapidly invaginates, forming a *lens pit* (Fig. 18–1D). The edges of these pits gradually approach each other and fuse to form *lens vesicles* (Fig. 18–1F). Meanwhile the optic vesicles invaginate and become double-layered *optic cups.*

The lens vesicles soon separate from the surface ectoderm and grooves, called *optic fissures,* develop on the inferior surfaces of the optic cups and along the optic stalks (Fig. 18–1E to H). Hyaloid blood vessels develop in the mesenchyme in these fissures. The *hyaloid artery* supplies the inner layer of the optic cup, the lens vesicle, and the mesenchyme within the optic cup. The hyaloid vein returns blood from these structures.

As the edges of the optic fissure come together and fuse, the hyaloid vessels are enclosed within the optic nerve (Fig. 18–2E and F). The distal portions of the hyaloid vessels eventually degenerate, but their proximal portions persist as the *central artery and vein of the retina.*

The Retina (Figs. 18–1, 18–3, 18–4, and 18–5). The retina develops from the walls of the optic cup, an outgrowth of the brain. The outer, thinner layer of the cup becomes the *retinal pigment epithelium,* and the inner, thicker layer differentiates into the *neural retina.*

During the embryonic and early fetal periods, the two retinal layers are separated by an *intraretinal space* representing the cavity of the original optic vesicle (Figs. 18–4 and 18–5). This space gradually disappears as the two layers of the retina fuse, but this fusion is never very firm. Hence, when an adult eyeball is dissected, the neural retina is often separated from the retinal pigment epithelium.

The retinal pigment epithelium becomes firmly fixed to the choroid, but its attachment to the neural retina is not so firm. Hence, detachment of the retina may also follow a blow to the eye. The detachment consists of separation of the retinal pigment epithelium from the neural retina, i.e., at the site of embryonic adherence of the outer and inner layers of the optic cup.

Because the optic cup is an outgrowth of the forebrain, the layers of the optic cup are continuous with the wall of the brain. Under the influence of the

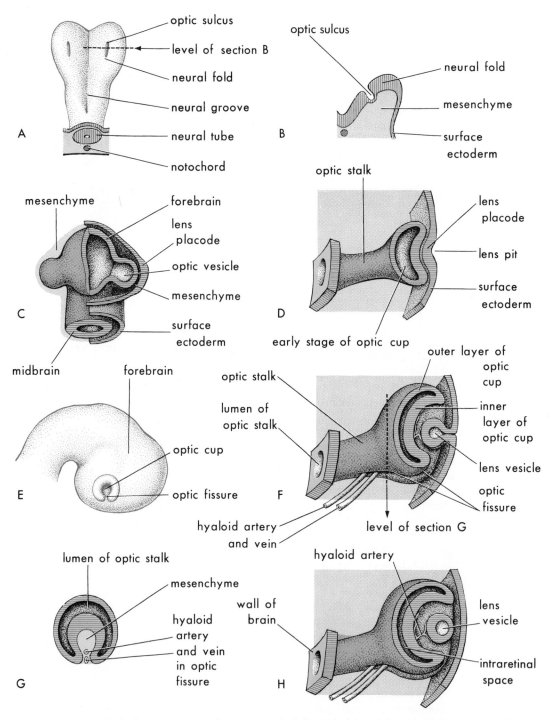

Figure 18–1. Drawings illustrating early eye development. *A*, Dorsal view of the cranial end of a 22-day embryo showing the first indication of eye development. *B*, Transverse section through a neural fold showing an optic sulcus. *C*, Schematic drawing of the forebrain and its covering layers of mesenchyme and surface ectoderm from an embryo of about 28 days. *D*, *F*, and *H*, Schematic sections of the developing eye illustrating successive stages in the development of the optic cup and the lens vesicle. *E*, Lateral view of the brain of an embryo of about 32 days showing the external appearance of the optic cup. *G*, Transverse section through the optic stalk showing the optic fissure and its contents.

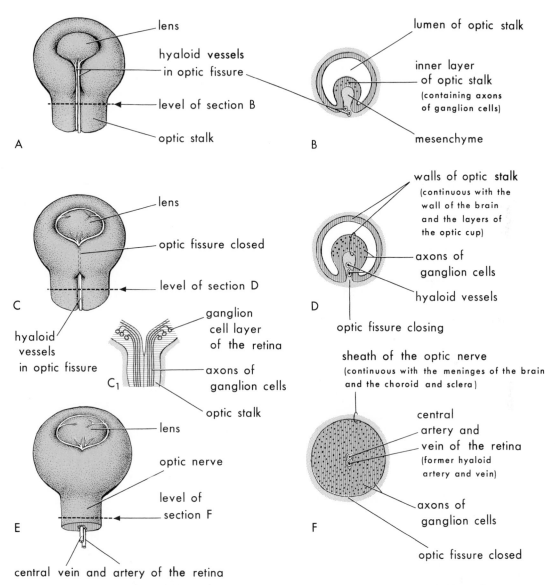

Figure 18–2. Diagrams illustrating closure of the optic fissure and formation of the optic nerve. *A, C,* and *E,* Views of the inferior surface of the optic cup and stalk showing progressive stages in the closure of the optic fissure. *C₁,* Schematic sketch of a longitudinal section of a portion of the optic cup and optic stalk showing axons of ganglion cells of the retina growing through the optic stalk to the brain. *B, D,* and *F,* Transverse sections through the optic stalk showing successive stages in the closure of the optic fissure and in formation of the optic nerve. The optic fissure normally closes during the sixth week. Defects of closure of the optic fissure result in a defect in the iris known as coloboma of the iris. Note that the lumen of the optic stalk is gradually obliterated as axons of ganglion cells accumulate in the inner layer of the optic stalk. Formation of the optic nerve occurs between the sixth and eighth weeks.

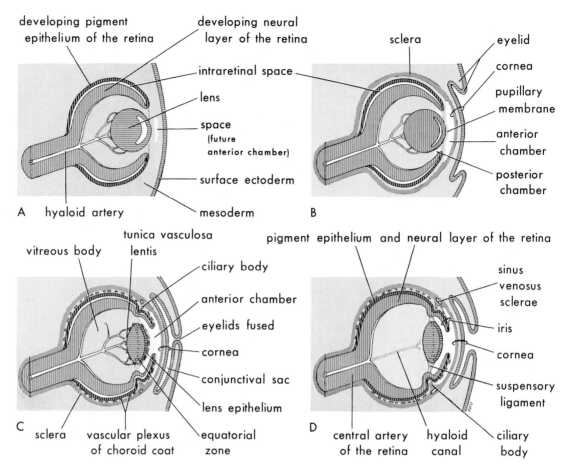

Figure 18–3. Drawings of sagittal sections of the eye showing successive developmental stages. *A,* Five weeks. *B,* Six weeks. *C,* 20 weeks. *D,* Newborn. Note that the layers of the optic cup are fused and form the retinal pigment epithelium and neural retina and that they extend anteriorly as the double epithelium of the ciliary and iridial parts of the retina. At the end of the fifth week the developing eye is completely surrounded by loose mesenchyme *(A).* This embryonic connective tissue soon differentiates into an inner layer continuous with the pia mater of the brain, and an outer layer which is continuous with the dura mater covering the brain. Observe that the cornea is formed (from outside in) by surface ectoderm; substantia propria or stroma which is continuous with the sclera; and an epithelial layer bordering the anterior chamber. At birth the eye is about three quarters of the adult size. Most growth occurs during the first year. After puberty, growth of the eye is negligible.

developing lens, the inner layer of the optic cup proliferates and forms a thick neuroepithelium, called the *neural retina.* Subsequently, the cells of this layer differentiate into the light-sensitive region of the eye, containing photoreceptors called rods and cones, bipolar cells, and ganglion cells.

The neural layer of the developing retina is continuous with the inner layer of the optic stalk (Figs. 18–1*F* and *G* and 18–2*D*). Consequently, axons of the ganglion cells pass into the inner wall of the optic stalk and gradually convert it into the *optic nerve* (Fig. 18–2*B, D,* and *F*).

The Ciliary Body (Fig. 18–3). Because the pigmented portion of the epithelium of the ciliary body

is derived from the outer layer of the optic cup, it is continuous with the retinal pigment epithelium. The nonpigmented portion of the ciliary epithelium represents the anterior prolongation of the neural retina in which no neural elements differentiate. The ciliary muscle, the smooth muscle responsible for focusing the lens, and connective tissue develop from mesenchyme at the edge of the optic cup.

The Iris (Fig. 18–3). The iris is derived from the anterior part or rim of the optic cup, which bends medially and partially covers the lens. In this area the two layers of the optic cup remain thin. The epithelium of the iris represents both layers of the optic cup and is continuous with the double-layered epithelium of

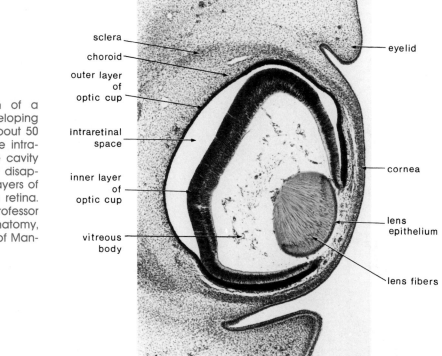

sclera
choroid
outer layer of optic cup
intraretinal space
inner layer of optic cup
vitreous body

eyelid
cornea
lens epithelium
lens fibers

Figure 18–4. Photomicrograph of a sagittal section through the developing eye of a human embryo at about 50 days (×75). The relatively large intraretinal space, representing the cavity of the optic vesicle, gradually disappears as the inner and outer layers of the optic cup fuse to form the retina. (See Figure 18–3.) (Courtesy of Professor Jean Hay, Department of Anatomy, Faculty of Medicine, University of Manitoba, Winnipeg, Canada.)

the ciliary body and the pigmented and neural layers of the retina (Fig. 18–3D).

The dilator and sphincter pupillae muscles of the iris are derived from the neuroectoderm of the optic cup. The vascular connective tissue of the iris is derived from mesenchyme located anterior to the rim of the optic cup.

The iris is bluish in most infants. It acquires its definitive color as pigmentation occurs during the first few months. It is the concentration and distribution of pigment-containing cells *(chromatophores)* in the spongy, vascular, loose connective tissue of the iris that determines eye color. If the melanin pigment is confined to the two-layered *pigmented epithelium* on the posterior surface of the iris, the eyes (irises) appear blue. If melanin is also distributed throughout the stroma of the irises, the eyes appear brown.

The Lens (Figs. 18–1 to 18–4). The lens develops from the lens vesicle. The anterior wall becomes the *anterior epithelium* of the adult lens; cells of the posterior wall lengthen to form *lens fibers* which grow into and gradually obliterate the cavity of the lens vesicle. New lens fibers are continuously added to the lens from epithelial cells at the *equatorial zone* of the lens.

The Aqueous Chambers and Cornea (Figs. 18–3 and 18–4). The anterior chamber develops from a space which forms in the mesenchyme located between the developing lens and the cornea.

The epithelium of the cornea and the conjunctiva are derived from surface ectoderm. The mesenchyme deep to this epithelium forms the substantia propria (dense connective tissue) of the cornea.

The posterior chamber develops from a space which forms in the mesenchyme posterior to the developing iris and anterior to the developing lens.

The Sclera and Choroid (Figs. 18–3 and 18–4). The mesenchyme surrounding the optic cup differentiates into an inner vascular layer, the choroid, and an outer fibrous layer, the sclera. Toward the rim (margin) of the optic cup, the choroid becomes modified to form the cores of the ciliary processes, consisting chiefly of capillaries supported by delicate connective tissue. The sclera is continuous with the substantia propria of the cornea.

The Eyelids (Figs. 18–3 and 18–4). The eyelids develop from two surface ectodermal folds that have cores of mesenchyme. The eyelids meet and adhere by about the tenth week and remain closed until about the twenty-sixth week (see Chapter 7). While the eyelids are adherent, a closed *conjunctival sac* exists anterior to the cornea. When the eyes open, the *conjunctiva* covers the "white" of the eye and lines the eyelids.

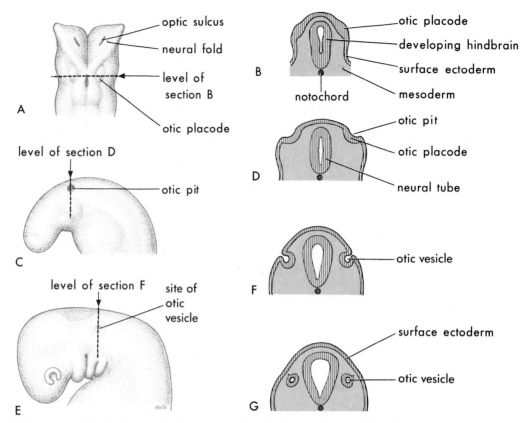

Figure 18–5. Drawings illustrating early development of the internal ear. *A*, Dorsal view of an embryo of 22 days showing the otic placodes. *B, D, F,* and *G,* Schematic sections illustrating successive stages in the development of the otic vesicles. *C* and *E,* Lateral views of the cranial region of embryos of about 24 and 28 days, respectively, showing the external appearance of the developing otic vesicle.

The eyelashes and glands are derived from the surface ectoderm in a manner similar to that described for other parts of the integument (*see* Chapter 19). The connective tissue and tarsal plates develop from mesenchyme in the cores of the eyelids. The *orbicularis oculi muscle* is derived from mesenchyme in the second branchial arch (*see* Chapter 11). As a result, it is supplied by the seventh cranial nerve (CN VII).

Congenital Malformations of the Eye

The critical period of human *eye* development is from about 22 to 50 days after fertilization. Most congenital abnormalities of the *eye* appear to be caused by genetic factors and intrauterine infections.

Most common congenital malformations of the *eye* are related to *defects of closure of the optic fissure* (choroid fissure). Usually it closes during the sixth week (*see* Fig. 18–2).

Congenital Cataract (*see* Fig. 9–17*A*). The lens is opaque and frequently appears grayish white in this condition. Many lens opacities are inherited, but some are caused by noxious agents which affect early lens development.

The developing lenses are vulnerable to the rubella virus between the fourth and seventh weeks of development, when the primary lens fibers are forming (*see* Figs. 18–3 and 18–4).

Congenital Glaucoma (*see* Fig. 9–17*B*). High intraocular pressure and enlargement of the *eye* in newborn infants usually results from abnormal development of the drainage mechanism of the aqueous humor.

Intraocular tension rises as a result of imbalance between production of aqueous humor and its outflow. This probably results from absence of or abnormal development of the *sinus venosus sclerae* or canal of Schlemm (Fig. 18–3*D*).

Congenital glaucoma is usually caused by recessive mutant genes, but the condition sometimes results from a rubella infection during early pregnancy.

THE EAR

The ear consists of internal, middle, and external parts. The external and middle ears are mainly concerned with the transference of sound waves from the exterior to the internal ear, which contains the *vestibulocochlear organ* concerned with equilibration and hearing.

The Internal Ear (Figs. 18–5 and 18–6). Early in the fourth week a thickened plate of surface ectoderm, the *otic placode,* appears on each side of the developing hindbrain. Each placode soon invaginates and forms an *otic pit.* The edges of the pit come together and fuse to form an *otic vesicle* (otocyst), the primordium of the *membranous labyrinth.* The otic vesicle soon loses its connection with the surface ectoderm.

Two regions of each otic vesicle soon become recognizable (Fig. 18–6A): a dorsal *utricular portion* from which the endolymphatic duct arises, and a ventral *saccular portion.* Three flat discoid diverticula grow out from the utricular portion, and soon the central portions of the walls of these diverticula fuse and disappear (Fig. 18–6B to E). The peripheral unfused portions of the diverticula become the *semicircular ducts,* which are later enclosed in the *semicircular canals.*

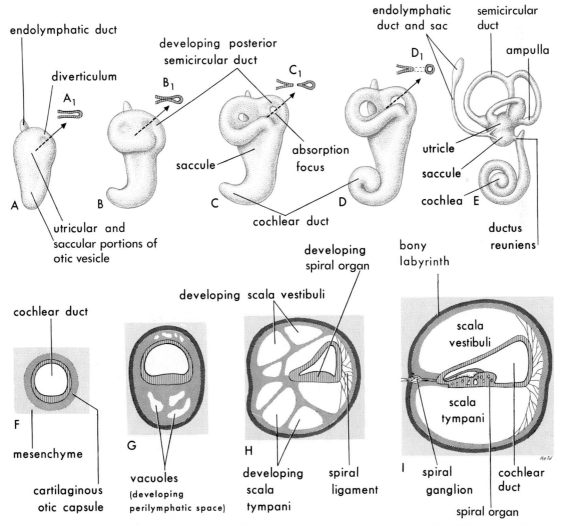

Figure 18–6. Diagrams showing development of the membranous and bony labyrinths of the internal ear. *A* to *E,* Lateral views showing successive stages in the development of the otic vesicle into the membranous labyrinth from the fifth to eighth weeks. *A₁* to *D₁,* Diagrammatic sketches illustrating the development of a semicircular duct. *F* to *I,* Sections through the cochlear duct showing successive stages in the development of the spiral organ (of Corti) and the perilymphatic space from the eighth to the twentieth weeks.

From the ventral saccular portion of the otic vesicle, a tubular diverticulum, the *cochlear duct,* grows and coils to form the *cochlea* (Fig. 18–6C to E).

The *spiral organ (of Corti)* differentiates from cells in the wall of the cochlear duct (Fig. 18–6F to I). Nerve processes grow from the *spiral ganglion* (cochlear ganglion) to the spiral organ where they terminate on hair cells.

The mesenchyme around the otic vesicle differentiates into a cartilaginous *otic capsule* (Fig. 18–6F). As the membranous labyrinth enlarges, vacuoles appear in the cartilaginous otic capsule that soon coalesce to form the *perilymphatic space.* The membranous labyrinth is soon suspended in a fluid, the *perilymph,* in the perilymphatic space. The perilymphatic space related to the cochlear duct develops in two divisions, the *scala tympani* and the *scala vestibuli* (Fig. 18–6H and I). The cartilaginous otic capsule later ossifies to form the *bony labyrinth* of the internal ear.

The Middle Ear (Fig. 18–7). The tubotympanic recess of the first pharyngeal pouch, described in Chapter 11, expands and becomes the *tympanic cavity.* The unexpanded portion becomes the *auditory tube.*

The *auditory ossicles* (malleus, incus, and stapes) develop by endochondral ossification of the cartilages of the first two pairs of branchial arches (see Fig. 11–4).

During the late fetal period, expansion of the tym-

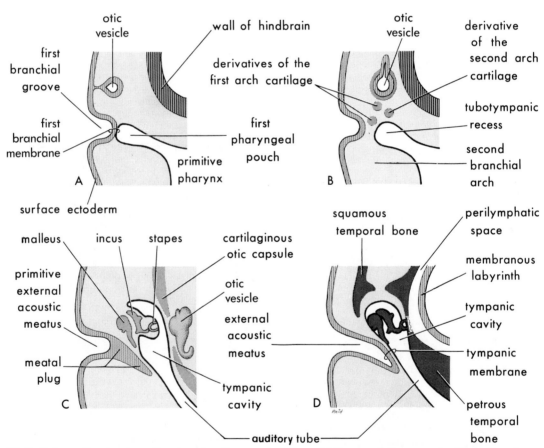

Figure 18–7. Schematic drawings showing development of the middle ear. *A,* Four weeks, illustrating the relation of the otic vesicle to the branchial apparatus. *B,* Five weeks, showing the tubotympanic recess and branchial arch cartilages. *C,* Later stage, showing the tubotympanic recess (future tympanic cavity and mastoid antrum) beginning to envelop the ossicles. *D,* Final stage of ear development, showing the relationship of the middle ear to the perilymphatic space and the external acoustic meatus. Observe that the epithelium lining the tympanic cavity is of endodermal origin and is derived from the first pharyngeal pouch. During late fetal life the tympanic cavity expands dorsally to form the mastoid antrum. Most mastoid cells develop after birth when the bone of the developing mastoid processes is invaded by the epithelium of the mastoid antrum.

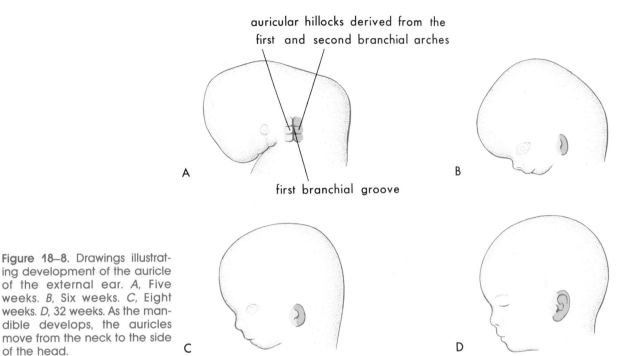

auricular hillocks derived from the
first and second branchial arches

A

B

first branchial groove

Figure 18–8. Drawings illustrating development of the auricle of the external ear. *A,* Five weeks. *B,* Six weeks. *C,* Eight weeks. *D,* 32 weeks. As the mandible develops, the auricles move from the neck to the side of the head.

C

D

panic cavity gives rise to the mastoid antrum. *No mastoid cells are present at birth.* By two years of age, the mastoid cells are well developed and they produce projections of the temporal bones, called the *mastoid processes.*

The External Ear (Figs. 18–7 and 18–8). The *external acoustic meatus* develops from the dorsal end of the first branchial groove. The cells at the bottom of this funnel-shaped tube proliferate and form a solid epithelial plate called the *meatal plug.* Late in the fetal period, the central cells of this plug degenerate, forming a cavity which becomes the inner part of the external acoustic meatus.

The *tympanic membrane* forms from the first branchial membrane (Fig. 18–7A). As development proceeds, mesenchyme extends between the two layers of the branchial membrane and differentiates into the collagenic fibers in the tympanic membrane. The external covering of very thin skin of the tympanic membrane is derived from the surface ectoderm, whereas its internal lining of very low cuboidal epithelium is derived from the endoderm of the tubotympanic recess.

The *auricle* or pinna develops from six swellings, called *auricular hillocks,* which develop around the first branchial groove (Fig. 18–8A). The auricles of the external ears begin to develop in the cranial part of the neck. As the mandible develops, the auricles ascend to the level of the eyes.

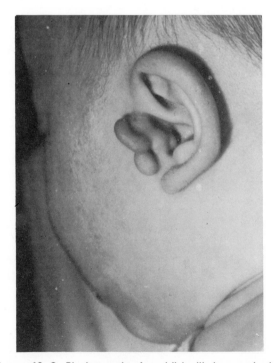

Figure 18–9. Photograph of a child with two auricular appendages or tags, which result from the development of accessory auricular hillocks. (From Swenson, O.: *Pediatric Surgery.* 1958. Courtesy of Appleton-Century-Crofts, Publishing Division of Prentice-Hall, Englewood Cliffs, NJ.)

Congenital Malformations of the Ear

There are many minor variations of the auricle of the external ear that are not clinically important. Major malformations of the auricle are associated with numerical chromosomal abnormalities (see Fig. 9–5) and with the *first arch syndrome* (see Fig. 11–9).

Congenital Deafness. Congenital impairment of hearing may be the result of maldevelopment of the sound-conducting apparatus of the middle ear or of the neurosensory or perceptive structures of the internal ear.

Most types of congenital deafness are caused by genetic factors. *Rubella infection* during the critical period of development of the internal ear can cause maldevelopment of the spiral organ (see Chapter 9).

Congenital fixation of the stapes results in congenital conductive deafness in an otherwise normal ear. Defects of two of the middle ear bones (malleus and incus) are often associated with the *first arch syndrome* (discussed in Chapter 11).

Auricular appendages or tags (Fig. 18–9) anterior to the auricle are common and result from the development of accessory auricular hillocks. Usually they consist of skin only, but they may contain some cartilage.

Atresia of the External Acoustic Meatus. Congenital blockage of the meatus results from failure of the meatal plug to canalize. Most cases are associated with the *first arch syndrome* (see Fig. 11–9).

SUMMARY

The eyes and ears begin to develop during the fourth week. These special sense organs are very sensitive to the teratogenic effects of infectious agents (e.g., cytomegalovirus and rubella virus). The most serious defects result from disturbances of development during the fourth to sixth weeks, but defects of sight and hearing may result from developmental disturbances by certain microorganisms during the fetal period.

The Eye. The first indications of the eyes are the *optic sulci*. Soon these sulci form an *optic vesicle* on each side of the forebrain. The optic vesicles contact the surface ectoderm and induce development of the *lens placodes*, the primordia of the lenses. As the lens placodes invaginate to form *lens vesicles*, the optic vesicles invaginate to form *optic cups*. The retina forms from both layers of the optic cup.

The retina, the optic nerve fibers, the muscles of the iris, and the epithelium of the iris and ciliary body are derived from the *neuroectoderm*. The lens, the epithelium of the lacrimal glands and ducts, the eyelids, the conjunctiva, and the cornea are derived from the *surface ectoderm*. The mesoderm gives rise to the eye muscles (except those of the iris) and all connective and vascular tissues of the eyelids, cornea, iris, ciliary body, choroid, and sclera.

There are many congenital ocular abnormalities, but most of them are uncommon. Most malformations are caused by defective closure of the optic fissure. During the sixth week *congenital cataract* and glaucoma may result from intrauterine *rubella infections*.

The Ear. The surface ectoderm gives rise to the *otic vesicle* during the fourth week. It develops into the *membranous labyrinth* of the internal ear. The bony labyrinth develops from the surrounding mesenchyme.

The epithelium lining the tympanic cavity, mastoid antrum, mastoid cells, and *auditory tube* is derived from endoderm of the tubotympanic recess of the first pharyngeal pouch.

The *otic vesicle* gives rise to the utricle, saccule, semicircular ducts, and the *spiral organ* (of Corti).

The middle ear bones or *auditory ossicles* develop from the cartilages of the first two branchial arches. The external acoustic meatus develops from ectoderm of the first branchial groove. The *tympanic membrane* develops from endoderm of the first pharyngeal pouch, ectoderm of the first branchial groove, and mesenchyme between these layers.

The auricle of the external ear develops from six *auricular hillocks* or swellings around the first branchial groove.

Congenital deafness may result from abnormal development of the membranous labyrinth or the bony labyrinth or both, as well as from abnormalities of the auditory ossicles. Recessive inheritance is the most common cause of congenital deafness, but prenatal rubella virus infection is a major environmental factor known to cause defective hearing. There are many minor anomalies of the auricle. Low-set malformed ears are often associated with numerical chromosomal abnormalities (e.g., trisomy 13).

Commonly Asked Questions

1. If a woman has *rubella* (German measles) during the first trimester of pregnancy, what are the chances that the embryo/fetus will be affected? What is the most common manifestation in babies of late fetal rubella infection?
2. I have heard that a good way of preventing congenital malformations caused by the rubella virus is by the purposeful exposure of young girls to rubella (German measles). Is this the best way of preventing a future mother from having a blind and deaf baby owing to rubella infection during pregnancy? If not, what can be done to provide *immunization against rubella infection?*
3. A nurse told me that deafness and blindness occurring during childhood can result from what she called "fetal syphilis." Is this true? If so, tell me how this could happen. Can these malformations be prevented?
4. I recently heard that blindness and deafness can result from *herpes virus* infections. Is this true, and if so, which herpes viruses are involved? What are the infants' chances of normal development?
5. I read in the paper that *methyl mercury exposure in utero* can cause mental retardation, deafness, and blindness. The mother had apparently been eating contaminated fish. Can you explain how these malformations could be caused by methyl mercury?

Answers

1. *The chance of significant damage to the embryo/ fetus depends primarily on the timing of the infection with the rubella virus.* With infection early in the first trimester, it is estimated that about 50 per cent of the pregnancies will end in spontaneous abortion, stillbirth, or severe congenital malformations (deafness, cataract, glaucoma, and mental retardation). When infection occurs at the end of the first trimester, the probability of congenital malformations is only slightly higher than for an uncomplicated pregnancy. However, infections occurring late in the first trimester may result in severe eye infections (e.g., chorioretinitis), which may affect visual development. *Deafness is the most common manifestation of late fetal rubella infection* (i.e., during the second and third trimesters).

2. The purposeful exposure of young girls to rubella (German measles) is not recommended. Although complications resulting from such infections are relatively uncommon, neuritis and arthritis occasionally occur. *Encephalitis* occurs in about 1 out of 6000 cases. Furthermore, the rubella infection is often subclinical (difficult to detect) and yet represents a risk to pregnant women. The chance of injury to embryos is possible because the danger period is greatest when the eyes and ears are developing. This occurs early enough in pregnancy that some women would be unaware that they are pregnant. A much better way of providing immunization against rubella is the use of *live-virus vaccine.* This is given to children over 15 months of age and to non-pregnant post-pubertal females who can be reasonably relied upon not to become pregnant within three months of immunization.

3. *Congenital syphilis* (fetal syphilis) results from the transplacental transmission of a microorganism called *Treponema pallidum.* The transmission from untreated pregnant women may occur throughout pregnancy but is most likely during the last trimester. Deafness and tooth deformities commonly develop in these children. These malformations can be prevented by treating the mother during pregnancy. The microorganism that causes syphilis is very sensitive to penicillin, an antibiotic that does not harm the fetus.

4. There are several viruses in the *herpes virus family* that can cause blindness and deafness during infancy. *Cytomegalovirus* can cross the placenta; it can be transmitted to the infant during birth, or it can be passed to the baby in the breast milk. Herpes simplex viruses (usually type 2, or genital, herpes) are usually transmitted just before or during birth. The chances for normal development of these infants is not good. Some of them develop microcephaly, seizures, deafness, and blindness.

5. *Methyl mercury has been shown to be teratogenic in human embryos,* especially to the developing brain. As the eyes and internal ears develop as outgrowths from the brain, it is understandable how their development could also be affected. Besides *the methyl mercury that passes from the mother to the embryo/fetus via the placenta,* the newborn infant may receive more methyl mercury from the breast milk. Sources of methyl mercury have included fish from contaminated water, flour made from methyl mercury–treated seed grain, and meat eaten from animals raised on such seed grain.

The Skin, Cutaneous Appendages, and Teeth

SKIN

The skin consists of two morphologically different layers, the *epidermis* and *dermis*. The epidermis is derived from surface *ectoderm* and the dermis from *mesoderm*.

Epidermis (Fig. 19–1). Initially the epidermis consists of a single layer of ectodermal cells. The surface ectodermal cells proliferate and form a protective layer, the *periderm*. Cells from this layer slough off and form part of the *vernix caseosa,* a cheeselike substance that protects the skin from constant exposure to amniotic fluid, which later contains fetal urine. In addition, it facilitates birth of the fetus owing to its slippery nature.

By about 11 weeks, cells from the basal layer, or *stratum germinativum,* have formed an intermediate layer. All layers of the adult epidermis are present at birth.

During the early fetal period, cells from the *neural crest* (see Fig. 17–8) migrate into the dermis and differentiate into *melanoblasts* (Fig. 19–1C). These cells soon enter the epidermis and differentiate into *melanocytes,* which lie at the epidermal-dermal junction (Fig. 19–1D). The melanocytes produce melanin and distribute it to the epidermal cells. Very few melanocytes develop in the skin of the palms and the soles. *Melanin pigment formation occurs mainly after birth* when the process is stimulated, e.g., by ultraviolet radiation.

Dermis (Fig. 19–1). The dermis is derived from the mesoderm underlying the surface ectoderm. By 11 weeks, the mesenchymal cells derived from the mesoderm have begun to produce collagenous and elastic connective tissue fibers. The dermis projects superficially into the epidermis and forms *dermal papillae.* Capillary loops develop in some dermal papillae and sensory nerve endings form in others.

Disorders of Keratinization. *Ichthyosis* (Gr. *ichthys,* fish) is a general term that is applied to a group of disorders resulting from *excessive keratinization.* They are characterized by dryness and *fishskin-like scaling of the skin.* Scaling is often pronounced, involving the entire body surface.

A *harlequin fetus* results from an uncommon keratinizing disorder that is inherited as an autosomal recessive trait. The skin is markedly thickened, ridged, and cracked. Affected infants have a grotesque appearance, and most of them die within the first week of life.

A *"collodion baby"* is covered at birth by a thick, taut membrane resembling collodion. This membrane cracks with the first respiratory efforts and begins to fall off in large sheets, but complete shedding may take several weeks.

HAIR

Hair begins to develop early in the fetal period, but it does not become easily recognizable until about the twentieth week.

A hair follicle begins as a solid downgrowth of the epidermis into the underlying dermis (Fig. 19–2A). The deepest part of the *hair bud* soon becomes club-shaped to form a *hair bulb* (Fig. 19–2B). The epithelial

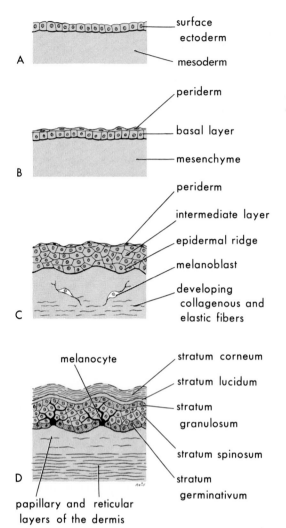

Figure 19-1. Drawings illustrating successive stages in the development of thick skin. *A*, Four weeks. *B*, Seven weeks. *C*, 11 weeks. *D*, Newborn. The epidermis is derived from the surface ectoderm and the dermis develops from mesenchyme that is derived from the somatic layer of mesoderm. Note the position of the melanocytes in the basal layer of the epidermis and the way their branching processes extend between the epidermal cells to supply them with melanin.

cells of the hair bulb constitute the *germinal matrix*, which later gives rise to the hair.

The hair bulb is soon invaginated by a small *mesenchymal hair papilla* (Fig. 19–2C). The peripheral cells of the developing hair follicle form the *epithelial root sheath*. The surrounding mesenchymal cells differentiate into the *dermal root sheath* (Fig. 19–2D). As cells in the *germinal matrix* proliferate, they are pushed toward the surface, where they become keratinized (hardened) to form the *hair shaft* (Fig. 19–2C). The hair grows, pierces the epidermis, and protrudes above the surface of the skin.

Hairs on the eyebrows and upper lip have developed by the end of the twelfth week. These initial hairs, called *lanugo* or *lanugo hairs*, are shed at birth or shortly thereafter.

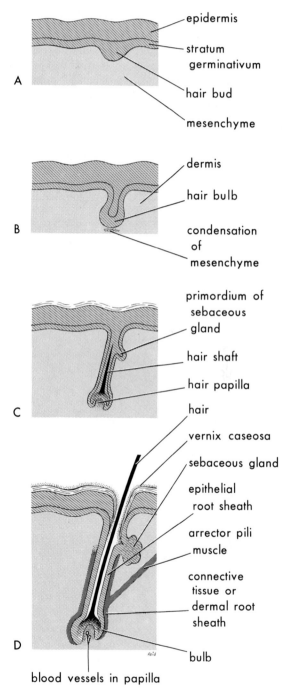

Figure 19–2. Drawings showing successive stages in the development of a hair and its associated sebaceous gland. *A*, 12 weeks. *B*, 14 weeks. *C*, 16 weeks. *D*, 18 weeks. Note that the sebaceous gland develops as an outgrowth from the side of the hair follicle.

Congenital Alopecia (Atrichia Congenita). Absence or loss of hair may occur alone or with other abnormalities of the skin and its derivatives. The hair loss may be caused by failure of hair follicles to develop, or it may result from follicles producing poor-quality hairs.

Hypertrichosis. Excessive hairiness results from the development of excess hair follicles, or from the persistence of hairs that normally disappear during the perinatal period. Localized hypertrichosis is often associated with *spina bifida occulta* (see Chapter 17).

SEBACEOUS GLANDS

These glands develop as buds from the sides of developing hair follicles (Fig. 19–2C). The glandular buds grow into the surrounding connective tissue and branch to form the primordia of several alveoli and their associated ducts (Fig. 19–2D).

The whitish, creamlike paste, called *vernix caseosa,* covering the skin of the fetus is formed from the mixture of the secretion of the sebaceous glands with degenerated epidermal cells and hairs. *Vernix caseosa protects the skin* against the macerating action of the amniotic fluid.

SWEAT GLANDS

These glands develop as solid epidermal downgrowths into the underlying dermis (Fig. 19–3). As the bud elongates, its end coils to form the primordium of the secretory portion of the gland. The epithelial attachment of the developing gland to the epidermis forms the primordium of the duct (Fig. 19–3C and D).

The distribution of *large sweat glands* in humans is very limited; they are mostly confined to the axillae, pubic region, and areolae of the breasts. They develop from the downgrowths of the stratum germinativum of the epidermis that give rise to hair follicles. As a result, the ducts of these glands open not onto the skin surface, as do ordinary sweat glands, but into hair follicles superficial to the openings of the sebaceous glands.

NAILS

The nails begin to develop at the tips of the digits at about 10 weeks. Development of fingernails precedes that of toenails. The nails first appear as thickened areas or fields of epidermis on the dorsal aspect of each digit (Fig. 19–4A). These *nail fields* are surrounded laterally and proximally by elevations of the epidermis called *nail folds.* Cells from the proximal nail fold grow over the nail field and become keratinized to form the *nail plate,* commonly called the *nail* (Fig. 19–4B and C).

The fingernails reach the fingertips by about 32 weeks; the toenails reach the toetips by about 36 weeks (see Fig. 7–9). Nails that have not reached the tips of the digits at birth are an indication of prematurity.

MAMMARY GLANDS

The mammary glands begin to develop during the sixth week as solid primary buds of the epidermis into the underlying mesenchyme (Fig. 19–5C). These primary buds occur along two thickened strips of ectoderm, the *mammary ridges* (Fig. 19–5A). Each primary mammary bud soon gives rise to several secondary buds which develop into the *lactiferous*

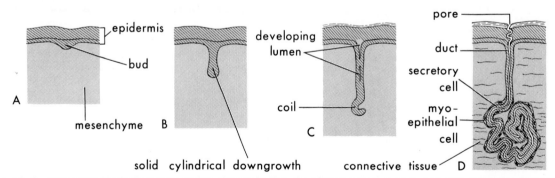

Figure 19–3. Diagrams illustrating successive stages in the development of a sweat gland. It begins to develop at about 20 weeks as a solid downgrowth of epidermal cells into the mesenchyme. The terminal part coils and forms the body of the gland. The central cells degenerate to form the lumen of the gland and the peripheral cells differentiate into secretory cells and contractile myoepithelial cells.

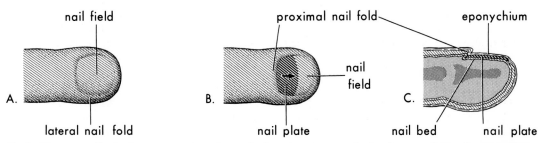

Figure 19–4. Diagrams illustrating successive stages in the development of a fingernail. The fingernails reach the fingertips by 32 weeks and extend beyond them in full-term infants. The first indication of a nail is a thickening of the epidermis, the nail field, at the tip of the digit. The nail field grows dorsally and proximally to occupy the normal position of the nail *(A)*. As the nail develops, it slowly grows toward the tip of the digit *(B)*, which it reaches before birth.

ducts and their branches that make up the *mammary gland* (Fig. 19–5F).

The epidermis at the origin of the mammary gland becomes depressed to form a shallow *mammary pit* (Fig. 19–5E). The nipples are poorly formed and depressed in newborn infants. Soon after birth, the nipples usually rise from the mammary pits owing to the proliferation of the surrounding connective tissues of the *areola,* the circular pigmented area of skin around the nipple.

The mammary glands of newborn males and females are often enlarged and may produce secretions

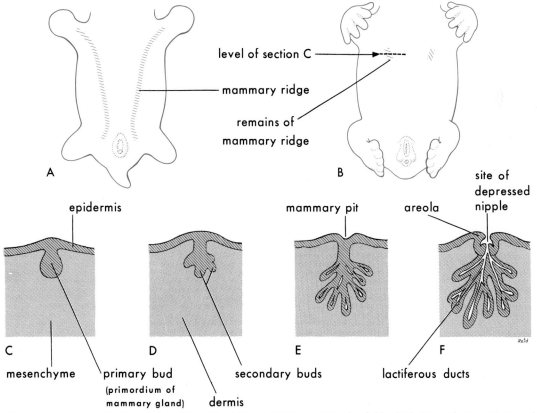

Figure 19–5. Drawings illustrating development of the mammary glands. *A,* Ventral view of an embryo of about 28 days showing the mammary ridges. *B,* Similar view at six weeks showing the remains of these ridges. *C,* Transverse section through the mammary ridge at the site of a developing mammary gland. *D, E,* and *F,* Similar sections showing successive stages of development between the twelfth week and birth.

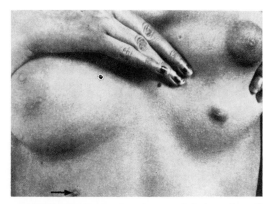

Figure 19–6. Photograph of an adult female with a supernumerary nipple on the right (arrow) and a supernumerary breast inferior to the normal left one. (From Haagensen, C. D.: *Diseases of the Breast,* rev. 2nd ed. Philadelphia, W. B. Saunders Company, 1974.)

(often called "witch's milk"). These transitory changes are caused by maternal hormones passing into the fetal circulation via the placenta.

Supernumerary Breasts and Nipples (Fig. 19–6). An extra breast *(polymastia)* or nipple *(polythelia)* occurs in about 1 per cent of the female population and is an inheritable condition. Supernumerary nipples may also occur in males.

An extra breast or nipple usually develops just inferior to the normal breast. In these positions, the extra nipples or breasts develop from extra mammary buds along the mammary ridges. Accessory breasts may have normal mammary gland tissue and become functional during pregnancy.

TEETH

Two sets of teeth normally develop: the *primary dentition,* or deciduous teeth (milk teeth), and the *secondary dentition,* or permanent teeth (Table 19–1).

The teeth develop from ectoderm and mesoderm. Enamel is derived from the ectoderm of the oral cavity; all other tissues differentiate from the surrounding mesoderm.

The Bud Stage (Figs. 19–7 and 19–8A and B). Tooth development begins early in the sixth week as linear U-shaped bands of oral epithelium, called **dental laminae,** form. Localized proliferations of cells in the dental laminae produce ten round or oval swellings called **tooth buds.** These buds grow into the underlying mesenchyme and develop into the deciduous teeth. The first teeth are called deciduous teeth because they are shed during childhood (Table 19–1). There are ten tooth buds in each jaw, one for each deciduous tooth.

The tooth buds for the permanent teeth with deciduous predecessors begin to appear at about 10 weeks (Fig. 19–8D). They develop as outgrowths from the dental lamina. The buds for the second and third permanent molars develop after birth.

The Cap Stage (Fig. 19–8C). The tooth bud becomes slightly invaginated by mesenchyme called the *dental papilla.* This gives the developing tooth a caplike appearance. The dental papilla gives rise to the *dentin* and *dental pulp.*

The developing tooth, now called an *enamel organ,* later produces enamel. As the enamel organ and dental papilla form, the mesenchyme surrounding them condenses to form a capsule-like structure called the *dental sac* (Fig. 19–8E and F). It gives rise to the cementum and *periodontal ligament.*

The Bell Stage (Fig. 19–8D). As invagination of the enamel organ continues, the developing tooth assumes the shape of a bell. Mesenchymal cells in the dental papilla adjacent to the inner enamel epithelium differentiate into **odontoblasts.** These cells produce *predentin* and deposit it adjacent to the inner enamel epithelium. Later the predentin calcifies and becomes *dentin.* As the dentin thickens, the odontoblasts regress toward the center of the dental papilla, but cytoplasmic processes, called *odontoblastic processes,* remain embedded in the dentin (Fig. 19–8F and I).

Cells of the inner enamel epithelium, adjacent to the dentin, differentiate into **ameloblasts.** These cells produce enamel prisms (rods) over the dentin (Fig. 19–8I). As the enamel increases, the ameloblasts regress toward the outer enamel epithelium.

Enamel and dentin formation begins at the tip (cusp) of the tooth and progresses toward the future root.

Table 19–1. Order and Time of Eruption of Teeth and Time of Shedding of Deciduous Teeth

Tooth	Eruption Time	Shedding Time
Deciduous		
Medial incisor	6–8 mo	6–7 yr
Lateral incisor	8–10 mo	7–8 yr
Canine	11–20 mo	10–12 yr
First molar	12–16 mo	9–11 yr
Second molar	20–24 mo	10–12 yr
Permanent		
Medial incisor	7–8 yr	
Lateral incisor	8–9 yr	
Canine	10–12 yr	
First premolar	10–11 yr	
Second premolar	11–12 yr	
First molar	6–7 yr	
Second molar	12 yr	
Third molar	13–25 yr	

From Moore, K. L.: *Clinically Oriented Anatomy,* 2nd ed. Baltimore, Williams & Wilkins, 1985.

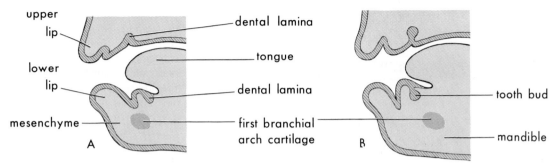

Figure 19-7. Diagrammatic sketches of sagittal sections through the developing jaws, illustrating early development of the teeth. *A*, Early in the sixth week, showing the dental laminae. *B*, Later in the sixth week, showing the tooth buds arising from the dental laminae.

The *root of the tooth* begins to develop after dentin and enamel formation is well advanced. The inner and outer enamel epithelia come together in the neck region of the tooth and form an epithelial fold called the *epithelial root sheath*. This sheath grows into the mesenchyme and *initiates root formation*. The odontoblasts adjacent to this sheath form dentin, which is continuous with that of the crown. As the dentin increases, it reduces the pulp cavity to a narrow *root canal* through which the vessels and nerves pass.

The inner cells of the dental sac differentiate into **cementoblasts** and produce cementum which is deposited over the dentin of the root.

As the teeth develop and the jaws ossify, the outer cells of the dental sac also become active in bone formation. Each tooth soon becomes surrounded by bone, except over its crown.

The tooth is held in its *alveolus* (bony socket) by the *periodontal ligament*, a derivative of the dental sac (Fig. 19–8G). Some fibers of this ligament are embedded in the cementum, others in the bony wall of the alveolus.

Tooth Eruption (Fig. 19–8 and Table 19–1). As the teeth develop, they begin a slow movement toward the exterior.

As the root grows, the crown gradually erupts through the oral mucosa. Eruption of the deciduous teeth usually occurs between the sixth and twenty-fourth months after birth.

The mandibular teeth usually erupt before the maxillary teeth, and girls' teeth usually erupt earlier than boys' teeth. *A child's dentition normally contains 20 deciduous teeth.*

The mandibular medial (central) incisors usually erupt six to eight months after birth (Table 19–1), but this process may not begin until 12 to 13 months in some normal children. Despite this, all 20 deciduous teeth are usually present by the end of the second year in healthy children.

Delayed eruption of all teeth may indicate systemic or nutritional disturbances such as *hypopituitarism* or *hypothyroidism.*

The permanent teeth develop in a manner similar to that previously described for deciduous teeth (Figs. 19–8 and 19–9). As a permanent tooth grows, the root of the corresponding deciduous tooth is gradually resorbed by osteoclasts. Consequently, when the deciduous tooth is shed, it consists only of the crown and uppermost portion of the root. The permanent teeth usually begin to erupt during the sixth year and continue appearing until early adulthood. The permanent teeth are not shed; however, if they are not properly cared for, or if disease of the gingiva (gum) develops, they may have to be extracted.

Malformations of the Teeth

Although most abnormalities of the teeth are genetic disorders, such as *dentinogenesis imperfecta,* environmental factors (e.g., rubella virus, syphilis, radiation, and tetracyclines) can cause tooth defects.

Enamel Hypoplasia (Fig. 19–10B). Defective enamel formation results in grooves, pits, or fissures on the enamel surface. These conditions result from a temporary disturbance in enamel formation. Various factors may injure the ameloblasts (e.g., nutritional deficiency, tetracycline therapy, and infections such as rubella).

All tetracyclines are extensively incorporated in the enamel and produce ugly brownish yellow discoloration and hypoplasia of the enamel. The primary teeth are affected if the tetracyclines are given from 18 weeks (prenatal) to 10 months (postnatal), and the permanent teeth are affected from 18 weeks (prenatal) to 12 years.

Tetracyclines should not be administered to pregnant women or to children, if they can be avoided, because these drugs adversely affect tooth development.

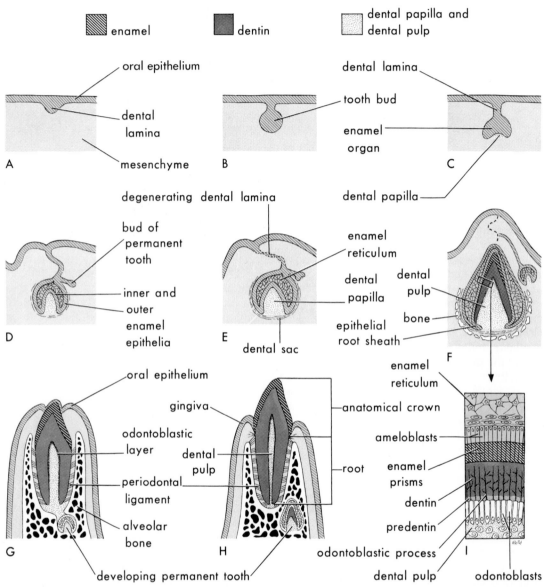

Figure 19–8. Schematic drawings of sagittal sections showing successive stages in the development and eruption of an incisor tooth. *A,* Six weeks, showing the dental lamina. *B,* Seven weeks, showing the tooth bud developing from the dental lamina. *C,* Eight weeks, showing the cap stage of tooth development. *D,* 10 weeks, showing the early bell stage of the enamel organ of the deciduous tooth and the bud stage of the developing permanent tooth. *E,* 14 weeks, showing the advanced bell stage of the enamel organ. Note that the connection (dental lamina) of the tooth to the oral epithelium is degenerating. *F,* 28 weeks, showing the enamel and dentin layers. *G,* Six months *postnatal,* showing early tooth eruption. *H,* 18 months *postnatal,* showing a fully erupted deciduous incisor tooth. The permanent incisor tooth now has a well-developed crown. *I,* Section through a developing tooth showing the ameloblasts (enamel producers) and the odontoblasts (dentin producers).

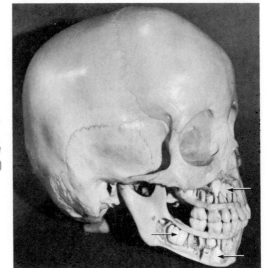

Figure 19–9. Photograph of the skull of a child in the fourth year. The bone of the jaws has been removed to show the relations of the developing permanent teeth (arrows) to the deciduous teeth. (From Moore, K. L.: *The Developing Human: Clinically Oriented Embryology*, 4th ed. Philadelphia, W. B. Saunders Company, 1988.)

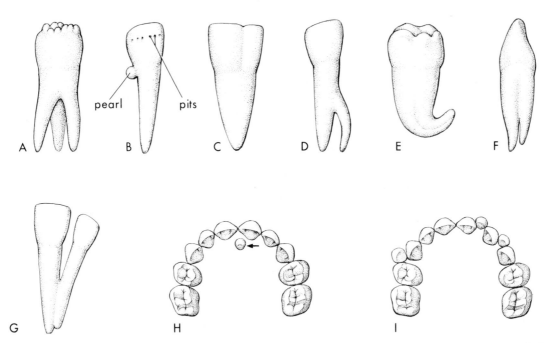

Figure 19–10. Drawings illustrating common abnormalities of teeth. *A*, Irregular raspberry-like crown. *B*, Enamel pearl and pits. *C*, Incisor tooth with a double crown. *D*, Abnormal division of root. *E*, Distorted root. *F*, Branched root. *G*, Fused roots. *H*, Hyperdontia, with a supernumerary incisor tooth in the anterior region of the palate (arrow). *I*, Hyperdontia, with 13 deciduous teeth in the maxilla (upper jaw) instead of the normal 10.

Rickets, a vitamin D deficiency disease, occurring during the critical period of permanent tooth development, is *the most common known cause of enamel hypoplasia.*

Abnormalities in Shape (Fig. 19–10*A* to *G*). Abnormally shaped teeth are relatively common. Occasionally, spherical masses of enamel, called *enamel pearls,* are attached to the tooth. They are formed by aberrant groups of ameloblasts.

Numerical Abnormalities (Fig. 19–10*H* and *I*).

One or more supernumerary teeth may develop, or teeth may not form.

Supernumerary teeth usually appear in the area of the maxillary incisors, where they disrupt the position and eruption of normal teeth. The extra teeth commonly erupt posterior to the normal ones.

Fused Teeth (Fig. 19–10*C* and *G*). Occasionally, a tooth bud divides or two buds partially fuse. In some cases the permanent tooth does not form.

SUMMARY

The skin and its appendages develop from ectoderm and mesoderm. The *epidermis* and its derivatives (hairs, nails, and glands) are derived from surface ectoderm and the *dermis* is derived from mesoderm.

Cast-off cells from the epidermis mix with secretions of the sebaceous glands to form a whitish, greasy coating for the skin known as *vernix caseosa.* It protects the epidermis, probably making it more waterproof, and facilitates birth owing to its slipperiness.

Hairs develop from downgrowths of the epidermis into the dermis. The sebaceous glands develop as outgrowths from the sides of hair follicles. The sweat and mammary glands develop from epidermal downgrowths. Supernumerary breasts *(polymastia)* or nipples *(polythelia)* are relatively common.

The teeth develop from ectoderm and mesoderm. The *enamel* is produced by cells called *ameloblasts,* which are derived from ectoderm; all other dental tissues develop from mesoderm. The *odontoblasts* produce *dentin* and the *cementoblasts* form *cementum.*

The common congenital malformations of teeth are defective formation of enamel and dentin, abnormalities in shape, and variations in number and position.

Commonly Asked Questions

1. I recently heard someone talking about a baby that was born without skin. Would it have any skin? Could such a baby survive? What is the cause of *congenital absence of skin?*
2. I once saw a dark-skinned person with patches of white skin on his face, chest, and limbs. He even had a white forelock. What is this condition called, and what is its developmental basis? Is there any treatment for these skin defects?
3. I was told that some male babies have enlarged breasts at birth. Is this an indication of abnormal sex development? I have also heard that some males develop breasts during puberty. Are they intersexes?
4. A nurse told me about a girl who developed a breast in her axilla during puberty. She also said that this girl had extra nipples on her trunk. What is the embryological basis of these abnormalities?
5. I recently read in the newspaper that a baby was born with four teeth. Would these be normal teeth? Is this a common occurrence?

Answers

1. *Congenital absence of skin is a very uncommon malformation.* Only patches of skin (several centimeters in diameter) are absent, most often from the scalp, but there may be patches of skin missing from the trunk and limbs. The skin defects are usually in the median plane of the scalp in the parietal and occipital areas. These infants usually survive because healing of the lesions is uneventful and takes one or two months. A hairless scar persists. The cause of congenital absence of hair, called *aplasia cutis congenita,* is usually unknown. Most cases are sporadic, but there are several well-documented pedigrees demonstrating *autosomal dominant transmission* of the defect.
2. The white patches of skin on a dark-skinned person result from a condition called *partial albinism* (piebaldism). This defect, which also affects light-skinned persons, is a *heritable disorder transmitted by an autosomal dominant gene.* Ultrastructural studies show that there is an *absence of melanocytes* in the depigmented areas of skin.

Presumably there is a genetic defect in the differentiation of melanoblasts (see Fig. 19–1). These skin and hair defects are not amenable to treatment, but they can be covered with cosmetics and hair dyes.

3. The breasts (including the mammary glands) of males and females are similar at birth. Breast enlargement *(gynecomastia)* in newborn male and female infants is a common occurrence owing to stimulation by maternal hormones. Hence, this is a normal occurrence in male infants and does not indicate abnormal sex development. Similar *physiological pubertal gynecomastia* occurs in some males during their early teens owing to decreased levels of testosterone. Usually the breast enlargement is transitory. *Familial gynecomastia* is an X-linked or autosomal dominant sex-limited trait. Gynecomastia also occurs in some males with the *Klinefelter syndrome* (XXY syndrome), as described in Chapter 9 and illustrated in Figure 9–7. *These men are not intersexes,* because their external and internal genitalia appear normal, except that their testes are small owing to degeneration of the seminiferous tubules.

4. An extra breast *(polymastia)* or nipple *(polythelia)* is common, as described in the text. The axillary breast may enlarge during puberty or it may not be noticed until pregnancy occurs. The embryological basis of these extra breasts and nipples is the presence of mammary ridges that extend from the axillary to the inguinal regions (see Fig. 19–5A). Usually only one pair of breasts and nipples develop, but they can develop anywhere along the mammary ridges. Usually the extra breast or nipple is just superior or inferior to the normal breast (see Fig. 19–6).

5. Teeth that are present at birth are called **natal teeth** (L. *natalis,* to be born). A more appropriate designation would be *congenital teeth* (L. *congenitus,* born with). Natal teeth are *erupted at birth* and are observed in about 1 in 2000 newborn infants. Usually there are two in the position of the mandibular medial (central) incisors. This usually suggests that early eruption of other teeth will occur. Obviously natal teeth may produce maternal discomfort owing to biting of the nipples during feeding. In addition, the infant's tongue may be lacerated or the teeth may detach and be aspirated into the lungs. For these reasons, natal teeth are sometimes extracted, but often they fall out on their own. Such teeth should not be considered supernumerary until they have been identified as such by x-ray examination. A natal tooth may be a prematurely erupted deciduous tooth, in which case early eruption of the other deciduous teeth may be expected.

References

Chapter 1

Meyer, A. W.: *The Rise of Embryology.* Stanford, Stanford University Press, 1939.

Moore, K. L.: A scientist's interpretation of references to embryology in the Qur'an. *JIMA* 18:15, 1986

Needham, J.: *A History of Embryology,* 2nd ed. Cambridge, Cambridge University Press, 1959.

O'Rahilly, R.: *Developmental Stages in Human Embryos, Part A: Embryos of the First Three Weeks.* Washington, DC, Carnegie Institution of Washington, 1973.

Persaud, T. V. N.: *Problems of Birth Defects: From Hippocrates To Thalidomide and After.* Baltimore, University Park Press, 1977.

Chapter 2

Cormack, D. H.: *Introduction to Histology.* Philadelphia, J. B. Lippincott Company, 1984.

Hafez, E. S. E.: *Human Ovulation. Mechanisms, Prediction, Detection and Induction.* Amsterdam, North Holland Publishing Company, 1979.

Moore, K. L.: *Clinically Oriented Anatomy,* 2nd ed. Baltimore, Williams & Wilkins Company, 1985.

Moore, K. L.: *The Developing Human: Clinically Oriented Embryology,* 4th ed. Philadelphia, W. B. Saunders Company, 1988.

Page, E. W., Villee, C. A., and Villee, D. B.: *Human Reproduction: Essentials of Reproductive and Perinatal Medicine,* 3rd ed. Philadelphia, W. B. Saunders Company, 1981.

Chapter 3

Biggers, J. D.: New observations on the nutrition of the mammalian oocyte and the preimplantation embryo. *In* Blandau, R. J. (Ed.): *The Biology of the Blastocyst.* Chicago, University of Chicago Press, 1971.

Carr, D. H., and Gedeon, M.: Population cytogenetics of human abortuses. *In* Hook, E. B., and Porter, I. H. (Eds.): *Population Cytogenetics: Studies in Humans.* New York, Academic Press, 1977.

Edwards, R. G., and Steptoe, P. C.: Current status of *in vitro* fertilization and implantation of human embryos. *Lancet* 2:1265, 1983.

Friedman, S.: Artificial donor insemination with frozen human semen. *Fertil. Steril.* 28:1230, 1977.

Hertig, A. T., Adams, E. C., and Menkin, M. C.: Thirty-four fertilized human ova, good, bad, and indifferent, recovered from 210 women of known fertility. *Pediatrics* 23:202, 1959.

Hertig, A. T., Adams, E. C., and Mulligan, W. J.: On the preimplantation stages of the human ovum: A description of four normal and four abnormal specimens ranging from the second to the fifth day of development. *Contrib. Embryol. Carnegie Inst.* 35:199, 1954.

Hertig, A. T., Rock, J., and Adams, E. C.: A description of human ova within the first seventeen days of development. *Am. J. Anat.* 98:435, 1956.

Moore, K. L.: *The Developing Human: Clinically Oriented Embryology,* 4th ed. Philadelphia, W. B. Saunders Company, 1988.

O'Rahilly, R.: *Developmental Stages in Human Embryos, Part A: Embryos of the First Three Weeks.* Washington, DC, Carnegie Institution of Washington, 1973.

Thompson, M. W.: *Medical Genetics,* 4th ed. Philadelphia, W. B. Saunders Company, 1986.

Trounson, A., and Mohr, L.: Human pregnancy following cryopreservations, thawing, and transfer of an eight-cell embryo. *Nature* 305:707, 1983.

Chapter 4

Blandau, R. J. (Ed.): *The Biology of the Blastocyst.* Chicago, University of Chicago Press, 1971.

Hertig, A. T., and Rock, J.: Two human ova of the pre-villous stage, having a developmental age of about eleven and twelve days respectively. *Contrib. Embryol. Carnegie Inst.* 29:127, 1941.

Hertig, A. T., and Rock, J.: Two human ova of the pre-villous stage, having a developmental age of about seven and nine days respectively. *Contrib. Embryol. Carnegie Inst.* 31:65, 1945.

Hertig, A. T., and Rock, J.: A description of 34 human ova within the first seventeen days of development. *Am. J. Anat.* 98:435, 1956.

Moore, K. L.: *The Developing Human: Clinically Oriented Embryology,* 4th ed. Philadelphia, W. B. Saunders Company, 1988.

Page, E. W., Villee, C. A., and Villee, D. B.: *Human Reproduction: Essentials of Reproductive and Perinatal Medicine,* 3rd ed. Philadelphia, W. B. Saunders Company, 1981.

Stander, R. W.: Abdominal pregnancy. *Clin. Obstet. Gynecol.* 5:1065, 1962.

Chapter 5

Boué, J., Boué, A., and Lazar, P.: Retrospective and prospective epidemiological studies of 1500 karyotyped spontaneous abortions. *Teratology* 12:11, 1975.

Carr, D. H.: Chromosomes and abortion. *Adv. Hum. Genet.* 2:201, 1971.

Depp, R.: How ultrasound is used by the perinatologist. *Clin Obstet. Gynecol.* 20:315, 1977.

Hertig. A. T.: Angiogenesis in the early human chorion and in the primary placenta of the macaque monkey. *Contrib. Embryol. Carnegie Inst.* 25:37, 1935.

Moore, K. L.: *The Developing Human: Clinically Oriented Embryology,* 4th ed. Philadelphia, W. B. Saunders Company, 1988.

Wilson, K. M.: A normal human ovum of 16 days development, the Rochester ovum. *Contrib. Embryol. Carnegie Inst.* 31:103, 1945.

Chapter 6

Moore, K. L.: *The Developing Human: Clinically Oriented Embryology,* 4th ed. Philadelphia, W. B. Saunders Company, 1988.

Nishimura, H., Tanimura, T., Semba, R., and Uwabe, C.: Normal development of early human embryos: observation of 90 specimens at Carnegie stages 7 to 13. *Teratology* 10:1, 1974.

O'Rahilly, R.: Guide to the staging of human embryos. *Anat. Anz.* 130:556, 1972.

O'Rahilly, R.: *Developmental Stages in Human Embryos. Part A: Embryos of the First Three Weeks (Stages 1 to 9).* Washington, DC, Carnegie Institution of Washington, 1973.

Sirlin, J. L., and Brahma, S. L.: Studies on embryonic induction using radioactive tracers. II. The mobilization of protein components during induction of the lens. *Dev. Biol.* 1:234, 1959.

Thompson, M. W.: *Genetics in Medicine,* 4th ed. Philadelphia, W. B. Saunders Company, 1986.

Wessels, N. K.: *Tissue Interactions in Development.* Menlo Park, CA, W. B. Benjamin Incorporated, 1977.

Chapter 7

Balsam, D., and Weiss, R. R.: Amniography in prenatal diagnosis. *Pediatr. Radiol.* 141:379, 1981.

Brock, D. H. J.: Prenatal diagnosis—chemical methods. *Br. Med. Bull.* 32:16, 1976.

Cadkin, A. V., Ginsberg, N. A., Pergament, E., and Verlinski, Y.: Chorionic villi sampling: A new technique for detection of genetic abnormalities in the first trimester. *Radiology* 151:159, 1984.

Chilcote, W. S., and Asokan, S.: Evaluation of first-trimester pregnancy by ultrasound. *Clin. Obstet. Gynecol.* 20:253, 1977.

Depp, R.: How ultrasound is used by the perinatologist. *Clin. Obstet. Gynecol.* 20:315, 1977.

Laurence, K. M., and Gregory, P.: Prenatal diagnosis of chromosome disorders, *Br. Med. Bull.* 32:9, 1976.

MacVicar, J.: Antenatal detection of fetal abnormality—physical methods. *Br. Med. Bull.* 32:4, 1976.

Moore, K. L.: *The Sex Chromatin.* Philadelphia, W. B. Saunders Company, 1966.

Persaud, T. V. N.: *Prenatal Pathology. Fetal Medicine.* Springfield, IL, Charles C Thomas, 1979.

Riis, P., and Fuchs, F.: Sex chromatin and antenatal sex diagnosis. *In* Moore, K. L. (ed.): *The Sex Chromatin.* Philadelphia, W. B. Saunders Company, 1966.

Sanders, R. C., and James, A. E. (Eds.): *The Principles and Practice of Ultrasonography in Obstetrics and Gynecology,* 2nd ed. New York, Appleton-Century-Crofts, 1980.

Shepard, T. H.: Normal and abnormal growth patterns. *In* Gardner, L. I. (Ed.): *Endocrine and Genetic Diseases of Childhood and Adolescence,* 2nd ed. Philadelphia, W. B. Saunders Company, 1975.

Stevenson, R. E.: *The Fetus and Newly Born Infant. Influences of the Prenatal Environment.* St. Louis, C. V. Mosby Company, 1973.

Chapter 8

Behrman, R. E., and Vaughan, V. C. III (Eds.): *Nelson Textbook of Pediatrics,* 13th ed. Philadelphia, W. B. Saunders Company, 1987.

Bulmer, M. G.: *The Biology of Twinning in Man.* Oxford, Clarendon Press, 1970.

Chamberlain, G., and Wilkinson, A. (Eds.): *Placental Transfer.* Baltimore, University Park Press, 1979.

Fox, H.: *Pathology of the Placenta.* Philadelphia, W. B. Saunders Company, 1978.

Moore, K. L.: *The Developing Human: Clinically Oriented Embryology,* 4th ed. Philadelphia, W. B. Saunders Company, 1988.

Page, E. W., Villee, C. A., and Villee, D. B.: *Human Reproduction: Essentials of Reproductive and Perinatal Medicine,* 3rd ed. Philadelphia, W. B. Saunders Company, 1981.

Ramsey, E. M.: The placenta and fetal membranes. *In* Greenhill, J. P. (Ed.): *Obstetrics,* 13th ed. Philadelphia, W. B. Saunders Company, 1972.

Smith, S. M., and Penrose, L. S.: Monozygotic and dizygotic twin diagnosis. *Ann. Hum. Genet.* 19:273, 1955.

Waisman, H. A., and Kerr, G.: *Fetal Growth and Development.* New York, McGraw-Hill Book Company, 1970.

Chapter 9

Amin-Zaki, L., Elhassani, S., Majeed, M. A., et al.: Intrauterine methylmercury poisoning in Iraq. *Pediatrics* 54:587, 1974.

Behrman, R. E., and Vaughan, V. C. III (Eds.): *Nelson Textbook of Pediatrics,* 13th ed. Philadelphia, W. B. Saunders Company, 1987.

Carr, D. H., Law, E. M., and Ekins, J. G.: Chromosome studies in selected spontaneous abortions. IV. Unusual cytogenetic disorders. *Teratology* 5:49, 1972.

Cooper, L. Z.: Congenital rubella in the United States. *In* Krugman, S., and Gershon, A. A. (Eds.): *Infections of the Fetus and Newborn Infant.* Progress in Clinical and Biological Research, Vol. 3. New York, Alan R. Liss, 1975.

Golbus, M. S.: Teratology for the obstetrician: Current status. *Obstet. Gynecol.* 55:269, 1980.

Holmes, L. B.: Bendectin. *In* Sever, J. L., and Brent, R. L. (Eds.): *Teratogen Update: Environmentally Induced Birth Defect Risks.* New York, Alan R. Liss, 1986.

Hook, E. B.: Rates of Down's syndrome in live births and at midtrimester amniocentesis. *Lancet* 1:1053, 1978.

Kalant, H., Roschlau, H. E., and Sellers, E. M. (Eds.): *Principles of Medical Pharmacology,* 4th ed. Toronto, University of Toronto Press, 1985.

Mole, R. H.: Consequences of pre-natal radiation exposure for post-natal development. *Int. J. Radiol. Biol.* 42:1, 1982.

Moore, K. L.: *The Developing Human: Clinically Oriented Embryology,* 4th ed. Philadelphia, W. B. Saunders Company, 1988.

Persaud, T. V. N.: *Problems of Birth Defects: From Hippocrates to Thalidomide and After.* Baltimore, University Park Press, 1977.

Persaud, T. V. N., and Moore, K. L.: Causes and prenatal diagnosis of congenital abnormalities. *J. Obstet. Gynecol. Nurs.,* 3:40, 1974.

Sever, J. L., and Brent, R. L. (Eds.): *Teratogen Update: Environmentally Induced Birth Defect Risks.* New York, Alan R. Liss, 1986.

Thompson, M. W.: *Genetics in Medicine,* 4th ed. Philadelphia, W. B. Saunders Company, 1986.

Chapter 10

Avery, M. E.: Disorders of the diaphragm. *In* Avery, M. E., and Taeusch, H. W. (Eds.): *Schaffer's Diseases of the Newborn,* 5th ed. Philadelphia, W. B. Saunders Company, 1984.

Bremer, J. L.: The diaphragm and diaphragmatic hernia. *Arch. Pathol.* 36:539, 1943.

Moore, K. L.: *The Developing Human: Clinically Oriented Embryology,* 4th ed. Philadelphia, W. B. Saunders Company, 1988.

Wells, L. J.: Development of the human diaphragm and pleural sacs. *Contr. Embryol. Carnegie Inst.* 35:107, 1954.

Chapter 11

Avery, M. E., and Taeusch, H. W. (Eds.): *Schaffer's Diseases of the Newborn,* 5th ed. Philadelphia, W. B. Saunders Company, 1984.

Behrman, R. E., and Vaughan, V. C. III (Eds.): *Nelson Textbook of Pediatrics,* 13th ed. Philadelphia, W. B. Saunders Company, 1987.

Fraser, F. C.: The genetics of cleft lip and palate: yet another look. *In* Pratt, R. M., and Christiansen, R. L. (Eds.): *Current Research Trends in Prenatal Craniofacial Development.* New York, Elsevier North-Holland, 1980.

Goodman, R. M., and Gorlin, R. J.: *The Face in Genetic Disorders.* St. Louis, C. V. Mosby Company, 1970.

Jones, K. L.: *Smith's Recognizable Patterns of Human Malformation,* 4th ed. Philadelphia, W. B. Saunders Company, 1987.

McKenzie, J.: The first arch syndrome. *Dev. Med. Child. Neurol.* 8:55, 1966.

Moore, K. L.: *Clinically Oriented Anatomy,* 2nd ed. Baltimore, Williams & Wilkins Company, 1985.

Moore, K. L.: *The Developing Human: Clinically Oriented Embryology,* 4th ed. Philadelphia, W. B. Saunders Company, 1988.

Noden, D. M.: The migration and cytodifferentiation of cranial neural crest cells. *In* Pratt, R. M., and Christiansen, R. L. (Eds.): *Current Research Trends in Prenatal Craniofacial Development.* New York, Elsevier North-Holland, 1980.

Ross, R. B., and Johnston, M. C.: *Cleft Lip and Palate.* Baltimore, Williams & Wilkins Company, 1972.

Sperber, G. H.: Development of the dentition (odontogenesis). *In* Sperber, G. H. (Ed.): *Craniofacial Embryology,* 2nd ed. Bristol, John Wright and Sons, Ltd. (distributed by Year Book Medical Publishers, Chicago), 1976.

Thompson, M. W.: *Genetics in Medicine,* 4th ed. Philadelphia, W. B. Saunders Company, 1986.

Chapter 12

Avery, M. E., Fletcher, B. D., and Williams, R.: *The Lung and Its Disorders in the Newborn Infant,* 4th ed. Philadelphia, W. B. Saunders Company, 1981.

Conen, P. E., and Balis, J. U.: Electron microscopy in study of lung development. *In* Emery, J. (Ed.): *The Anatomy of the Developing Lung.* London, William Heinemann, Ltd., 1969, p. 18.

Cormack, D. H.: *Introduction to Histology.* Philadelphia, J. B. Lippincott Company, 1984.

Crelin, E. S.: Development of the lower respiratory system. *Clin. Symp.* 27(4):3–28, 1975.

Crelin, E. S.: Development of the upper respiratory system. *Clin. Symp.* 28(3):3–26, 1976.

Emery, J.: *The Anatomy of the Developing Lung.* London, William Heinemann, Ltd., 1969, pp. 1–8.

Hast, H. M.: Developmental anatomy of the larynx. *In* Hinchcliffe, R., and Harrison, D. (Eds.): *Scientific Foundations of Otolaryngology.* London, William Heinemann Medical Books, Ltd., 1976.

Moore, K. L.: *The Developing Human: Clinically Oriented Embryology,* 4th ed. Philadelphia, W. B. Saunders Company, 1988.

O'Rahilly, R., and Boyden, E.: The timing and sequence of events in the development of the human respiratory system during the embryonic period proper. *Z. Anat. Entwicklungsgesch.* 141:237, 1973.

Chapter 13

Avery, M. E., and Taeusch, H. W. (Eds.): *Schaffer's Diseases of the Newborn,* 5th ed. Philadelphia, W. B. Saunders Company, 1984.

Crelin, E. S.: Development of the gastrointestinal tract. *Clin. Symp.* 13:67, 1961.

Ladd, W. E., and Gross, R. E.: Congenital malformations of the anus and rectum. *Am. J. Surg.* 23:167, 1934.

Moore, K. L.: *The Developing Human: Clinically Oriented Embryology,* 4th ed. Philadelphia, W. B. Saunders Company, 1988.

Stephens, F. D.: *Congenital Malformations of the Rectum, Anus and Genito-Urinary Tracts.* Edinburgh, E. & S. Livingstone, Ltd., 1963.

Chapter 14

Barr, M. L.: Correlations between sex chromatin patterns and sex chromosome complexes in man. *In* Moore, K. L.: *The Sex Chromatin.* Philadelphia, W. B. Saunders Company, 1966.

Behrman, R. E., and Vaughan, V. C. III (Eds.): *Nelson Textbook of Pediatrics,* 13th ed. Philadelphia, W. B. Saunders Company, 1987.

Federman, D. D.: *Abnormal Sexual Development: A Genetic and Endocrine Approach to Differential Diagnosis.* Philadelphia, W. B. Saunders Company, 1967.

Jones, H. H., and Scott, W. W.: *Hermaphroditism, Genital Anomalies and Related Endocrine Disorders.* Baltimore, Williams & Wilkins Company, 1958.

Moore, K. L.: The development of clinical sex chromatin tests. *In* Moore, K. L.: *The Sex Chromatin.* Philadelphia, W. B. Saunders Company, 1966.

Moore, K. L.: Sex determinations, sexual differentiation and intersex development. *Can. Med. Assoc. J.* 7:292, 1967.

Moore, K. L.: *The Developing Human: Clinically Oriented Embryology,* 4th ed. Philadelphia, W. B. Saunders Company, 1988.

Simpson, J. L.: *Disorders of Sexual Differentiation: Etiology and Clinical Delineation.* New York, Academic Press, 1976.

Chapter 15

Anderson, R. H., and Taylor, I. M.: Development of atrioventricular specialized tissue in human heart. *Br. Heart J.* 34:1205, 1972.

Behrman, R. E., and Vaughan, V. C. III (Eds.): *Nelson Textbook of Pediatrics,* 13th ed. Philadelphia, W. B. Saunders Company, 1987.

Keith, J. D., Rowe, R. D., and Vlad, P.: *Heart Disease in Infancy and Childhood,* 3rd ed. New York, The Macmillan Company, 1978.

Moore, K. L.: *The Developing Human: Clinically Oriented Embryology,* 4th ed. Philadelphia, W. B. Saunders Company, 1988.

O'Rahilly, R.: The timing and sequence of events in human cardiogenesis. *Acta Anat.* 79:70, 1971.

Chapter 16

Blechschmidt, E.: The early stages of human limb development. *In* Swinyard, C. A. (Ed.): *Limb Development and Deformity: Problems of Evaluation and Rehabilitation.* Springfield, IL, Charles C Thomas, 1969.

Dubowitz, V.: *Muscle Disorders in Childhood.* Philadelphia, W. B. Saunders Company, 1978.

Ford, E. H. R.: The growth of the foetal skull. *J. Anat.* 90:63, 1956.

Gasser, R. F.: The development of the facial muscles in man. *Am. J. Anat.* 120:357, 1967.

Gray, D. J., Gardner, E., and O'Rahilly, R.: The prenatal development of the skeleton and joints of the human hand. *Am. J. Anat.* 101:169, 1957.

Lenz, W., and Knapp, K.: Foetal malformations due to thalidomide. *Ger. Med. Mon.* 7:253, 1962.

Moore, K. L.: *The Developing Human: Clinically Oriented Embryology,* 4th ed. Philadelphia, W. B. Saunders Company, 1988.

O'Rahilly, R., and Gardner, E.: The timing and sequence of events in the development of the limbs in the human embryo. *Anat. Embryol.* 148:1, 1975.

Sperber, G. H.: *Craniofacial Embryology,* 2nd ed. Chicago, Year Book Medical Publishers, 1976.

Chapter 17

Clayton, B. E. (Ed.): *Mental Retardation: Environmental Hazards.* London, Butterworth & Company, 1973.

Crelin, E. S.: *Development of the Nervous System. A Logical Approach to Neuroanatomy.* Clin. Symp. 26(2):2–32, 1974.

Kalter, H.: *Teratology of the Central Nervous System.* Chicago, University of Chicago Press, 1968.

Laurence, K. M., and Weeks, R.: Abnormalities of the central nervous system. *In* Norman, A. P. (Ed.): *Congenital Abnormalities in Infancy,* 2nd ed. Oxford, Blackwell Scientific Publications, 1971.

Mole, R. H.: Consequences of pre-natal radiation exposure for post-natal development. *Int. J. Radiat. Biol.* 42:1, 1982.

Moore, K. L.: *The Developing Human: Clinically Oriented Embryology,* 4th ed. Philadelphia, W. B. Saunders Company, 1988.

O'Rahilly, R., and Gardner, E.: The timing and sequence of events in the development of the human nervous system during the embryonic period proper. *Z. Anat. Entwicklungsgesch.* 134:1, 1971.

Wald, N. J.: Neural tube defects and vitamins: The need for a randomized clinical trial. *Br. J. Obstet. Gynecol.* 91:516, 1984.

Chapter 18

Brown, C. A.: Abnormalities of the eyes and associated structures. *In* Norman, A. P. (Ed.): *Congenital Abnormalities in Infancy,* 2nd ed. Oxford, Blackwell Scientific Publications, 1971.

Fraser, G. R.: A study of causes of deafness amongst 2,355 children in special schools. *In* Fisch, L. (Ed.): *Research in Deafness in Children.* Oxford, Blackwell Scientific Publications, 1964.

Gray, J. E.: Rubella in pregnancy; fetal pathology in the internal ear. *Ann. Otol.* 68:170, 1959.

Langman, J.: The first appearance of specific antigens during induction of the lens. *J. Embryol. Exp. Morphol.* 7:264, 1959.

Mann, I. C.: *The Development of the Human Eye,* 3rd ed. London, British Medical Association, 1974.

Moore, K. L.: *The Developing Human: Clinically Oriented Embryology,* 4th ed. Philadelphia, W. B. Saunders Company, 1988.

O'Rahilly, R.: The prenatal development of the human eye. *Exp. Eye Res.* 21:93, 1975.

Chapter 19

Behrman, R. E., and Vaughan, V. C. III (Eds.): *Nelson Textbook of Pediatrics,* 13th ed. Philadelphia, W. B. Saunders Company, 1987.

Butler, P. M., and Joysey, K. A. (Eds.): *Development, Function and Evolution of Teeth.* New York, Academic Press, 1978.

Cormack, D. H.: *Ham's Histology,* 9th ed. Philadelphia, J. B. Lippincott Company, 1987.

Kalant, H., Roschlau, H. E., and Sellers, E. M. (Eds.): *Principles of Medical Pharmacology,* 4th ed. Toronto, University of Toronto Press, 1985.

Moore, K. L.: *The Developing Human: Clinically Oriented Embryology,* 4th ed. Philadelphia, W. B. Saunders Company, 1988.

Sperber, G. H.: Development of the dentition. *In* Sperber, G. H.: *Craniofacial Embryology,* 2nd ed. Chicago, Year Book Medical Publishers, 1976.

Index

Note: Page numbers in *italics* refer to illustrations; page numbers followed by (t) refer to tables.